Wearable Sensors & Gait

Wearable Sensors & Gait

Editors

Felipe García-Pinillos
Luis Enrique Roche-Seruendo
Diego Jaén-Carrillo

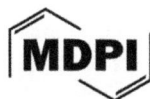

Editors
Felipe García-Pinillos
University of Granada
Granada
Spain

Luis Enrique Roche-Seruendo
Universidad San Jorge
Zaragoza
Spain

Diego Jaén-Carrillo
University of Innsbruck
Innsbruck
Austria

Editorial Office
MDPI
St. Alban-Anlage 66
4052 Basel, Switzerland

This is a reprint of articles from the Special Issue published online in the open access journal *Sensors* (ISSN 1424-8220) (available at: https://www.mdpi.com/journal/sensors/special_issues/WSG).

For citation purposes, cite each article independently as indicated on the article page online and as indicated below:

Lastname, A.A.; Lastname, B.B. Article Title. *Journal Name* **Year**, *Volume Number*, Page Range.

ISBN 978-3-0365-8642-7 (Hbk)
ISBN 978-3-0365-8643-4 (PDF)
doi.org/10.3390/books978-3-0365-8643-4

© 2023 by the authors. Articles in this book are Open Access and distributed under the Creative Commons Attribution (CC BY) license. The book as a whole is distributed by MDPI under the terms and conditions of the Creative Commons Attribution-NonCommercial-NoDerivs (CC BY-NC-ND) license.

Contents

About the Editors vii

Diego Jaén-Carrillo, Santiago A. Ruiz-Alias, Jose M. Chicano-Gutiérrez, Emilio J. Ruiz-Malagón, Luis E. Roche-Seruendo and Felipe García-Pinillos
Test-Retest Reliability of the MotionMetrix Software for the Analysis of Walking and Running Gait Parameters
Reprinted from: *Sensors* **2022**, *22*, 3201, doi:10.3390/s22093201 1

Mario Fernández-Gorgojo, Diana Salas-Gómez, Pascual Sánchez-Juan, David Barbado, Esther Laguna-Bercero and María Isabel Pérez-Núñez
Clinical–Functional Evaluation and Test–Retest Reliability of the G-WALK Sensor in Subjects with Bimalleolar Ankle Fractures 6 Months after Surgery
Reprinted from: *Sensors* **2022**, *22*, 3050, doi:10.3390/s22083050 11

Marija M. Gavrilović and Milica M. Janković
Temporal Synergies Detection in Gait Cyclograms Using Wearable Technology
Reprinted from: *Sensors* **2022**, *22*, 2728, doi:10.3390/s22072728 27

Zanru Yang, Le Chung Tran and Farzad Safaei
Step Length Estimation Using the RSSI Method in Walking and Jogging Scenarios
Reprinted from: *Sensors* **2022**, *22*, 1640, doi:10.3390/s22041640 45

Emiri Gondo, Saiko Mikawa and Akito Hayashi
Using a Portable Gait Rhythmogram to Examine the Effect of Music Therapy on Parkinson's Disease-Related Gait Disturbance
Reprinted from: *Sensors* **2021**, *21*, 8321, doi:10.3390/s21248321 63

Antonio Martínez-Serrano, Elena Marín-Cascales, Konstantinos Spyrou, Tomás T. Freitas and Pedro E. Alcaraz
Electromyography, Stiffness and Kinematics of Resisted Sprint Training in the Specialized SKILLRUN® Treadmill Using Different Load Conditions in Rugby Players
Reprinted from: *Sensors* **2021**, *21*, 7482, doi:10.3390/s21227482 77

Vânia Guimarães, Inês Sousa and Miguel V. Correia
Orientation-Invariant Spatio-Temporal Gait Analysis Using Foot-Worn Inertial Sensors
Reprinted from: *Sensors* **2021**, *21*, 3940, doi:10.3390/s21113940 89

Víctor Rodríguez-Rielves, José Ramón Lillo-Beviá, Ángel Buendía-Romero, Alejandro Martínez-Cava, Alejandro Hernández-Belmonte, Javier Courel-Ibáñez and Jesús G. Pallarés
Are the Assioma Favero Power Meter Pedals a Reliable Tool for Monitoring Cycling Power Output?
Reprinted from: *Sensors* **2021**, *21*, 2789, doi:10.3390/s21082789 109

Juan Pardo Albiach, Melanie Mir-Jimenez, Vanessa Hueso Moreno, Iván Nácher Moltó and Javier Martínez-Gramage
The Relationship between VO_2max, Power Management, and Increased Running Speed: Towards Gait Pattern Recognition through Clustering Analysis
Reprinted from: *Sensors* **2021**, *21*, 2422, doi:10.3390/s21072422 119

José Torreblanca González, Beatriz Gómez-Martín, Ascensión Hernández Encinas, Jesús Martín-Vaquero, A. Queiruga-Dios, Araceli Queiruga-Dios and Alfonso Martínez-Nova
The Use of Infrared Thermography to Develop and Assess a Wearable Sock and Monitor Foot Temperature in Diabetic Subjects
Reprinted from: *Sensors* **2021**, *21*, 1821, doi:10.3390/s21051821 133

**Antonio Cartón-Llorente, Felipe García-Pinillos, Jorge Royo-Borruel,
Alberto Rubio-Peirotén, Diego Jaén-Carrillo and Luis E. Roche-Seruendo**
Estimating Functional Threshold Power in Endurance Running from Shorter Time Trials Using
a 6-Axis Inertial Measurement Sensor
Reprinted from: *Sensors* **2021**, *21*, 582, doi:10.3390/s21020582 153

**Stephanie R. Moore, Christina Kranzinger, Julian Fritz, Thomas Stöggl, Josef Kröll
and Hermann Schwameder**
Foot Strike Angle Prediction and Pattern Classification Using LoadsolTM Wearable Sensors:
A Comparison of Machine Learning Techniques
Reprinted from: *Sensors* **2020**, *20*, 6737, doi:10.3390/s20236737 167

**Iván Nacher Moltó, Juan Pardo Albiach, Juan José Amer-Cuenca, Eva Segura-Ortí,
Willig Gabriel and Javier Martínez-Gramage**
Wearable Sensors Detect Differences between the Sexes in Lower Limb Electromyographic
Activity and Pelvis 3D Kinematics during Running
Reprinted from: *Sensors* **2020**, *20*, 6478, doi:10.3390/s20226478 181

**Javier Martínez-Gramage, Juan Pardo Albiach, Iván Nacher Moltó, Juan José Amer-Cuenca,
Vanessa Huesa Moreno and Eva Segura-Ortí**
A Random Forest Machine Learning Framework to Reduce Running Injuries in
Young Triathletes
Reprinted from: *Sensors* **2020**, *20*, 6388, doi:10.3390/s20216388 195

Lauren C. Benson, Anu M. Räisänen, Christian A. Clermont and Reed Ferber
Is This the Real Life, or Is This Just Laboratory? A Scoping Review of IMU-Based Running
Gait Analysis
Reprinted from: *Sensors* **2022**, *22*, 1722, doi:10.3390/s22051722 207

About the Editors

Felipe García-Pinillos

Felipe García Pinillos gained a degree in Sports Sciences at the University of Granada (2010) and a master's degree in Research and Teaching in Physical Activity and Health at the University of Jaen (2011). His academic background also includes a master's degree in Injury Prevention and Return to Sport (2017, University of Jaen) and a Master Degree in High Performance in Endurance Sports (2020, University of Murcia).

He started his PhD project as a fellow researcher at the University of Jaen (2013–2016). Thereafter, his main research interest is related to performance optimization in endurance athletes by determining the metabolic, physiological, neuromuscular, and biomechanical impact of different programs. Related to this topic, he stayed at different laboratories (e.g., Liverpool John Moores University, the Sport & Health Institute at the University of Granada, and the Sport Physiology Laboratory at the University of La Frontera) and finally attained his PhD degree (2016) at the University of Jaen (awarded with Extraordinary Mention by the University of Jaen, 2019).

When he finished his PhD studies, he started working for the University of La Frontera (Temuco, Chile) as a postdoctoral researcher. He stayed there for 2.5 years, investigating and teaching about training and its application to different contexts (from performance optimization to injury management). Finally, in February 2020, he started teaching as an Associate Professor at the Faculty of Sport Sciences (University of Granada).

From 2013 to today, he has published 183 papers, including 168 documents published in journals indexed in the JCR: 49 papers published in Q1 journals, 41 in Q2, 36 in Q3, and 42 in Q4. In 136 out of those 168 papers, he is the first or last author. According to Google Scholar's citation index, these papers have been cited 3172 times since 2018, and Felipe has an H-INDEX of 32.

Luis Enrique Roche-Seruendo

Ph.D. in Biomedicine and Professor of Human Biomechanics and Sports Physiotherapy in the Physiotherapy Degree Program at University San Jorge, Zaragoza, Spain.

Currently, he leads the research group UNLOC (Unlimited Locomotion), which aims to establish the limiting factors of performance, as well as the factors that contribute to the development of injuries associated with human locomotion. In particular, his research focuses on the analysis of human movement, with efforts concentrated on the characterization of locomotion (standing, walking, running, and jumping). His recent research articles have focused on understanding the factors involved the way we run and the extent to which they influence it, primarily in the modulation of the so-called mass–spring model. The latest studies have already shifted towards more specific parameters at the joint, tendon, and muscular levels.

He is the author of over 40 JCR articles focused on locomotion biomechanics, especially in running, a chapter in a book on cycling foot mechanics, and 1 book in the form of a doctoral thesis on "Analysis of Influential Variables in the Mass-Spring Model Applied to Long-Distance Running".

Luis has published numerous articles on running biomechanics and foot biomechanics in specialized works and scientific journals. He has participated in national and international conferences on lower extremity biomechanics and motion analysis.

Diego Jaén-Carrillo

Diego was born in Murcia, Spain and completed his undergraduate degree in Sport Science (BSc) at the Catholic University San Antonio of Murcia (UCAM), Spain, in 2009. After that, Diego completed an MA in Teaching Proficiency at the University of Granada, Spain (2010) and a BA in English Studies at the University of Murcia, Spain, in 2014. During this time, he also received a funded scholarship at the UCAM Research and High-Performance Center as an MSc student to complete an MSc in High Performance Sport: Strength and Conditioning. His work during that time focused on the mechanisms of ACL rupture during landing after jumping in different sports. After spending some time working in Spain and Germany as a Sports Teacher in secondary schools, Diego started a Graduate Teaching Assistant position at Universidad San Jorge, Zaragoza (2018-2019) and completed his PhD in Health Sciences in 2020 at the same university. Immediately after that, he took the role of Assistant Professor of Sport Biomechanics and Sport Therapy at Universidad San Jorge, Zaragoza until December 2022. Since January 2023, Diego has acted as a Postdoc Researcher at the Department of Sports Science of the University of Innsbruck, Austria.

Since 2021, Diego has also collaborated as a Visiting Associate Professor of Sport Biomechanics in the MSc in High Performance in Cyclic Sports: running, swimming and cycling at the University of Murcia, Spain.

Diego's research focuses on human locomotion (i.e., gait and running), movement analysis, and motor control. He also has ongoing projects on Running with Power that aim to assess the validity and reliability of power-related metrics to quantify training load in order to prescribe training and racing accurately for both road and trail running.

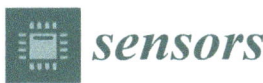

Article

Test-Retest Reliability of the MotionMetrix Software for the Analysis of Walking and Running Gait Parameters

Diego Jaén-Carrillo [1], Santiago A. Ruiz-Alias [2,3], Jose M. Chicano-Gutiérrez [3], Emilio J. Ruiz-Malagón [2,3], Luis E. Roche-Seruendo [1] and Felipe García-Pinillos [2,3,4,*]

[1] Faculty of Health Sciences, Campus Universitario, Universidad San Jorge, Autov A23 km 299, Villanueva de Gállego, 50830 Zaragoza, Spain; djaen@usj.es (D.J.-C.); leroche@usj.es (L.E.R.-S.)
[2] Department of Physical Education and Sport, University of Granada, 18071 Granada, Spain; aljruiz@ugr.es (S.A.R.-A.); emiliorm@ugr.es (E.J.R.-M.)
[3] Sport and Health Research Institute (iMUDS), University of Granada, 18007 Granada, Spain; jchicano@ugr.es
[4] Department of Physical Education, Sports and Recreation, Universidad de La Frontera, Temuco 1145, Chile
* Correspondence: fgpinillos@ugr.es; Tel.: +34-678638967

Abstract: The use of markerless motion capture systems is becoming more popular for walking and running analysis given their user-friendliness and their time efficiency but in some cases their validity is uncertain. Here, the test-retest reliability of the MotionMetrix software combined with the use of Kinect sensors is tested with 24 healthy volunteers for walking (at 5 km·h^{-1}) and running (at 10 and 15 km·h^{-1}) gait analysis in two different trials. All the parameters given by the MotionMetrix software for both walking and running gait analysis are tested in terms of reliability. No significant differences ($p > 0.05$) were found for walking gait parameters between both trials except for the phases of loading response and double support, and the spatiotemporal parameters of step length and step frequency. Additionally, all the parameters exhibit acceptable reliability (CV < 10%) but step width (CV > 10%). When analyzing running gait, although the parameters here tested exhibited different reliability values at 10 km·h^{-1}, the system provided reliable measurements for most of the kinematic and kinetic parameters (CV < 10%) when running at 15 km·h^{-1}. Overall, the results obtained show that, although some variables must be interpreted with caution, the Kinect + MotionMetrix system may be useful for walking and running gait analysis. Nevertheless, the validity still needs to be determined against a gold standard system to fully trust this technology and software combination.

Keywords: analysis; biomechanics; gait; markerless; testing

1. Introduction

In both research and diagnosis, the use of marker-based motion capture technologies has been expanded dramatically. However, inherent limits in data collecting may restrict its use in contexts such as patient homes, sports fields, or public spaces where the use of a large number of cameras is impractical. Here, a markerless motion capture system has been offered as one possible solution [1,2].

Markerless systems do not require any markers or sensors to be attached to the body, reducing clinical feasibility and testing time significantly. The lack of markers, on the other hand, may have an impact on measuring accuracy. Thus, investigations examining the validity of such systems under different conditions are crucial. In this context, doctors, sports practitioners, and researchers have been paying close attention to a markerless motion capture system [1,3–7].

The validity of the Kinect™ sensor, created first for interacting with video games on the Microsoft Xbox™ platform by using body movements, for the analysis of gait parameters has been previously evaluated [1,3–7]. Various pieces of software, including various filters and calibrations, have been studied in these works. Whereas Schmitz et al. [1] analyzed the validity of the Kinect™ system with the KinectFusion software for kinematic data assessment, Dolatabadi et al. [3] identified the concurrent validity of the Kinect™ for Windows to measure gait spatiotemporal variables. Then, the validity of the Kinect™ for gait kinematics analysis in comparison with a "gold standard" motion capture system was assessed, operating both systems under Cartesian calibration [4]. Likewise, concurrent validity of the Kinect system for spatiotemporal gait parameters was also assessed [6]. However, none of the mentioned studies considered the MotionMetrix™ software, which might affect measuring accuracy.

As far as the authors' concern, only one study took into account the Kinect + MotionMetrix combination [8]. Here, the absolute reliability and concurrent validity of the Kinect + MotionMetrix combination was evaluated for spatiotemporal parameters when running at a comfortable velocity by comparing data between the combination system and two widely used systems (i.e., high-speed video analysis and OptoGait). It was found that contact time (CT) was overestimated by the system, whereas flight time (FT) was underrated. However, it resulted to be a valid tool for step frequency (SF) and step length (SL) measures [8]. Although concurrent validity has been assessed, the reliability of the Kinect + MotionMetrix system for either walking or running parameters has not been evaluated.

To identify whether findings are attributable to changes in gait pattern or merely systematic measurement errors, a gait analysis system's reliability is critical. Therefore, the aim of this study is to analyze the test–retest reliability of both walking and running gait on a treadmill running at 5, 10 and 15 km·h^{-1} by comparing inter-session data obtained from the Kinect + MotionMetrix system.

2. Materials and Methods

This study follows the STROBE recommendations for reporting observational studies [9].

2.1. Subjects

A group of 16 men and 8 women recreationally active (age = 22.7 ± 2.6 years; body mass = 69.1 ± 11.7 kg; height = 1.72 ± 0.10 m; weekly training = 6.9 ± 2.4 h/week) [10] and familiar with treadmill running voluntarily took part in the study. All of them were free from injuries and reported no physical limitations or health problems. An informed consent was signed by each participant after being informed of the objectives and procedures. It was made clear that they were free to leave at any point. The study followed the Declaration of Helsinki (2013) and was approved by the Ethics Board of the local university (No. 2546/CEIH/2022).

2.2. Procedures

Each participant attended the laboratory only once. The participants were instructed to refrain from strenuous activity for, at least, 48 h before data collection [11]. During the test, they wore their usual running clothes and shoes. A treadmill (WOODWAY Pro XL, Woodway, Inc., Waukesha, WI, USA) walking and running protocol was completed. An accommodation period on the treadmill of, at least, 8 min was completed at a self-selected velocity [12]. Thereafter, a protocol where 1-min bouts at 5, 10 and 15 km·h^{-1} was completed. After a 5-min break to avoid fluctuations in the running pattern caused by fatigue, all the participants completed the protocol again. Data were collected during the last 30 s of each bout to guarantee participant adaptation to the running speed

2.3. Materials and Testing

Participants body mass (kg) and height (m) were obtained using a bioimpedance scale (Inbody 230, Inbody, Seul, Korea) and a stadiometer (SECA 222, SECA, Corp., Hamburg, Germany), respectively.

Table 1 shows the definition of all the parameters provided by the MotionMetrix software (MotionMetrix AB). It offers different kinetic and kinematic variables depending on gait velocity used during analysis. The combination Kinect + MotionMetrix was employed to measure such parameters and all the additional variables that the software provides for walking and running gait. To control potential influencing factors for temporal parameters, only the right leg of the participants was analyzed (i.e., asymmetry) [11]. Through the use of a depth sensor, the Microsoft KinectTM sensor (version 1.0, Microsoft, Redmond, WA, USA) can monitor 3-D motions. It can locate 20 body joints in 3D space at 30 Hz. Here, two Microsoft KinectTM sensors were placed on either side of a treadmill in a certain configuration (170 cm from the treadmill's center in forward direction and 190 cm in the perpendicular direction, according to manufacturer recommendations) and utilized in conjunction with MotionMetrixTM software (Figure 1). The Microsoft KinectTM sensors can reach 60 Hz when both sensors can track the same point at the same time (according to the manufacturer). For data collection, manufacturer recommendations were considered (i.e., software calibration, tight clothes, no shiny black fabric or reflexes, no moving shoelaces, no moving hair, no sunlight, and no treadmill parts blocking the entire view of the participant).

Table 1. Definitions of the variables provided by the MotionMetrix software.

Gait Variables	Definition
Stance phase (% gait cycle)	Period when the foot is in contact with the floor
Swing phase (% gait cycle)	Period when the foot is not in contact with the floor
Load response (ms)	Period of initial double limb support
Pre-swing (ms)	Last phase of stance
Doble support (ms)	Stance with both feet in contact with the floor
Step time (ms)	Interval between initial contacts of the contralateral foot
Step length (cm)	Distance between initial contacts of the contralateral foot
Step frequency (spm)	Step rate per minute
Hip frontal angle (deg)	Hip angle at the coronal plane at the initial single support stage
Knee frontal angle (deg)	Knee angle at the coronal plane at the initial single support stage
Step width (cm)	Distance between the heels of the two feet during double stance
Running Variables	**Definition**
Stride time (ms)	Time between initial contacts of the same foot
Stride length (cm)	Distance between initial contacts of the same foot
Step frequency (spm)	Step rate per minute
Step time (ms)	Interval between initial contacts of the contralateral foot
Step length (cm)	Distance between initial contacts of the contralateral foot
Contact time (ms)	Time between initial contact to toe-off
Flight time (ms)	Time between toe off and initial contact of the contralateral foot
Foot strike angle (deg)	Angle between foot and ground at initial contact
Ankle landing (deg)	Angle between foot and shank at initial contact
Center of mass vertical displacement (cm)	Center of mass vertical displacement between steps
Spine angle (deg)	Forward lean
Thigh flexion (deg)	Maximum thigh flexion during the swing phase
Thigh extension (deg)	Maximum thigh extension during the swing phase
Shank angle (deg)	Shank angle at initial contact with respect the vertical axis at a sagittal plane
Landing knee flexion (deg)	Knee flexion at initial contact
Stance knee flexion (deg)	Maximum knee flexion during the stance phase
Swing knee flexion (deg)	Maximum knee flexion during the swing phase
Knee rotation (deg)	Axial rotation of the knee
Step width (cm)	Distance between the heel and the projection of the center of mass
Vertical force (BW)	Maximum vertical force during the stance phase
Brake force (% of max vertical force)	Maximum brake force during the initial contact phase
Lateral force (% of max vertical force)	Maximum lateral force during the stance phase
Maximal loading rate (BW/s)	Speed at which maximum vertical force is achieved
Maximal propulsion rate (BW/s)	Speed at which maximum propulsion force is achieved
External work (Joules/kg/m)	Work done to accelerate the center of mass with respect the environment
Internal work (Joules/kg/m)	Work done to accelerate the body segments with respect the center of mass
Leg-spring stiffness (BW/m)	Vertical leg length in response to the maximum vertical force of a step
Leg length difference at stance phase (cm)	Vertical leg length change during the stance phase

Table 1. *Cont.*

Running Variables	Definition
Elastic exchange (%)	Fraction of total work stored and released as elastic energy
Knee mediolateral force (BW)	Maximum medial force at the knee
Knee vertical force (BW)	Maximum vertical force at the knee
Knee frontal moment (BW/m)	Maximum adduction torque at the knee
Knee sagittal moment (BW/m)	Maximum propulsive torque at the knee
Hip mediolateral force (BW)	Maximum medial force at the hip
Hip vertical force (BW)	Maximum vertical force at the hip
Hip frontal moment (BW/m)	Maximum adduction torque at the hip
Hip sagittal moment (BW/m)	Maximum propulsive torque at the hip

ms: milliseconds; cm: centimeters; spm: steps per minute; deg: degrees; BW: bodyweight; %: percentage; BW/s: bodyweight per second; Joules/kg/m: joules per kilogram per meter; BW/m: bodyweight per meter.

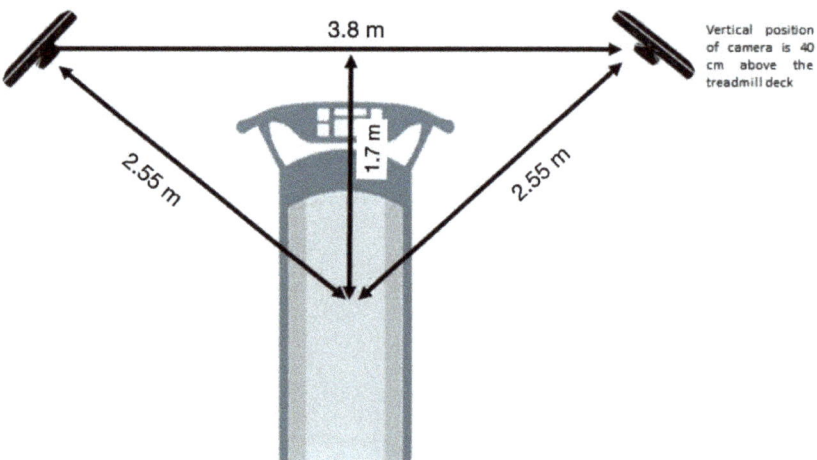

Figure 1. Experimental set-up including treadmill and the positioning of the kinect cameras.

2.4. Statistical Analysis

Data are shown as mean, standard deviation (SD), and ranges. Shapiro-Wilk test confirmed the assumption of data normal distribution ($p > 0.05$). A mean comparison analysis (i.e., dependent samples T-test) was applied between variables from both trials of each participant (i.e., test-retest) for magnitude comparison. Cohen's d effect size (ES) was adopted to interpret the magnitude of the differences following the next criterion: trivial (<0.20), small (0.20–0.59), moderate (0.60–1.19), large (1.20–2.00) and very large (>2.00) [13]. By means of standard error (SE) and coefficient of variation (CV in %, confidence interval (CI): 95%) reliability was assessed [13] and identified as acceptable when CV < 10% [14]. Moreover, intraclass correlation coefficient (ICC, model 3.1) between both trials and for each of the variables analyzed was provided after recommendations by Koo and Li [15]. ICC was interpreted considering the following cut-off values [16]: poor (ICC < 0), trivial (0–0.2), small (0.21–0.40), moderate (0.41–0.60), substantial (0.61–0.80), and almost perfect (>0.81). The 95% CI for these ICCs was also described. Custom spreadsheets were used to assess reliability [17]. The criterion alpha level was set at $\alpha = 0.05$.

3. Results

3.1. Test-Retest Reliability and ICC Interpretation during Walking Gait

The test-retest reliability data for the kinematic parameters reported by the Kinect + MotionMetrix system during walking at 5 km·h^{-1} are shown in Table 2.

Table 2. Descriptive data (means, ±SD) and inter-session reliability of kinematic parameters obtained from Kinect + MotionMetrix software walking at 5 km·h^{-1}.

Variable	Measure 1 (±SD)	Measure 2 (±SD)	p-Value (Cohen's d)	CV (%) (95% CI)	ICC (95% CI)	Typical Error
StP (% gait cycle)	65.079 (0.67)	65.054 (0.71)	0.849 (−0.04)	0.70 (0.54–0.98)	0.59 (0.25–0.80)	0.45 (0.35–0.64)
SwP (% gait cycle)	34.92 (0.67)	34.94 (0.71)	0.849 (0.04)	1.30 (1.01–1.82)	0.59 (0.25–0.80)	0.45 (0.35–0.64)
LR (ms)	147.72 (8.9)	151.29 (8.3)	0.016 (0.42) *	3.18 (2.47–4.46)	0.71 (0.44–0.86)	4.75 (3.69–6.67)
PSw (ms)	152 (8.9)	153.5 (7.5)	0.287 (0.18)	3.09 (2.40–4.34)	0.69 (0.40–0.85)	4.72 (3.67–6.62)
DS (ms)	299.73 (14.1)	304.83 (13.4)	0.014 (0.37) *	2.20 (1.71–3.09)	0.78 (0.56–0.90)	6.65 (5.17–9.33)
ST (ms)	520.65 (21)	523.25 (23.7)	0.108 (0.12)	1.03 (0.80–1.45)	0.95 (0.88–0.98)	5.39 (4.19–7.56)
SL (cm)	72.68 (3.4)	73.59 (4)	0.002 (0.12) *	1.24 (0.96–1.74)	0.94 (0.88–0.98)	0.74 (0.58–1.04)
SF (spm)	115.1 (4.8)	114.2 (5.4)	0.008 (−0.17) *	0.91 (0.71–1.27)	0.96 (0.92–0.98)	1.04 (0.81–1.46)
HFA (deg)	−0.32 (2.12)	0.18 (2.08)	0.548 (0.24)	-	−0.85 (−0.93–−0.69)	2.85 (2.22–4.00)
KFA (deg)	0.30 (2.16)	−0.62 (2.13)	0.293 (−0.43)	-	−0.92 (−0.97–−0.83)	2.97 (2.31–4.17)
SW (cm)	15.72 (3.92)	16.06 (4.28)	0.545 (0.08)	12.12 (9.42–17.01)	0.79 (0.58–0.91)	1.93 (1.50–2.70)

StT: stance phase; SwT: swing phase; LR: load response; PSw: pre-swing; DS: double support; ST: step time; SL: step length SF: step frequency; HFA: hip frontal angle; KFA: knee frontal angle; SW: step width; ms: milliseconds; spm: steps per minute; deg: degrees; cm: centimeters; SD: Standard deviation; CV: coefficient of variation; %: percentage, ICC: intraclass coefficient; CI: confidence interval; * $p < 0.05$.

When analyzing walking gait, significant differences were exhibited only for load response (LR) and double support (DS) phases ($p = 0.016$ and 0.014, respectively) showing a small magnitude of differences (ES = 0.42 and 0.37, respectively) when evaluating both measurements. Moreover, SL and SF showed significant differences ($p = 0.002$ and 0.008, respectively) with a trivial magnitude of differences (ES ≤ 0.12). For the rest of variables, no significant differences were identified.

Walking gait measures showed acceptable reliability for all variables (i.e., CV < 4%) except step width (SW) (CV = 12.12%). The ICC values obtained with markerless system for ST, SL and SF exhibited an almost perfect correlation (ICC = 0.95, 0.94, and 0.96, respectively). Pre-swing phase (PSw), LR, DS and SW showed substantial correlation (ICC < 0.80). Moreover, whereas ICCs for both StP and SwP were interpreted as moderate (<0.60), ICCs for hip frontal angle (HFA) and knee frontal angle (KFA) were considered as poor (ICC < 0).

3.2. Test-Retest Reliability and ICC Interpretation during Running Gait

Tables 3 and 4 show the test-retest reliability data for the kinetic and kinematic variables reported by the Kinect + MotionMetrix system during running at both 10 and 15 km·h^{-1}, respectively.

When analyzing running gait at 10 km·h^{-1}, significant differences were found between both measures for stride time (StrT), stride length (StrL), SF, SL, maximal thigh flexion (ThighFlex), maximal knee flexion during swing (KFSw), knee rotation (KRot) and SW ($p < 0.05$). The magnitude of the differences for these variables was interpreted as either trivial (ES < 0.20 for SF, ThighFlex, KFSw, KRot, and SW) or small (ES < 0.60 for StrT, StrL, and SL). However, no significant differences for the rest of the variables provided by the system when running at 10 km·h^{-1} (see Table 3).

Table 4 displays running analysis at 15 km·h^{-1} using Kinect + MotionMetrix system. Here, no significant differences between trials were found when analyzing kinematic parameters ($p > 0.05$) except when assessing vertical displacement (Vdisp) and KRot ($p < 0.03$), which also show a small (ES = 0.22) and trivial (ES = 0.17) magnitude of the differences, respectively. When examining kinetic variables, significant differences ($p < 0.05$) were found for vertical force (VertF), maximal loading rate (LRmax), maximal propulsion rate (PRmax), external work (ExW), leg-spring stiffness (LSS), knee vertical force (KFv), knee frontal moment (KMf), hip vertical force (HFv), and hip frontal moment (HMf). The magnitude of the differences for all the parameters mentioned above were identified as small (ES < 0.60) except PRmax, KFv, and HFv that were identified as trivial (ES < 0.20).

The rest of the variables show no significant differences when analyzing running gait at 15 km·h^{-1} (see Table 4).

When assessing reliability for running gait analysis at 10 km·h^{-1}, all variables seemed to show acceptable reliability (CV < 10%) except when evaluating reliability for foot strike angle (FSA), ankle landing (AL), spine angle (SpA), ThighFlex, knee flexion when landing (KFL), and SW (CV > 10%). The ICCs obtained revealed moderate correlation for thigh extension (ThighExt) and CT (ICC = 0.44 and 0.51, respectively), substantial correlation for ThighFlex, shank angle (ShA), KFL, knee flexion during stance phase (KFS), and knee flexion during swing phase (KFSw) (ICC = 0.67–0.78), and an almost perfect correlation (ICC > 0.81) for the rest of variables at a running speed of 10 km·h^{-1}.

Then, when running velocity was set at 15 km·h^{-1}, although all the kinematic variables provided by the system show acceptable reliability (CV < 10%), AL, SpA, and SW exhibited CV > 10% for their measures. When kinetic variables were considered, all the parameters show acceptable reliability (CV < 10%) except lateral force (LatF) and elastic exchange EEx showing CV = 13.97% and 21.4%, respectively. The ICC values obtained revealed almost perfect correlation for most of the kinetic and kinematic parameters (ICC > 0.83) except the kinematic parameters of ShA, SpA, and CT (ICC = 0.69, 0.76, 0.80, respectively) and the kinetic parameters of VertF, LRmax, Prmax, KFv, and HFv (ICC = 0.79, 0.71, 0.65, 0.80, and 0.79, respectively). Furthermore, the kinetic variable of elastic exchange (Eex) shows moderate correlation (ICC = 0.58).

Table 3. Descriptive data (means, ±SD) and inter-session reliability of the kinematic parameters obtained from Kinect + MotionMetrix software running at 10 km·h^{-1}.

Variable	Measure 1 (±SD)	Measure 2 (±SD)	p-Value (Cohen's d)	CV (%) (95% CI)	ICC (95% CI)	Typical Error
StrT (ms)	733.39 (45.0)	744.70 (40.0)	0.023 (0.27) *	2.17 (1.69–3.04)	0.87 (0.72–0.94)	16.04 (12.47–22.50)
StrL (cm)	203.72 (12.5)	206.86 (1.11)	0.023 (0.27) *	2.17 (1.69–3.04)	0.87 (0.72–0.94)	4.46 (3.46–6.25)
SF (spm)	164.23 (10.3)	161.58 (8.71)	0.030 (−0.28) *	2.43 (1.89–3.41)	0.84 (0.67–0.93)	3.96 (3.07–5.55)
ST (ms)	366.69 (22.5)	372.35 (20)	0.023 (0.27) *	2.17 (1.69–3.04)	0.87 (0.72–0.94)	8.02 (6.23–11.25)
SL (cm)	101.86 (6.2)	103.43 (5.6)	0.023 (0.27) *	2.17 (1.69–3.04)	0.87 (0.72–0.94)	2.23 (1.73–3.13)
CT (ms)	279.23 (23.4)	285.23 (21.5)	0.207 (0.27)	5.67 (4.40–7.95)	0.51 (0.14–0.75)	15.99 (12.43–22.44)
FT (ms)	87.46 (30.2)	87.12 (28.6)	0.925 (−0.01)	14 (10.88–19.64)	0.84 (0.66–0.93)	12.22 (9.50–17.14)
FSA (deg)	9.94 (4.1)	9.45 (4.1)	0.276 (−0.12)	15.90 (12.36–22.31)	0.87 (0.72–0.94)	1.54 (1.20–2.16)
AL (deg)	0.066 (0.03)	0.064 (0.03)	0.343 (−0.12)	17.46 (13.57–24.49)	0.84 (0.67–0.93)	0.45 (0.35–0.64)
Vdisp (cm)	8.21 (2.0)	8.46 (1.6)	0.206 (0.13)	7.86 (6.11–11.02)	0.88 (0.75–0.95)	0.55 (0.43–0.77)
SpA (deg)	6.78 (2.2)	6.52 (2)	0.261 (−0.13)	11.98 (9.31–16.81)	0.87 (0.72–0.94)	0.80 (0.62–1.12)
ThighFlex (deg)	24.91 (8.0)	22.38 (6.2)	0.032 (−0.35) *	16.26 (12.64–22.81)	0.73 (0.47–0.87)	3.85 (2.99–5.39)
ThighExt (deg)	−26.42 (4.3)	−27.29 (3.1)	0.306 (−0.23)	-	0.44 (0.05–0.71)	2.85 (2.21–3.99)
ShA (deg)	−5.18 (2.6)	−5.5 (2.8)	0.424 (−0.12)	-	0.76 (0.53–0.89)	1.35 (1.05–1.89)
KFL (deg)	18.93 (3.9)	19.39 (3.6)	0.425 (0.12)	10.14 (7.88–14.23)	0.75 (0.51–0.88)	1.94 (1.51–2.73)
KFS (deg)	44.84 (4.7)	43.88 (4.4)	0.145 (−0.21)	4.97 (3.86–6.97)	0.78 (0.56–0.90)	2.20 (1.71–3.09)
KFSw (deg)	92.98 (16.9)	87.48 (13.2)	0.043 (−0.36) *	9.89 (7.69–13.87)	0.67 (0.38–0.84)	8.92 (6.94–12.52)
KRot (deg)	−0.13 (2.5)	−0.74 (2)	0.037 (−0.27) *	-	0.83 (0.65–0.92)	0.96 (0.75–1.35)
SW (cm)	5.29 (2.1)	4.95 (2.4)	0.047 (−0.15) *	10.72 (8.33–15.04)	0.94 (0.88–0.98)	0.55 (0.43–0.77)

StrT: Stride time; StrL: stride length; SF: step frequency; ST: step time; SL: step length; CT: contact time; FT: flight time; FSA: foot strike angle; AL: ankle landing; Vdisp: vertical displacement of the center of mass; SpA: spine angle; ThighFlex: thigh flexion; thighExt: thigh extension; ShA: Shank angle; KFL: knee flexion when landing; KFS: knee flexion stance; KFSw: knee flexion swing; Krot: knee rotation; SW: step width; spm: steps per minute; cm: centimeters; deg: degrees; CV: coefficient of variation; %: percentage, ICC: intraclass coefficient; CI: confidence interval. * p < 0.05.

Table 4. Descriptive data (means, ±SD) and inter-session reliability of the kinematic and kinetic parameters obtained from Kinect + Motion-Metrix software running at 15 km·h^{-1}.

	Variable	Measure 1 (±SD)	Measure 2 (±SD)	p-Value (Cohen's d)	CV (%) (95% CI)	ICC (95% CI)	Typical Error
Kinematics	StrT (ms)	668.97 (47.2)	675.02 (42.4)	0.051 (0.13)	1.51 (1.18–2.12)	0.95 (0.89–0.98)	10.18 (7.91–14.28)
	StrL (cm)	281.74 (19.7)	281.26 (17.7)	0.051 (0.13)	1.51 (1.18–2.12)	0.95 (0.89–0.98)	4.24 (3.30–5.95)
	SF (spm)	179.43 (11.2)	178.43 (11)	0.223 (−0.09)	1.55 (1.20–2.17)	0.94 (0.87–0.97)	2.77 (2.15–3.89)
	ST (ms)	335.69 (21.8)	337.51 (21.2)	0.224 (0.08)	1.50 (1.16–2.10)	0.95 (0.89–0.98)	5.04 (3.92–7.07)
	SL (cm)	139.87 (9.1)	140.63 (8.8)	0.224 (0.08)	1.50 (1.16–2.10)	0.95 (0.89–0.98)	2.10 (1.63–2.95)
	CT (ms)	223.83 (11.4)	223.14 (11.8)	0.657 (−0.06)	2.38 (1.85–3.34)	0.80 (0.60–0.91)	5.32 (4.14–7.47)
	FT (ms)	111.86 (23.2)	114.37 (22.6)	0.250 (0.11)	6.52 (5.06–9.14)	0.90 (0.79–0.96)	7.37 (5.73–10.34)
	FSA (deg)	12.99 (5.5)	13.11 (5.2)	0.680 (0.02)	7.52 (5.85–10.55)	0.97 (0.93–0.99)	0.98 (0.76–1.38)
	AL (deg)	0.067 (0.03)	0.063 (0.03)	0.343 (−0.12)	17.46 (13.57–24.49)	0.84 (0.67–0.93)	0.01 (0.01–0.02)
	Vdisp (cm)	7.18 (1.9)	7.58 (1.7)	0.029 (0.22) *	8.09 (6.29–11.35)	0.90 (0.78–0.96)	0.60 (0.46–0.84)
	SpA (deg)	6.6 (3.3)	7.14 (3)	0.257 (0.17)	23.27 (18.09–32.64)	0.76 (0.52–0.89)	1.60 (1.24–2.24)
	ThighFlex (deg)	33.93 (5.97)	33.3 (6.28)	0.177 (−0.10)	4.72 (3.67–6.62)	0.94 (0.86–0.97)	1.59 (1.23–2.23)
	ThighExt (deg)	−35.35 (3.66)	−36.19 (2.91)	0.4 (−0.25)	–	0.85 (0.69–0.93)	1.33 (1.03–1.86)
	ShA (deg)	−0.5 (2.6)	−1.4 (2.8)	0.057 (−0.33)	–	0.69 (0.40–0.85)	1.54 (1.20–2.17)
	KFL (deg)	17.02 (4.07)	17.53 (4.06)	0.241 (0.13)	8.51 (6.62–11.94)	0.88 (0.74–0.95)	1.47 (1.14–2.06)
	KFS (deg)	40.9 (4.5)	40.6 (4.3)	0.35 (−0.07)	2.84 (2.21–3.98)	0.94 (0.86–0.97)	1.16 (0.90–1.62)
	KFSw (deg)	113.16 (11.5)	113.24 (10.36)	0.93 (0.01)	2.74 (2.13–3.84)	0.93 (0.84–0.97)	3.10 (2.41–4.35)
	Krot (deg)	−0.07 (2.6)	0.35 (2.4)	0.01 (0.17) *	–	0.96 (0.91–0.98)	0.53 (0.41–0.74)
	SW (cm)	4.39 (2.98)	4.43 (2.65)	0.88 (0.02)	22.22 (17.27–31.17)	0.89 (0.76–0.95)	0.98 (0.76–1.38)
Kinetics	VertF (BW)	2.44 (0.3)	2.52 (0.2)	0.017 (0.35) *	4.78 (3.71–6.70)	0.79 (0.58–0.91)	0.12 (0.09–0.17)
	BrakeF (Fv)	0.112 (0.02)	0.114 (0.03)	0.319 (0.10)	7.56 (5.88–10.61)	0.89 (0.77–0.95)	0.01 (0.01–0.01)
	Lrmax (BW/s)	30.04 (4.7)	31.98 (4.3)	0.013 (0.43) *	8.07 (6.27–11.31)	0.71 (0.44–0.86)	2.50 (1.94–3.51)
	Prmax (BW/s)	−27.14 (4.6)	−29.08 (3.9)	0.017 (−0.45) *	–	0.65 (0.34–0.83)	2.60 (2.02–3.65)
	ExW (Joules/kg/m)	0.42 (0.1)	0.44 (0.1)	0.034 (0.22) *	8.68 (6.75–12–17)	0.89 (0.77–0.95)	0.04 (0.03–0.05)
	IntW (Joules/kg/m)	0.69 (0.08)	0.7 (0.07)	0.58 (0.05)	3.05 (2.37–4.28)	0.92 (0.83–0.97)	0.02 (0.02–0.03)
	ExWg (Joules/kg/m)	1.12 (0.28)	1.17 (0.25)	0.079 (0.2)	8.58 (6.62–11.95)	0.87 (0.73–0.94)	0.1 (0.08–0.14)
	LSS (BW/m)	52.91 (10)	56.79 (11.8)	0.007 (0.35) *	8.31 (6.46–11.65)	0.84 (0.66–0.93)	4.56 (3.54–6.39)
	ΔLegSt (cm)	4.5 (0.9)	4.4 (0.9)	0.23 (0.11)	7.02 (5.46–9.85)	0.91 (0.80 − 0.96)	0.31 (0.24–0.44)
	LatF (Fv)	0.0337 (0.01)	0.0331 (0.01)	0.62 (−0.05)	13.97 (10.86–19.6)	0.87 (0.73–0.94)	0.00 (0.00–0.01)
	EEx (%)	31.06 (11.9)	31.32 (8)	0.89 (0.03)	21.40 (16.63–30.01)	0.58 (0.25–0.80)	6.67 (5.19–9.36)
	KFm (BW)	−0.092 (0.03)	−0.093 (0.03)	0.53 (−0.06)	–	0.90 (0.79–0.96)	0.01 (0.01–0.01)
	KFv (BW)	−2.29 (0.25)	−2.38 (0.22)	0.01 (−0.38) *	–	0.80 (0.58–0.91)	0.11 (0.09–0.15)
	KMf (BW/m)	0.12 (0.02)	0.13 (0.02)	0.002 (0.32) *	6.02 (4.68–8.44)	0.91 (0.80–0.96)	0.01 (0.01–0.01)
	KMs (BW/m)	0.41 (0.08)	0.42 (0.08)	0.33 (0.11)	7.11 (5.53–9.98)	0.87 (0.72–0.94)	0.03 (0.02–0.04)
	HFm (BW)	−0.097 (0.03)	−0.097 (0.03)	0.95 (−0.01)	–	0.90 (0.78–0.96)	0.01 (0.01–0.01)
	HFv (BW)	−2.07 (0.24)	−2.15 (0.20)	0.01 (−0.38) *	–	0.79 (0.58–0.90)	0.10 (0.08–0.15)
	HMf (BW/m)	0.24 (0.03)	0.25 (0.03)	0.016 (0.28) *	4.42 (3.44–6.2)	0.87 (0.73–0.94)	0.01 (0.01–0.02)
	HMs (BW/m)	0.54 (0.09)	0.55 (0.09)	0.34 (0.12)	7.07 (5.5–9.9)	0.84 (0.66–0.93)	0.04 (0.03–0.05)

StrT: stride time; StrL: stride length; SF: step frequency; ST: step time; SL: step length; CT: contact time; FT: flight time; FSA: foot strike angle; AL: ankle landing; Vdisp: vertical displacement of the center of mass; SA: spine angle; ThighFlex: thigh flexion; ThighExt: thigh extension; ShA: shank angle; KFL: knee flexion landing; KFS: knee flexion stance; KFSw: knee flexion swing; KRot: knee rotation; SW: step width; VertF: vertical force; VertImp: vertical impulse; BrakeF: brake force; LRmax: maximal loading rate; PRmax: maximal propulsion rate; ExW: velocity-normalized external work; IntW: internal work; ExWg: gravity-normalized external work; LSS: leg-spring stiffness; ΔLegSt: leg length difference at stance phase; LatF: lateral force; EEx: elastic exchange (i.e., fraction of total work stored and released as "free" elastic energy in muscle and tendons); KFm: knee mediolateral force; KFv: knee vertical force; KMf: knee frontal moment; KMs: knee sagittal moment; HFm: hip mediolateral force; HFv: hip vertical force; HMf: hip frontal moment; HMs: hip sagittal moment; spm: steps per minute; cm: centimeters; deg: degrees; BW: body weight; BW/m: body weight per meter; CV: coefficient of variation; %: percentage, ICC: intraclass coefficient; CI: confidence interval. * $p < 0.05$.

4. Discussion

This study aimed to determine the test–retest (inter-trial) reliability of the Kinect + MotionMetrix system for the analysis of both walking and running gait parameters (i.e., kinetic and kinematic variables) on a treadmill. Here, twenty-four participants were tested to assess the inter-trial reliability of such markerless system. Our results show that, although there were significant differences between both measurements for both LR and DS phases, and the spatiotemporal parameters of SL and SF, the system seems to provide reliable measurements when analyzing walking gait at 5 km·h^{-1}. Then, when considering reliability when running at 10 km·h^{-1}, no significant differences were found for most of the variables except when assessing StrT, StrL, SF, SL, ThighFlex, (KFSw), Krot, and SW. The system apparently provides reliable measures for all the variables apart from FSA, AL, SpA, ThighFlex, KFL, and SW. During running at 15 km·h^{-1}, no significant differences were found when evaluating kinematic parameters for both trials besides Vdisp and Krot obtaining, additionally, reliable measures from the system for all the kinematic parameters excepting AL, SpA, and SW. If kinematic parameters (i.e., running velocity) are considered, only Vdisp and Krot showed significant differences between both trials, providing the system reliable measurements for all these parameters except when assessing AL, SpA, and SW. For kinetic variables, although the system seems to be reliable when analyzing such parameters (excepting LatF and Eex), significant differences between trials were found for the measures of VertF, Lrmax, Prmax, ExW, LSS, KFv, KMf, HFv, and HMf. The results expose not only the overall intersession reliability of the system when assessing kinematics in walking and running gait, but also its inaccuracy when considering some kinetic parameters.

Research on validity and reliability of markerless motion capture systems for biomechanical analysis during either walking or running on a treadmill is limited. Although the validity of the Kinect™ sensor for walking gait analysis has been assessed [1,3–5], the findings reported are controversial. A previous study [3] stated that the Kinect™ sensor used for Windows is a valid tool for measuring walking gait spatiotemporal parameters. Others [5,6] have reported important differences when comparing spatiotemporal parameters measured by the Kinect™ sensor and such parameters by a three-dimensional motion capture system. Particularly, Clark et al. [6] determined that walking gait parameters obtained employing the Kinect™ were lower (i.e., −16% ST, −19% StrT, −1.7% SL) than those acquired utilizing the three-dimensional system. Similarly, Xu et al. [5] claimed that the Kinect™ system reported valid ST and StrT values, but shorter stance time (i.e., −9%) regarding the three-dimensional system when walking. Seemingly, the accuracy of the Kinect™ system in measuring spatiotemporal characteristics is mainly reliant on factors such as the software and filter settings used, the gold standard or reference system examined, or the procedure followed as well as target variables. It is worth noting that the treadmill protocol used in the present study was intended to reduce any potential gait and running variability caused by either treadmill inexperience or fatigue [18,19]. It has been reported that a minimum time of 6 to 8 min is required for healthy young adults and novice treadmill runners to accommodate their locomotion on the treadmill. Thus, it remains unknown whether the Kinect™ system would perform in greater variability conditions.

As treadmill running has been shown to have certain biomechanical variations from running on the ground [12], readers must be cautious when interpreting the results here reported. Some of the investigations that looked into the validity of the Kinect™ system were done on the ground [3,6], whereas just three studies were completed on a treadmill [4,5,7]. This is key as validity or reliability data obtained while walking should not be transferred to running situations since the magnitude of the parameters changes and other phases emerge (i.e., FT does not exist during walking, while there is no double-support time during running). Pfister and colleagues [7] investigated sagittal plane gait kinematics at different walking and running velocities (i.e., 4.8 to 8.8 km·h^{-1}), which are lower than the velocity in the current study (i.e., 5, 10 and 15 km·h^{-1}), without mentioning kinetic and kinematic parameters, and concluded that the measurement accuracy of the Kinect™ system was not acceptable for clinical measurement analysis (i.e., the system did not provide consistent hip or knee measurements as compared to a three-dimensional system). It is worth mentioning that Pfister [7] employed an older software (i.e., Brekel Kinect) combined with the Kinect™ sensor, which might explain the variations between the studies. The Brekel software operated at 30 Hz, but the software utilized in this study (i.e., MotionMetrix™) can operate at 60 Hz, implying a better level of precision. Indeed, the values obtained in the present study for knee and hip measures present lower CV at the different velocities (<~10%). However, when assessing ankle and spine angles, the CV were greater (>~12%) regardless running velocity.

To the best of the authors' knowledge, only one study [8] has examined the validity of the Kinect + MotionMetrix system during running. Here, absolute reliability and concurrent validity of this system for measuring CT, FT, SF, and SL was assessed when running at 12 km·h^{-1}. It was determined that the Kinect + MotionMetrix system provides valid SF and SL values, but CT and FT are overestimated and underestimated, respectively [8]. Our study complements the aforementioned study by assessing the reliability of the system not only for the spatiotemporal parameters previously mentioned, but for all the parameters (i.e., kinetic and kinematic variables) that the system provides as well. Of note, the MotionMetrix system offers different parameters depending on the walking or running velocity during analysis.

The lack of studies either assessing MotionMetrix™ reliability or employing the system for walking and/or running gait analysis has made the discussion section a challenge, being this the main limitation of the study. At the same time, this study offers evidence-based knowledge to fill such gap and to provide future studies support in the use of Kinect + MotionMetrix system. However, it is worth mentioning that the validity of the kinetics and kinematics variables still needs to be determined against a gold standard system to fully trust this technology and software combination. Furthermore, the sample recruited were active healthy subjects remaining therefore unknown how the system would perform in greater variability conditions such as (i.e., patients with gait disorders)

To sum up, the results indicate that the Kinect + MotionMetrix software provides reliable measures when analyzing walking gait at 5 km·h^{-1} for all the parameters that the software acquires except for SW (CV = 12.12%). Moreover, it provides reliable measurements for all the variables acquired in running at 10 km·h^{-1} except for FSA and AL (CV = 15.90% and 17.46%, respectively), ThighFlex, KFL and SW (CV = 16.26%, 10.14% and 10.72%, respectively). Finally, when running at 15 km·h^{-1}, the software also provides reliable values for all the kinematic parameters excepting AL, SpA, and SW (CV = 17.46%, 23.27% and 22.22%, respectively). However, when considering kinetic parameters in running at 15 km·h^{-1}, all the acquired values seem to be reliable apart from EEx (CV = 21.40%).

5. Conclusions

The results obtained show that, although some variables should be interpreted with caution, the Kinect + MotionMetrix system may be useful for walking and running gait analysis after a simple 30 s calibration. Both researchers and clinicians must be aware of the characteristics of the measures depending on either the walking or running velocity as the reliability of the parameters may fluctuate. The use of the MotionMetrix software offers practitioners a low-cost, time-efficient, and user-friendly motion analysis system for assessing and monitoring both walking and running gait at different velocities. Despite these promising results, the validity of the Kinect + MotionMetrix system still needs to be determined against a gold standard system to fully trust this technology and software combination.

Author Contributions: Conceptualization, S.A.R.-A. and F.G.-P.; methodology, D.J.-C. and E.J.R.-M.; software, L.E.R.-S. and J.M.C.-G.; validation, S.A.R.-A. and F.G.-P.; formal analysis, D.J.-C.; investigation, L.E.R.-S.; resources, E.J.R.-M. and J.M.C.-G.; data curation, L.E.R.-S.; writing—original draft preparation, D.J.-C.; writing—review and editing, F.G.-P.; visualization, S.A.R.-A.; supervision, L.E.R.-S.; project administration, F.G.-P.; funding acquisition, F.G.-P. and L.E.R.-S. All authors have read and agreed to the published version of the manuscript.

Funding: The authors declare no funding has been received for this research.

Institutional Review Board Statement: The study was conducted in accordance with the Declaration of Helsinki, and approved by the Institutional Review Board (or Ethics Committee) of University of Granada (protocol code 2546/CEIH/2022, 18th January 2022).

Informed Consent Statement: Informed consent was obtained from all subjects involved in the study.

Data Availability Statement: The data presented in this study are available on request from the corresponding author. The data are not publicly available due to the participants privacy.

Conflicts of Interest: The authors declare no conflict of interest.

References

1. Schmitz, A.; Ye, M.; Shapiro, R.; Yang, R.; Noehren, B. Accuracy and repeatability of joint angles measured using a single camera markerless motion capture system. *J. Biomech.* **2014**, *47*, 587–591. [CrossRef] [PubMed]
2. van der Kruk, E.; Reijne, M.M. Accuracy of human motion capture systems for sport applications; state-of-the-art review. *Eur. J. Sport Sci.* **2018**, *18*, 806–819. [CrossRef] [PubMed]
3. Dolatabadi, E.; Taati, B.; Mihailidis, A. Concurrent validity of the Microsoft Kinect for Windows v2 for measuring spatiotemporal gait parameters. *Med. Eng. Phys.* **2016**, *38*, 952–958. [CrossRef] [PubMed]
4. Lamine, H.; Bennour, S.; Laribi, M.; Romdhane, L.; Zaghloul, S. Evaluation of calibrated kinect gait kinematics using a vicon motion capture system. *Comput. Methods Biomech. Biomed. Eng.* **2017**, *20*, S111–S112. [CrossRef] [PubMed]
5. Xu, X.; McGorry, R.W.; Chou, L.-S.; Lin, J.-H.; Chang, C.-C. Accuracy of the Microsoft Kinect™ for measuring gait parameters during treadmill walking. *Gait Posture* **2015**, *42*, 145–151. [CrossRef] [PubMed]
6. Clark, R.A.; Bower, K.J.; Mentiplay, B.F.; Paterson, K.; Pua, Y.-H. Concurrent validity of the Microsoft Kinect for assessment of spatiotemporal gait variables. *J. Biomech.* **2013**, *46*, 2722–2725. [CrossRef] [PubMed]
7. Pfister, A.; West, A.M.; Bronner, S.; Noah, J.A. Comparative abilities of Microsoft Kinect and Vicon 3D motion capture for gait analysis. *J. Med. Eng. Technol.* **2014**, *38*, 274–280. [CrossRef] [PubMed]
8. García-Pinillos, F.; Jaén-Carrillo, D.; Hermoso, V.S.; Román, P.L.; Delgado, P.; Martinez, C.; Carton, A.; Seruendo, L.R. Agreement Between Spatiotemporal Gait Parameters Measured by a Markerless Motion Capture System and Two Reference Systems—A Treadmill-Based Photoelectric Cell and High-Speed Video Analyses: Comparative Study. *JMIR Mhealth Uhealth* **2020**, *8*, e19498. [CrossRef] [PubMed]
9. von Elm, E.; Altman, D.G.; Egger, M.; Pocock, S.J.; Gøtzsche, P.C.; Vandenbroucke, J.P. The Strengthening the Reporting of Observational Studies in Epidemiology (STROBE) statement: Guidelines for reporting observational studies. *Ann. Intern. Med.* **2007**, *147*, 573–577. [CrossRef] [PubMed]
10. McKay, A.K.; Stellingwerff, T.; Smith, E.S.; Martin, D.T.; Mujika, I.; Goosey-Tolfrey, V.L.; Sheppard, J.; Burke, L.M. Defining Training and Performance Caliber: A Participant Classification Framework. *Int. J. Sports Physiol. Perform.* **2022**, *17*, 317–331. [CrossRef] [PubMed]
11. Radzak, K.N.; Putnam, A.M.; Tamura, K.; Hetzler, R.K.; Stickley, C.D. Asymmetry between lower limbs during rested and fatigued state running gait in healthy individuals. *Gait Posture* **2017**, *51*, 268–274. [CrossRef] [PubMed]
12. van Hooren, B.; Fuller, J.T.; Buckley, J.D.; Miller, J.R.; Sewell, K.; Rao, G.; Barton, C.; Bishop, C.; Willy, R.W. Is Motorized Treadmill Running Biomechanically Comparable to Overground Running? A Systematic Review and Meta-Analysis of Cross-Over Studies. *Sports Med.* **2020**, *50*, 785–813. [CrossRef] [PubMed]
13. Hopkins, W.G.; Marshall, S.W.; Batterham, A.M.; Hanin, J. Progressive statistics for studies in sports medicine and exercise science. *Med. Sci. Sports Exerc.* **2009**, *41*, 3. [CrossRef] [PubMed]
14. Atkinson, G.; Nevill, A.M. Statistical methods for assessing measurement error (reliability) in variables relevant to sports medicine. *Sports Med.* **1998**, *26*, 217–238. [CrossRef] [PubMed]
15. Koo, T.K.; Li, M.Y. A guideline of selecting and reporting intraclass correlation coefficients for reliability research. *J. Chiropr. Med.* **2016**, *15*, 155–163. [CrossRef] [PubMed]
16. Landis, J.R.; Koch, G.G. The measurement of observer agreement for categorical data. *Biometrics* **1977**, *33*, 159–174. [CrossRef] [PubMed]
17. Hopkins, W.G. Spreadsheets for analysis of validity and reliability. *Sportscience* **2017**, *21*, 36–44.
18. Lavcanska, V.; Taylor, N.F.; Schache, A.G. Familiarization to treadmill running in young unimpaired adults. *Hum. Mov. Sci.* **2005**, *24*, 544–557. [CrossRef] [PubMed]
19. Schieb, D.A. Kinematic accommodation of novice treadmill runners. *Res. Q. Exerc. Sport* **1986**, *57*, 1–7. [CrossRef]

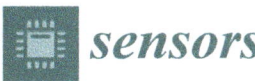

Article

Clinical–Functional Evaluation and Test–Retest Reliability of the G-WALK Sensor in Subjects with Bimalleolar Ankle Fractures 6 Months after Surgery

Mario Fernández-Gorgojo [1,2], Diana Salas-Gómez [1,*], Pascual Sánchez-Juan [1,3], David Barbado [4,5], Esther Laguna-Bercero [1,6] and María Isabel Pérez-Núñez [1,6]

1. Escuelas Universitarias Gimbernat (EUG), Physiotherapy School Cantabria, Movement Analysis Laboratory, University of Cantabria, 39005 Torrelavega, Spain; mario.fernandez@eug.es (M.F.-G.); psanchezjuan@fundacioncien.es (P.S.-J.); mesther.laguna@scsalud.es (E.L.-B.); isabel.perez@unican.es (M.I.P.-N.)
2. International Doctoral School, Rey Juan Carlos University (URJC), 28032 Madrid, Spain
3. Alzheimer's Centre Reina Sofia-CIEN Foundation, 28031 Madrid, Spain
4. Sports Research Centre, Department of Sport Science, Miguel Hernández University of Elche, 03202 Elche, Spain; dbarbado@umh.es
5. Alicante Institute for Health and Biomedical Research (ISABIAL), 03550 Alicante, Spain
6. Traumatology Service and Orthopedic Surgery, University Hospital "Marqués de Valdecilla" (UHMV), 39008 Santander, Spain
* Correspondence: diana.salas@eug.es

Abstract: Ankle fractures can cause significant functional impairment in the short and long term. In recent years, gait analysis using inertial sensors has gained special relevance as a reliable measurement system. This study aimed to evaluate the differences in spatiotemporal gait parameters and clinical–functional measurements in patients with bimalleolar ankle fracture and healthy subjects, to study the correlation between the different variables, and to analyze the test–retest reliability of a single inertial sensor in our study population. Twenty-two subjects with bimalleolar ankle fracture six months after surgery and eleven healthy subjects were included in the study. Spatiotemporal parameters were analyzed with the G-WALK sensor. Functional scales and clinical measures were collected beforehand. In the ankle fracture group, the main differences were obtained in bilateral parameters (effect size: $0.61 \leq d \leq 0.80$). Between-group differences were found in cadence, speed, stride length, and stride time (effect size: $1.61 \leq d \leq 1.82$). Correlation was moderate ($0.436 < r < 0.554$) between spatiotemporal parameters and clinical–functional measures, explaining up to 46% of gait performance. Test–retest reliability scores were high to excellent ($0.84 \leq ICC \leq 0.98$), with the worst results in the gait phases. Our study population presents evident clinical–functional impairments 6 months after surgery. The G-WALK can be considered a reliable tool for clinical use in this population.

Keywords: malleolar fractures; inertial sensor unit; wearable sensor; walking; spatiotemporal parameters; gait analysis; functional scales; clinical measurement; agreement of measurements

1. Introduction

Ankle fractures represent 10% of all bone fractures, with bimalleolar or lateral malleolus fractures being the most common according to the selection criteria used in studies [1,2]. The incidence has been increasing over the last two decades to between 71 and 187 fractures per 100,000 people depending on age, sex, and geographic region [3]. Surgical treatment of these fractures is necessary when joint congruence cannot be restored by conservative treatment, as instability, misalignment, and residual displacements will lead to short- and long-term functional impairment [4–9].

The importance of the severity of the injury, the surgical intervention, and the immobilization time ranging from 6 to 9 weeks implies significant biomechanical alterations.

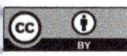

These consequences are reflected by decreased range of motion of the ankle joint, soft tissue impairments, proprioception, and loss of muscle strength, which indirectly affects functional activities such as walking, balance, jumping, and running [10–13].

Several studies have reported short- and long-term outcomes after surgery [14–16]. A meta-analysis researching the time course of physical recovery after ankle fracture with data from 23 studies concluded that adults, on average, recovered rapidly from activity limitation in the first 3 months after fracture, improved little between 3 and 6 months, and stabilized, without reaching full recovery, at 24 months [5].

Usually, different scores such as the American Orthopedic Foot and Ankle Society Ankle Hindfoot Score (AOFAS) [17] and the Olerud–Molander Ankle Score (OMAS) [18] can be used for the assessment of outcomes after surgery in terms of function and pain. Although these scores can provide a good assessment of function and patient-reported outcome measures (PROMs), they remain quite subjective [19,20].

After an ankle fracture, in addition to assessing functional capacity, it is important to identify clinical parameters that may be conditioning the recovery of these patients. Parameters such as lower extremity strength and range of motion have been studied as good predictors of functional capacity in the short term [10,13]. However, most studies focus on the assessment of ankle strength and do not evaluate other muscle groups of the lower extremity that may be affected after ankle surgery [10,21].

The analysis of spatiotemporal parameters of gait has been widely used to characterize functional performance in different populations [22,23].

This analysis is of particular importance in clinical practice, either to evaluate a rehabilitation process or after surgery [24]. It quantitatively describes the main gait events and thus reflects the patient's ability to meet the general gait requirements [25]. The most advanced technologies used for gait analysis make use of plantar pressures or 3D motion capture systems to detect changes in gait characteristics; these systems have been validated and are highly reliable for clinical use [26–28]. However, despite their advantages, they are expensive and must be operated by specialized personnel. With the advent of inertial measurement systems (IMUs) for spatiotemporal and kinematic assessments came a technological breakthrough in the field of biomechanics, as they are relatively inexpensive and allow the assessment of a virtually unlimited number of steps. In addition, they offer the possibility of assessing gait and movement disorders outside the restricted environments of the clinic and research laboratory [29].

A recent systematic review and meta-analysis provides encouraging results regarding the concurrent validity and reliability of IMUs for measuring step and stride length/time, with small differences depending on their placement on the body. However, measures of spatiotemporal asymmetry present inconsistent results that could be biased by the difference in protocols used for gait analysis or algorithms used for event detection [30]. Based on these results, individual reliability studies of these devices in different populations are needed before recommendations for their clinical use can be made.

Finally, some studies in healthy subjects [31,32] and with lower limb pathology [33] conclude that the individual use of a single IMU placed in the lumbar-sacral spine allows us to obtain reliable information based on trunk acceleration and angular velocity algorithms to estimate the spatiotemporal gait parameters [32,34,35]. Only a small number of studies have focused on gait analysis in patients with ankle malleolar fractures [6–10,19,36–38], but to date, none use a single IMU to record these spatiotemporal parameters.

The aims of this study were (1) to evaluate differences in spatiotemporal gait parameters and clinical measures in patients with ankle fracture 6 months after surgery (operated and non-operated ankle) and a control group of healthy subjects, (2) to study the association of gait parameters with clinical measures and functional scales in the ankle fracture group, and (3) to analyze the intra-session test–retest reliability and agreement of measurements from a single inertial sensor, placed on the lumbar-sacral spine, for the spatiotemporal parameters of gait in this population.

2. Materials and Methods

2.1. Type of Study

This cross-sectional study was carried out in the movement analysis laboratory of the University Schools of Physiotherapy and Speech Therapy Gimbernat-Cantabria attached to the University of Cantabria.

2.2. Participants

The population was composed of twenty-two participants (ten women/twelve men) who underwent surgery after a bimalleolar ankle fracture at the Trauma Unit of the University Hospital "Marqués de Valdecilla" (UHMV) in Santander. The surgical technique used was open reduction and internal fixation (ORIF), and the time elapsed from injury to surgery was 4.8 ± 7.6 days. After the immobilization period (3.4 ± 1.2 weeks), progressive and variable rehabilitation was carried out depending on the individual improvement of each case (13 ± 2.4 weeks) 5 days a week by the physiotherapy service of the UHMV. Inclusion criteria were established as 6 months after surgery and age between 18 and 55 years. Patients with previous surgery on the lower limb, bilateral ankle involvement, neurological, and rheumatic pathology were excluded.

Subjects were selected through medical records registered at the UHMV and with the collaboration of the Trauma Unit. After the Informed Consent was approved in writing by the Cantabrian Research Ethics Committee (CEIC) (Reference: 2017.072), they were invited to participate by telephone or email, where they were informed of the objective of the study and the procedure to be followed for its realization.

In this study, we also had a control group (CG) of eleven healthy subjects (six women/five men), consisting of university faculty and staff who agreed to participate on a voluntary basis. These participants were chosen on the basis of characteristics similar to the ankle fracture group in age and sex. All of them were currently free of musculoskeletal pathology of the lower extremity, neurological or rheumatological problems, and with no history of such pathologies.

2.3. Procedure

Data collection was carried out in a single individual visit 6 months after surgery, and, after a brief explanation of the procedure to be followed, the Informed Consent was signed. The control group was assessed during the same period as the data collection. Sociodemographic and clinical information regarding the surgery and the rehabilitation process was extracted from the medical records. The clinical data collected were firstly the American Orthopaedic Foot and Ankle Society (AOFAS) Ankle Hindfoot score [39] and the Olerud Molander Ankle Score (OMAS) [18] questionnaires, which assess the functional status of the patients. Subsequently, physical examination of both legs was performed by anthropometric measurement, bimalleolar/calf perimeters, ankle dorsiflexion range of motion (ADF ROM), and hip abductor (ABD)/adductor (ADD) muscle strength. The protocol performed for the clinical measurements was described in detail in our previous study [13].

The gait cycle (GC) analysis was performed with the subject barefoot on a walkway 8 m long and 2.5 m wide where they had to perform 4 laps (32 m) at their normal walking speed. We considered normal speed to be the speed previously preferred by each subject after a brief trial at different speeds following the recommendations of some authors for gait analysis on level ground [40]. Two valid trials were collected for each subject, discarding in the processing the first and last step of each lap. For gait analysis, a wireless inertial sensor system BTS G-WALK (BTS Bioengineering S.p.A., Milan, Italy) weighing 37 g and measuring $70 \times 40 \times 18$ mm was used, placed by means of a semi-elastic belt at the level of the fifth lumbar vertebra (L5) and the first two sacral vertebrae (S1–S2). This inertial system is equipped with 4-Sensor Fusion technology that integrates a triaxial accelerometer (16 bits/axis, ± 8 g), a triaxial magnetometer (13 bits, ± 1200 uT), a triaxial gyroscope (16 bits/axis, $\pm 250\,°/s$), and a GPS receiver. All data were collected at a frequency of 100 Hz and transmitted through a Bluetooth 3.0 connection to the computer. A specific software (BTS G-Studio) allows processing the information and calculating the spatiotemporal gait parameters and the percentage of symmetry for these parameters between both legs. The exact algorithms of the G-WALK are unknown and are part of the internal organization of the BTS company. However, some studies validate its use in different populations [34,35,41], although it has not been validated in subjects after ankle fracture.

The general spatiotemporal parameters collected were cadence (strides/min), speed (m/s), stride length (m) (this length was normalized by the length of the legs, trochanter-floor distance), and stride time (s). Bilateral spatiotemporal parameters (leg differences expressed as a percentage of the gait cycle) were step length (% stride length), stance phase (%GC), swing phase (%GC), double support (%GC), single support (%GC), and propulsion index (m/s^2) (the difference in anterior/posterior acceleration of the body barycenter during the single support phase of the right and left side's gait cycle) [30].

2.4. Statistical Analysis

First, participants in the ankle fracture group (AFG) were classified according to their operated and non-operated ankle. For the CG, the dominant leg was taken as the reference. Sociodemographic and clinical variables were described. For categorical variables, percentages with their corresponding 95% confidence intervals (95%CI) were estimated, and for continuous variables, means were estimated with their standard deviation or, if they did not follow a normal distribution, their median and range. The Shapiro–Wilk test was performed to analyze the normality of the variables.

In the AFG, the results of the different variables were obtained for both ankles (operated/non-operated). The difference between them was analyzed using Student's *t*-test for paired samples (expressed as mean difference) or its non-parametric equivalent Wilcoxon matched-pairs signed-ranks test (expressed with the Z-value typed for comparison with that of a standardized normal distribution). Differences between groups (AFG/CG) were performed using the Student's *t*-test for independent samples or its equivalent non-parametric Mann–Whitney U test. Likewise, the effect size was calculated using Cohen's *d* or Hodges' *g*, whose values are quantified as follows: 0.2 small, 0.5 medium, and 0.8 large [42].

The relationship between clinical measurements and functional scales with spatiotemporal gait parameters was analyzed using Pearson's correlation coefficient (r) or Spearman's rank correlation (Rho) (non-parametric). A regression model (simple and multiple linear regression, r^2), expressed together with the value of the F-statistic, was then applied to the variables that showed a significant correlation to determine the extent to which clinical measurements or functional scale scores could predict the results of the gait analysis. Intra-session test–retest reliability of spatiotemporal gait parameters measured with the G-WALK in the AFG was calculated using two valid trials. For relative reliability, an ICC$_{2,1}$ model with a 95% CI was used following the recommendations described in the literature [43]. The ICC values were classified as follows: excellent (0.90 to 1.00), high (0.70 to 0.89), moderate (0.50 to 0.69) and low (<0.50) [44]. Absolute reliability was obtained with the standard error of measurement (SEM) calculated as SEM = SD × $\sqrt{(1 - ICC)}$ [45]. The SEM values were expressed in the same units as the mean value and in a percentage (SEM%) to facilitate interpretation and extrapolation of the results to other individuals.

Finally, Bland–Altman plots analysis with 95% limits of agreement (LoA; mean differences: ±1.96 SD) were generated to visualize the degree of agreement between the measurements reported. Systematic error (bias) was obtained using the mean of the differences.

Statistical analysis of the data was performed using SPSS 20.0 software (Statistical Product and Service Solutions IBM SPSS Statistics 19.0 2010).

3. Results

A total of twenty-two patients with bimalleolar ankle fractures and 6 months after surgery participated in the present study. The mean age was 43.5 ± 10.2 years, with ages ranging from 21 to 55 years. Eleven healthy subjects with a mean age of 39.9 ± 8.6 were in the control group (CG). Table 1 describes the demographic and anthropometric characteristics of both groups, as well as the functional status of the AFG.

Table 1. Demographic, anthropometric, and functional characteristics of patients with bimalleolar ankle fractures 6 months after surgery and the control group.

Type (n = 22)	AFG (n = 22) Mean ± SD	95%CI	CG (n = 11) Mean ± SD	95%CI
Age (years)	43.5 ± 10.2	39.0; 48.0	39.9 ± 8.6	34.1; 45.7
Sex Women (%); Men (%)	45% (W); 55% (M)		55% (W); 45% (M)	
Height (cm)	169.3 ± 9.5	164.8; 173.7	170.5 ± 7.9	165.2; 175.8
Weight (kg)	77.8 ± 10.6	73.1; 82.5	74.0 ± 9.1	67.9; 80.1
Operated Limb Length	85.6 ± 5.9	82.9; 88.2	86.2 ± 5.5 *	82.6; 89.9 *
Healthy Limb Length (cm)	85.6 ± 5.9	82.9; 88.2		
Days from injury to surgery	4.8 ± 7.6	1.4; 8.1		
Immobilization (weeks)	3.4 ± 1.2	2.8; 3.9		
AOFAS Ankle Hindfoot score	73.6 ± 11.4	71.9; 75.3		
OMAS	57.3 ± 22.0	54.1; 60.6		

AFG: ankle fracture group; CG: control group; SD: standard deviation; CI: confidence interval; AOFAS: American Orthopedic Foot and Ankle Society; OMAS: Olerud Molander Ankle Score; Dominant leg CG * cm.

The difference between the operated and non-operated ankle in the spatiotemporal gait parameters showed a significant difference in step length (-3.8%; $p = 0.009$; $d = 0.61$), stance phase ($Z = -2.9$; $p = 0.004$; $g = 0.76$), swing phase ($Z = -2.9$; $p = 0.004$; $g = 0.76$), single support ($Z = -3.0$; $p = 0.002$; $g = 0.80$), and propulsion index (-0.8 m/s^2; $p = 0.010$; $d = 0.62$). We also found differences in clinical measurements except for ADD strength with an effect size between $0.15 \leq d \leq 2.30$ (Table 2).

Table 2. Difference between the operated and non-operated ankle in clinical measurements, spatial–temporal gait parameters, and dynamic plantar pressure.

	Type (n = 22)	Operated Ankle Mean ± SD/Median (Range)	Non-Operated Ankle Mean ± SD/Median (Range)	Differences between Ankles Mean (95% CI)/Z [1]	Cohen's d/Hedges' g	p Value *
Clinical measurements	Calf perimeter (cm)	34.2 ± 4.0	35.5 ± 4.4	−1.3 (−2.0; −0.5)	0.78	0.001 *
	Bimalleolar perimeter (cm)	25.1 ± 2.1	24.1 ± 2.1	1.0 (0.8; 1.2)	2.30	<0.001 *
	ADF ROM (degrees)	22.8 ± 7.7	35.4 ± 5.3	−12.7 (−15.1; −10.3)	2.23	<0.001 *
	Strength ABD (%)	25.5 ± 7.2	29.3 ± 8.6	−3.8 (−6.4; −1.2)	0.62	0.006 *
	Strength ADD (%)	26.3 ± 9.1	25.8 ± 8.6	0.6 (−1.1; −2.2)	0.15	0.491
Spatiotemporal parameters	Cadence (step/min)	99.9 ± 9.8				
	Speed (m/s)	0.94 ± 0.1				
	Stride length (m)	1.28 ± 0.1				
	Stride time (s)	1.21 ± 0.1				
	Step length % SL	48.1 ± 3.1	51.9 ± 3.1	−3.8 (−6.7; −1.1)	0.61	0.009 *
	Stance % GC [1]	63.4 (20.3)	67.4 (17.9)	−2.9	0.76	0.004 *
	Swing % GC [1]	36.6 (20.3)	32.6 (17.9)	2.9	0.76	0.004 *
	Double support % GC	15.0 ± 4.3	16 ± 2.1	−1.0 (−2.8; −0.8)	0.25	0.267
	Single support % GC [1]	32.6 (17.6)	36.7 (20.6)	−3.0	0.80	0.002 *
	Propulsion index (m/s^2)	5.2 ± 1.8	6.0 ± 1.4	−0.8 (−0.2; −1.2)	0.62	0.010 *

SD: standard deviation; CI: confidence interval; ADF ROM: ankle dorsiflexion range of movement; ABD: hip abductor muscle (normalized by body mass); ADD: hip adductor muscle (normalized by body mass); ROM: range of movement; GC: gait cycle; SL: stride length; Cohen's d: size effect; Hedges' g: size effect (non-parametric); [1] Wilcoxon matched-pairs signed-ranks test (non-parametric; expressed with the typed Z-value); * Significance level $p < 0.05$.

In the comparative analysis between AFG and CG of spatiotemporal gait parameters (Table 3), we found a significant difference and a high effect size in cadence (−13.8 p/m; $p < 0.001$; $d = 1.61$); speed (−0.24 m/s; $p < 0.001$; $d = 1.71$), stride length (−0.18 m; $p = 0.003$; $d = 1.82$); stride time (0.16 s; $p < 0.001$; $d = 1.65$); single support (−3.0%; $p = 0.045$; $d = 0.71$), and propulsion index (−1.7 m/s^2; $p = 0.013$; $d = 0.98$). The differences found in clinical measurements were significant for bimalleolar perimeter (3.2 cm; $p < 0.001$; $d = 1.64$), ADF ROM (−19.1°; $p < 0.001$; $d = 2.71$), and ABD strength (−8.6%; $p = 0.005$; $d = 1.12$).

Table 3. Difference between bimalleolar ankle fracture patients and the control group in clinical measurements and spatiotemporal gait parameters.

	Type	AFG (n = 22) Mean ± SD/Median (Range)	CG (n = 11) Mean ± SD/Median (Range)	Differences between Ankles Mean (95% CI)/Z [1]	Cohen's d/Hedges' g	p Value *
Clinical measurements	Calf perimeter (cm)	34.2 ± 4.0	33.7 ± 2.5	0.5 (3.1; −2.3)	−0.14	0.76
	Bimalleolar perimeter (cm)	25.1 ± 2.1	21.9 ± 1.6	3.2 (4.6; 1.7)	−1.64	<0.001 *
	ADF ROM (degrees)	22.8 ± 7.4	41.9 ± 6.1	−19.1 (−13.8; −24.4)	2.71	<0.001 *
	Strength ABD (%)	25.5 ± 7.2	34.2 ± 8.8	−8.6 (−2.7; −14.5)	1.12	0.005 *
	Strength ADD (%)	26.3 ± 9.1	32.7 ± 9.2	−6.4 (0.5; −13.2)	0.72	0.06
Spatiotemporal parameters	Cadence (step/min)	99.9 ± 9.8	113.7 ± 5.2	−13.8 (−8.4; −19.1)	1.61	<0.001 *
	Speed (m/s)	0.94 ± 0.1	1.18 ± 0.2	−0.24 (−0.12; −0.36)	1.71	<0.001 *
	Stride length (m)	1.28 ± 0.1	1.46 ± 0.1	−0.18 (−0.06; −0.27)	1.82	0.003 *
	Stride time (s)	1.21 ± 0.1	1.05 ± 0.1	0.16 (0.23; 0.08)	−1.65	<0.001 *
	Step length % SL	48.1 ± 3.1	49.2 ± 1.2	−1.1 (0.6; −2.8)	0.42	0.196
	Stance % GC [1]	63.4 (20.3)	63.6 (9.5)	−0.2	0.03	0.834
	Swing % GC [1]	36.6 (20.3)	36.4 (10.3)	−0.4	−0.02	0.688
	Double support % GC	15.0 ± 4.3	14.3 ± 3.3	0.7 (−2.3; 3.7)	−0.17	0.612
	Single support % GC	32.6 ± 4.5	35.6 ± 3.6	−3.0 (−0.1; −6.2)	0.71	0.045 *
	Propulsion index (m/s^2)	5.2 ± 1.8	6.9 ± 1.6	−1.7 (−1.1; −2.3)	0.98	0.013 *

AFG: ankle fracture group; CG: control group; SD: standard deviation; CI: confidence interval; ADF ROM: ankle dorsiflexion range of movement; ABD: hip abductor muscle (normalized by body mass); ADD: hip adductor muscle (normalized by body mass); ROM: range of movement; GC: gait cycle; SL: stride length; Cohen´s d: size effect; Hedges' g: size effect (non-parametric); [1] Wilcoxon matched-pairs signed-ranks test (non-parametric; expressed with the typed Z-value); * Significance level $p < 0.05$.

Correlation analysis between clinical measurements and spatiotemporal gait parameters in the operated ankle showed statistically significant results and a moderate to large effect size (Table 4). Regression model analysis showed that both ADF ROM, ABD strength, and calf perimeter scores can explain the variability of gait analysis results between 20% and 46%. Specifically, cadence increased with increasing ADF ROM r = 0.552 (F (1, 21) = 8.7, $r^2 = 0.30$, $p = 0.009$); speed increased with increasing ADF ROM r = 0.533 and increasing ABD strength r = 0.436 (F (1, 21) = 6.6, $r^2 = 0.25$, $p = 0.018$); stride length increased with increasing ABD strength r = 0.444 (F (1, 21) = 4.9; $r^2 = 0.20$); stride time decreased with increasing ADF ROM r = −0.554 (F (1, 21) = 8.8; $r^2 = 0.26$); propulsion index was greater the higher the ADF ROM r = 0.523 and calf perimeter r = 0.447 (F (1, 21) = 10, $r^2 = 0.46$, $p = 0.001$). Finally, with respect to the AOFAS scores, the correlation was positive with cadence (r = 0.540), speed (r = 0.428) and stride time (r = 0.547). Simple linear regression analysis showed that the AOFAS score could only explain the variability of cadence (F (1, 21) = 8.2, $r^2 = 0.29$, $p = 0.009$) and stride time (F (1, 21) = 8.5, $r^2 = 0.30$, $p = 0.008$) by 30%.

The intra-session test–retest reliability analysis, including ICC$_{2,1}$, SEM, and SEM% values, are shown in Table 5. Excellent relative reliability scores ($0.95 \leq ICC \leq 0.98$) were found for the general parameters of gait analysis, as well as low absolute reliability values between $1.56\% \leq SEM\% \leq 2.47\%$. For the bilateral parameters, a good to excellent ICC score was found with values between 0.84 and 0.95. The worst SEM% values were for double support (11.20%) in the operated ankle and propulsion index (7.88%) in the non-operated ankle.

Table 4. Correlation between clinical measurements and functional scales with the spatiotemporal gait parameters in operated ankle.

Spatiotemporal Gait Parameters	Clinical Measurements and Functional Scales					
	ADF ROM	Strength ABD	Bimalleolar Perimeter	Calf Perimeter	AOFAS	OMAS
Cadence (step/min) [1]	0.552 **	0.405	0.230	0.177	0.540 **	0.415
Speed (m/s) [1]	0.533 *	0.436 *	0.335	−0.124	0.428 *	0.247
Stride length (m) [1]	0.413	0.444 *	0.070	−0.289	0.247	0.083
Stride time (s) [1]	−0.554 **	−0.393	−0.263	−0.205	−0.547 **	−0.398
Step length % SL [1]	−0.001	0.231	0.056	−0.144	0.163	0.205
Stance % GC [2]	−0.054	−0.178	−0.112	0.144	0.115	0.172
Swing % GC [2]	0.054	0.178	0.112	−0.144	−0.115	−0.172
Double support % GC [1]	−0.224	−0.303	−0.060	0.222	−0.069	0.036
Single support % GC [2]	0.318	0.491 *	−0.001	−0.076	0.402	0.284
Propulsion index (m/s²) [1]	0.516 *	−0.052	0.122	0.449 *	0.407	0.261

[1] Pearson's correlations (r); [2] Spearman's rank correlation coefficient (Rho) (non-parametric); * $p < 0.05$; ** $p < 0.01$.

Table 5. Intra-session test–retest reliability spatiotemporal gait parameters with the G-WALK sensor. Limits of agreement (Bland–Altman analysis) and mean of the differences (bias) between two trials.

	Spatiotemporal Gait Parameters	ICC (95%CI)	SEM (95% CI)	SEM%	LoA (Lower; Upper)	Bias
	Cadence (step/min)	0.95 (0.89; 0.97)	2.21 (0.79; −3.64)	2.21	−3.91; 2.12	−0.89
	Speed (m/s)	0.97 (0.93; 0.98)	0.02 (0.01; 0.05)	2.12	−0.06; 0.04	−0.01
	Stride length (m)	0.98 (0.97; 0.99)	0.02 (0.01; 0.03)	1.56	−0.07; 0.06	0.01
	Stride time (s)	0.95 (0.70 0.98)	0.03 (0.01; 0.05)	2.47	−0.06; 0.10	0.02
Operated Ankle	Step length % SL	0.90 (0.82; 0.94)	1.01 (0.55; 1.46)	2.09	−2.17; 1.92	−0.12
	Stance phase % GC	0.91 (0.84; 0.94)	1.43 (0.75; 2.12)	2.25	−5.02; 4.51	−0.26
	Swing phase % GC	0.86 (0.75; 0.91)	1.79 (1.10; 2.47)	4.89	−4.51; 5.02	0.26
	Double support % GC	0.85 (0.74; 0.91)	1.68 (1.06; 2.31)	11.20	−6.80; 7.74	0.47
	Single support % GC	0.84 (0.74; 0.91)	1.82 (1.17; 2.48)	5.58	−9.21; 5.63	−1.79
	Propulsion index (m/s²)	0.90 (0.83; 0.94)	0.45 (0.24; 0.65)	7.50	−1.79; 1.89	0.05
Non-operated Ankle	Step length % GC	0.90 (0.84; 0.95)	1.01 (0.55; 1.46)	1.94	−1.92; 2.17	0.12
	Stance phase % GC	0.94 (0.89; 0.96)	1.12 (0.46; 1.77)	1.66	−2.96; 4.50	0.77
	Swing phase % GC	0.92 (0.86; 0.95)	1.29 (0.63; 1.95)	3.95	−4.50; 2.96	−0.77
	Double support % GC	0.84 (0.73; 0.90)	1.06 (0.68; 1.44)	6.62	−5.57; 7.83	1.13
	Single support % GC	0.84 (0.73; 0.91)	1.90 (1.22; 2.58)	5.17	−7.59; 8.17	0.29
	Propulsion index (m/s²)	0.95 (0.92; 0.97)	0.41 (0.15; 0.68)	7.88	−1.89; 1.20	−0.34
	Propulsion index (m/s²)	0.95 (0.92; 0.97)	0.41 (0.15; 0.68)	7.88	−1.89; 1.20	−0.34

CI: confidence interval; ICC: intraclass correlation coefficient; SEM: standard error of the measurement; LoA: limits of agreement; Bias: mean of the differences.

Figures 1 and 2 show the Bland–Altman plots comparing the results of the spatiotemporal gait parameters. The horizontal line represents the mean of the differences, while the dotted lines represent the confidence interval. The Bland–Altman plot analysis showed an excellent degree of agreement between measurements for speed (bias = −0.01; LoA = −0.06; 0.04) and stride length (bias = 0.01; LoA = −0.07; 0.06). Single support (bias = −1.79; LoA = −9.21; 6.63) in the operated ankle and double support (bias = 1.13; LoA = −5.57; 7.83) in the non-operated ankle showed the lowest degrees of agreement. The mean error and limits of agreement for the remaining variables are reported in Table 5.

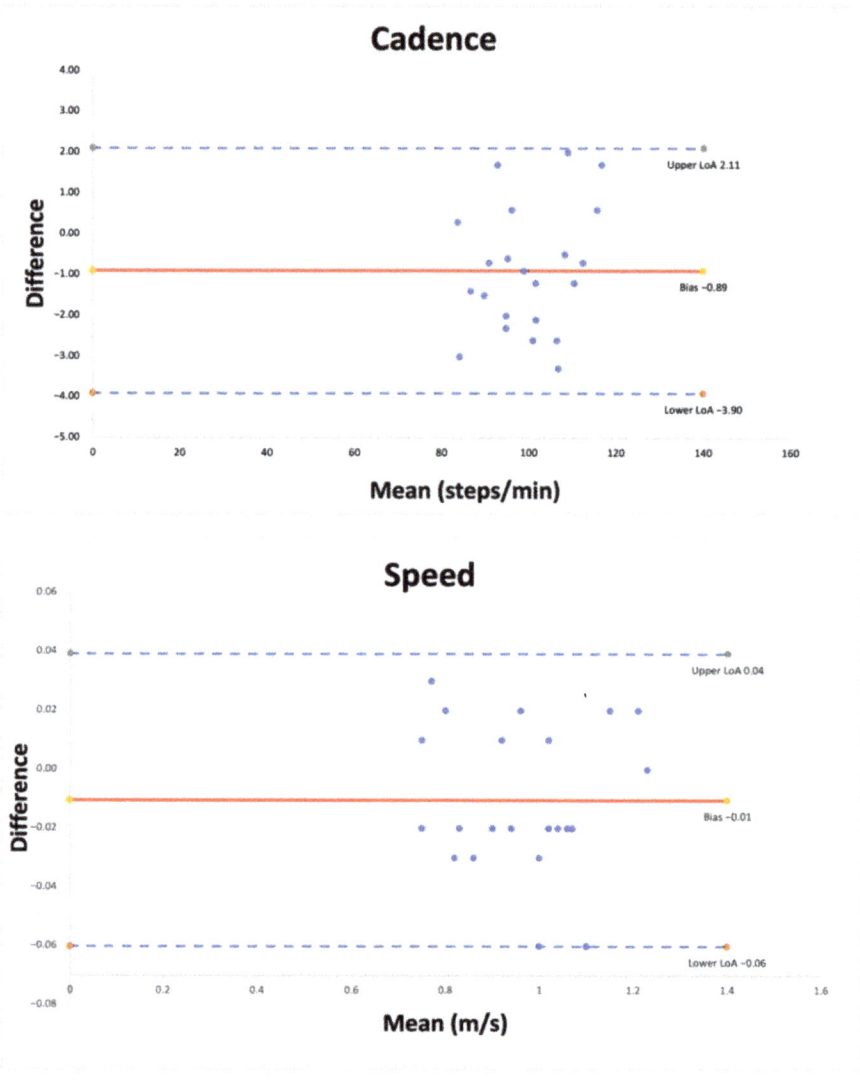

Figure 1. Bland-Altman plots for cadence and speed. Each graph presents the mean difference (solid line) and 1.96-fold standard deviation of difference (dashed line) indicating the limits of agreement between the measurement.

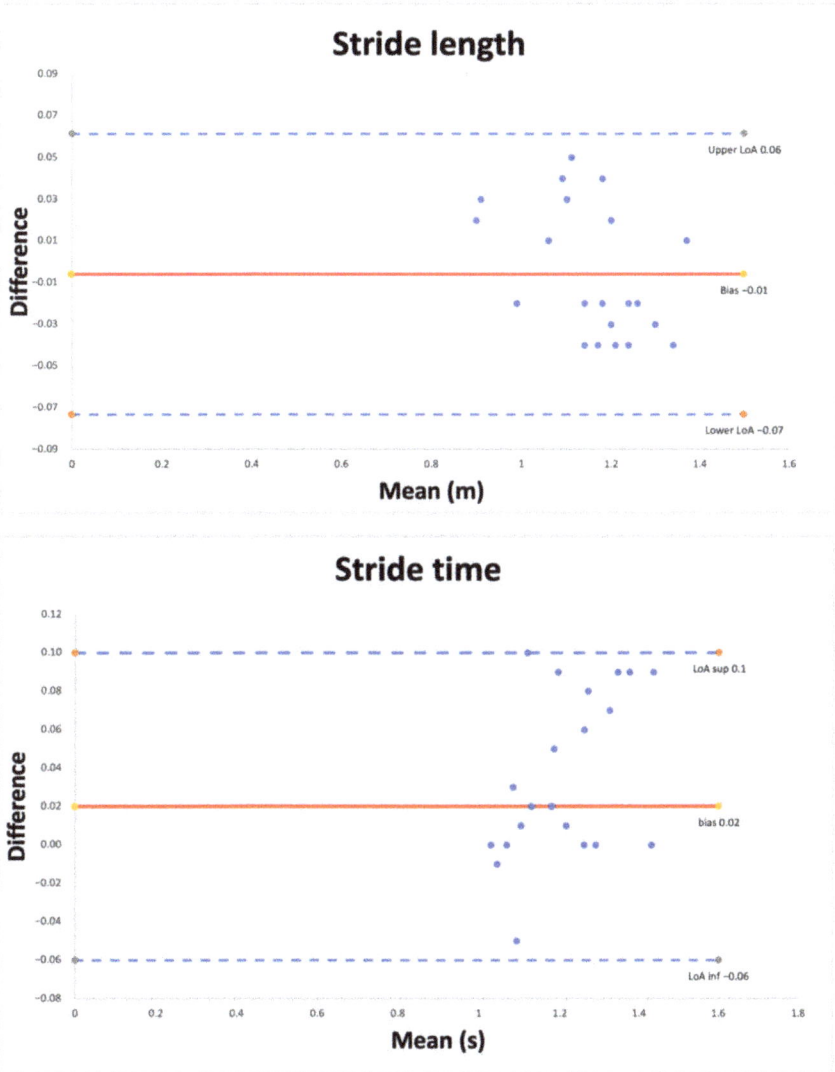

Figure 2. Bland-Altman plots for stride length and stride time. Each graph presents the mean difference (solid line) and 1.96-fold standard deviation of difference (dashed line) indicating the limits of agreement between the measurement.

4. Discussion

One of the aims of our study was to evaluate the spatiotemporal gait parameters in patients with bimalleolar ankle fractures 6 months after surgery and compare them with healthy subjects.

In the AFG, we found a clear difference between both legs in the gait phases. In particular, the double support was the only parameter where no differences were obtained. Regarding the comparative analysis with the CG, the main differences were obtained in cadence, speed, stride length, stride time, and single support in the operated ankle. Our results are in agreement with a study by Suciu et al. [37] in thirty patients with bimalleolar ankle fractures and twenty-one healthy subjects, in which they found differences between both ankles in step time, step length, swing phase, stance phase, and single support after

12 weeks of specific rehabilitation. Compared to the control group they found differences in stride length and speed. However, in contrast to our findings, they found no differences in cadence or stride time. Aspects that may determine the differences between the two studies include the measurement system used and the type of rehabilitation performed. On the other hand, half of the participants in their study were over 50 years of age, and the results were considerably different from younger adults whose recovery process was very rapid. Another study conducted on patients with trimalleolar ankle fractures 6 months after surgery found similar results to ours when compared to healthy subjects in speed, cadence, stride length, and stride time [46]. In contrast, our patients with bimalleolar fractures had a stride length 18 cm longer than that obtained in their study, which we believe to be a clinically important difference. However, other studies conclude that there are no short-term differences in gait characteristics between bimalleolar and trimalleolar ankle fractures [6,7]. Segal et al. [7], in their study of forty-one subjects with ankle fracture and seventy-two healthy subjects, found in the bimalleolar fracture group (n = 15) differences between the two ankles in step length (−29.2% SL) and single support (−15.9% GC). In our patients, we also found this asymmetry in step length (−3.8% SL) and single support (−4.1% GC), although the difference was not as large. In addition, the speed was only 0.48 m/s, very different from what we found (0.94 m/s). The differences in the results seem to be justified by the period of the measurements, as the Segal et al. study was performed from the 12th week after surgery, just when weight-bearing on the operated ankle was allowed.

As we have just seen, the decrease in speed and stride length is very much conditioned by the time of recovery in which the patients find themselves. In this sense, another study carried out at the beginning of the rehabilitation process on twenty-four patients with ankle fractures and twenty-four healthy controls found a difference between groups of −40 cm in stride length, greater than the difference found in our study [6]. In contrast, if we look at what happens in the long term, some authors find that even one year after surgery, the spatiotemporal gait parameters are not yet normalized. In particular, gait speed is significantly lower in patients with malleolar fractures compared to healthy subjects [8,38]. Other authors, however, only found a reduced gait speed but did not consider this to be clinically relevant [9].

Specific and individualized rehabilitation is fundamental in ankle recovery, and no less important is to keep a functional and clinical record throughout the recovery process [47]. A good way to estimate the patient's functional capacity is by assessing ankle mobility or lower extremity strength. These clinical parameters allow prediction of performance in functional tasks such as gait [10].

In this regard, in our work, we evaluated ADF ROM, ABD/ADD hip muscle strength, and bimalleolar/calf perimeter in both study groups and additionally studied the degree of correlation, including regression models, between-gait parameters, and clinical measurements in the AFG.

ADF ROM is one of the most studied variables after ankle injury [48]. Despite rehabilitation efforts to improve ankle motion, short- and medium-term studies conclude that the gain is only 6–12% [48]. Such a low gain in range of motion is a major barrier to acquiring pre-injury status. Some authors put a cut-off point of 30° of weight-bearing dorsiflexion as the minimum to be able to perform tasks such as descending stairs or squatting without problems [15]. In our study, we found in the AFG a difference between the operated and non-operated ankle in the ADF ROM of −12.7° and −19.1° concerning the CG. Using a measurement methodology similar to ours, Nilsson et al. 2009 [36], in a sample of 105 patients with ankle fractures 6 months after surgery, obtained similar results to ours. In our work, the measurement was performed before the gait analysis to correlate it with the different spatiotemporal parameters. This ankle motion quantification system obtained excellent intra- and inter-test reliability [49]. Studies analyzing the kinematics of gait show the restrictions of the ADF ROM during the different phases of gait [9,38,50]; however, they do not relate this decrease in the movement to the spatiotemporal parameters. In our study, we were able to observe how ankle ADF ROM and ABD strength had a moderate association with cadence, speed, stride length, and stride time; moreover, they predicted up to 30% of the variability of their values.

The muscle atrophy observed in the calf perimeter could influence the gait pattern of patients with ankle fractures. In our study, only 24 weeks after surgery, the calf musculature of the operated ankle had a smaller calf perimeter (-1.3 cm; $p = 0.002$) compared to the non-operated ankle. Human studies quantifying the effect of disuse on muscle morphology show that in only 8 weeks of immobilization, the cross-sectional area measured with MRI shows decreases of 19% and 24% in the anterior and posterior calf muscle compartments [51]. The strength and activation of the plantar flexor muscles also suffer a significant loss [52], and their improvement after a period of rehabilitation has already been studied [10,36]. In our research, we did not directly assess the strength of the plantar flexors; however, we analyzed the propulsion index that could be associated with the strength of this muscle group during single support [53]. In reference to this parameter, we found that the propulsion index was significantly lower (-0.8 m/s^2) when comparing the operated and non-operated ankle of the AFG, and even lower (-1.7 m/s^2) when compared to the CG. Furthermore, we found a positive and significant correlation between calf perimeter and propulsion index ($r = 0.447$), and together with ADF ROM ($r = 0.523$), it could predict 46% of the propulsion index score. These results reflect the importance of having a good range of motion and calf muscle volume to be able to propel yourself adequately during gait.

Among the questions raised before conducting this study were the consequences that non-weight-bearing immobilization after surgery might have on the hip musculature. In this regard, there is a lack of studies identifying this impact on gait, although it has been studied in dynamic balance [13]. In the present study, we found a significant difference in ABD strength of both legs within and between groups. Furthermore, the correlation was positive and moderate with speed ($r = 0.436$), stride length ($r = 0.444$) and individual support ($r = 0.491$). Despite these results, ABD strength alone was not a significant predictor of any of the gait parameters. Based on these results, we could think that, despite the ABD strength deficit, gait is not a task that requires the recruitment of this musculature as balance or running could be.

Quantitative information on the evolution of recovery of physical function after an ankle fracture is essential for adequate patient care. Professionals can make use of prognostic data to understand the course of recovery and make the right decisions throughout the rehabilitation process. In our study where we assessed functional condition using the OMAS and AOFAS scales, we found that 6 months after surgery, patients still had pain and impaired function. A meta-analysis studying the short-, medium-, and long-term prognosis of function improvement in patients operated on after an ankle fracture tells us that improvement in the first 6 months is rapid but incomplete, with only 78% of function recovered [5]. In our research, we even found worse results on the OMAS subjective functional scale (57.3 ± 22.0), which was used in most of the studies included in the meta-analysis. The reason for this low score could lie in the subjectivity of the scale due to its characteristics or the state of health of the patients at the time of surgery [54]. We obtained better results on the AOFAS scale (73.6 ± 11.4); in addition, we found that a higher cadence ($r = 0.540$) and speed ($r = 0.428$), as well as a shorter stride time ($r = -0.547$), were moderately correlated with better scores. However, this correlation was not found with the OMAS scale. This is in line with the results of other studies in which this correlation also did not exist [37] or was weak [8,9].

The final aim of this study was to assess the test–retest reliability and agreement of measurements from a single inertial sensor, placed on the lumbar-sacral spine, in this population.

In our results, we found high to excellent intra-session test–retest reliability, with ICC scores between 0.84 and 0.98; the worst ICC values were obtained for the variables single support and double support at both ankles. Our results are consistent with those found by De Ridder et al. [35] in a group of thirty healthy subjects, in which they obtained high to excellent reliability values (0.84 ≤ ICC ≤ 0.99) for the spatiotemporal gait parameters after five valid trials. In line with our findings and those of Rider et al., another study conducted on a large healthy population and with different neurological pathologies, finds ICC values between 0.82 and 0.97, with the worst result for the stance and swing phase [55]. Despite the similarities in our results, the two previous studies only assess relative reliability but do not provide data on absolute reliability that would allow us to see the degree of variation of repeated measurements in individuals. In our investigation, the lowest SEM was obtained for stride length (0.02 m), which represents only 1.56% of the SEM%. Furthermore, the degree of agreement between the two trials was excellent for speed, stride length, and stride time, with bias values close to 0 and a small range in LoA. Bravi et al. [33], on a sample of twenty subjects with lower limb pathology, found moderate to excellent inter-rater reliability (0.59 ≤ ICC ≤ 0.95), with the lowest values corresponding to the phases of the gait cycle. In our work, we did not find such low ICC values in the gait phases; however, we found a higher SEM% in double support and propulsion index of both ankles, although they represent less than 11% of the SEM%. Concerning the limits of agreement and estimated bias, the single support of the operated ankle obtained the worst accuracy (bias = −1.79; LoA = −9.21; 5.63), probably due to the presence of three outliers. Bravi et al. justify the low reliability of gait phase recognition to the reduced pelvic motion in their study population. This is in agreement with that described by Zijlstra and Hof [31], who report the influence of the pelvis in differentiating normal and pathological gait patterns. In relation to this, the differences between our study population and the characteristics of the Bravi et al. sample, with subjects who have undergone hip or knee replacement with subjects having undergone hip or knee repositioning and possibly presenting greater functional limitations, may justify the differences obtained.

Based on our results and the previously mentioned studies in different populations, it seems to indicate that the estimation of gait phases may be affected by an asymmetric gait cycle. Gait speed is another point to consider, as it has been shown to be a parameter that affects the validity of wearable sensors [56]. However, the ICC and SEM results obtained in our research, as well as the low bias values and limits of agreement, we consider to be within clinically acceptable limits.

Our study has some limitations. Firstly, the characteristics of a cross-sectional study. However, we believe that this type of study, carried out 6 months after surgery, is necessary because of the importance of an objective and global identification of functional problems that can guide a more specific rehabilitation. Secondly, we have a small sample size for the control group. However, the sample size calculation based on the differences in gait speed between groups indicates adequate power to detect a minimal clinically important difference. Finally, in our research, we did not use a gold-standard system for the concurrent validity of the G-WALK. Although it has not been studied in patients with ankle fractures, there are already studies in different populations where moderate to excellent levels of agreement and reliability were obtained, with the lowest values corresponding to the gait phases [33–35,41].

5. Conclusions

In our sample of patients with bimalleolar ankle fracture, 6 months after surgery, the analysis of the spatiotemporal gait parameters shows a clear asymmetry between both legs in the different gait phases. Furthermore, compared to healthy subjects, there is a decrease in cadence, speed, and stride length, as well as an increase in stride time. The decrease in clinical parameters such as ADF ROM, ABD hip muscle strength, and calf perimeter influence gait performance and may even explain 20–46% of the results in certain gait parameters. The low scores obtained at 6 months on the AOFAS and OMAS scales reveal a slow recovery of function and symptomatology; furthermore, better scores on the AOFAS scale are associated with better cadence and stride time. Finally, test–retest reliability and agreement analysis of the measurements made with the G-WALK sensor shows good to excellent results in our study population. Therefore, it can be considered a reliable gait analysis system, and its use could be justified in the clinical setting, although being cautious with the interpretation of the results in the identification of gait phases.

Author Contributions: Conceptualization, M.F.-G. and D.S.-G.; methodology, M.F.-G. and D.S.-G.; formal analysis, M.F.-G.; investigation, M.F.-G. and D.S.-G.; writing—original draft preparation, M.F.-G.; writing—review and editing, M.F.-G. and D.S.-G.; supervision, P.S.-J., D.B., E.L.-B., M.I.P.-N. All authors have read and agreed to the published version of the manuscript.

Funding: This research received no external funding.

Institutional Review Board Statement: The study was conducted in accordance with the Declaration of Helsinki and approved by the Cantabria Research Ethics Committee (CEIC) (reference: 2017.072) for studies involving humans.

Informed Consent Statement: Informed consent was obtained from all subjects involved in the study.

Data Availability Statement: Not applicable.

Acknowledgments: The authors would like to acknowledge the excellent cooperation of the patients in this project. We thank Vanesa Pérez and the institution for their continued support during this project.

Conflicts of Interest: The authors declare no conflict of interest.

References

1. Shibuya, N.; Davis, M.L.; Jupiter, D.C. Epidemiology of Foot and Ankle Fractures in the United States: An Analysis of the National Trauma Data Bank (2007 to 2011). *J. Foot Ankle Surg.* **2014**, *53*, 606–608. [CrossRef] [PubMed]
2. Elsoe, R.; Ostgaard, S.E.; Larsen, P. Population-based epidemiology of 9767 ankle fractures. *Foot Ankle Surg.* **2018**, *24*, 34–39. [CrossRef] [PubMed]
3. Juto, H.; Nilsson, H.; Morberg, P. Epidemiology of Adult Ankle Fractures: 1756 cases identified in Norrbotten County during 2009–2013 and classified according to AO/OTA. *BMC Musculoskelet. Disord.* **2018**, *19*, 441. [CrossRef]
4. Stufkens, S.A.S.; van den Bekerom, M.P.J.; Kerkhoffs, G.M.M.J.; Hintermann, B.; van Dijk, C.N. Long-term outcome after 1822 operatively treated ankle fractures: A systematic review of the literature. *Injury* **2011**, *42*, 119–127. [CrossRef]
5. Beckenkamp, P.R.; Lin, C.-W.C.; Chagpar, S.; Herbert, R.D.; van der Ploeg, H.P.; Moseley, A.M. Prognosis of physical function following ankle fracture: A systematic review with meta-analysis. *J. Orthop. Sports Phys. Ther.* **2014**, *44*, 841–851. [CrossRef]
6. Elbaz, A.; Mor, A.; Segal, G.; Bar, D.; Monda, M.K.; Kish, B.; Nyska, M.; Palmanovich, E. Lower Extremity Kinematic Profile of Gait of Patients After Ankle Fracture: A Case-Control Study. *J. Foot Ankle Surg.* **2016**, *55*, 918–921. [CrossRef]
7. Segal, G.; Elbaz, A.; Parsi, A.; Heller, Z.; Palmanovich, E.; Nyska, M.; Feldbrin, Z.; Kish, B. Clinical outcomes following ankle fracture: A cross-sectional observational study. *J. Foot Ankle Res.* **2014**, *7*, 50. [CrossRef]
8. Losch, A.; Meybohm, P.; Schmalz, T.; Fuchs, M.; Vamvukakis, F.; Dresing, K.; Blumentritt, S.; Stürmer, K.M. Functional results of dynamic gait analysis after 1 year of hobby-athletes with a surgically treated ankle fracture. *Sportverletz. Sportschaden Organ Ges. Orthopadisch-Traumatol. Sportmed.* **2002**, *16*, 101–107. [CrossRef]
9. Wang, R.; Thur, C.K.; Gutierrez-Farewik, E.M.; Wretenberg, P.; Broström, E. One year follow-up after operative ankle fractures: A prospective gait analysis study with a multi-segment foot model. *Gait Posture* **2010**, *31*, 234–240. [CrossRef]
10. Shaffer, M.A.; Okereke, E.; Esterhai, J.L.; Elliott, M.A.; Walter, G.A.; Yim, S.H.; Vandenborne, K. Effects of Immobilization on Plantar-Flexion Torque, Fatigue Resistance, and Functional Ability Following an Ankle Fracture. *Phys. Ther.* **2000**, *80*, 769–780. [CrossRef]
11. Hong, C.C.; Roy, S.P.; Nashi, N.; Tan, K.J. Functional outcome and limitation of sporting activities after bimalleolar and trimalleolar ankle fractures. *Foot Ankle Int.* **2013**, *34*, 805–810. [CrossRef] [PubMed]
12. Dudek, K.; Drużbicki, M.; Przysada, G.; Śpiewak, D. Assessment of standing balance in patients after ankle fractures. *Acta Bioeng. Biomech. Wroc. Univ. Technol.* **2014**, *16*, 59–65.
13. Salas-Gómez, D.; Fernández-Gorgojo, M.; Sanchez-Juan, P.; Bercero, E.L.; Perez-Núñez, M.I.; Barbado, D. Quantifying balance deficit in people with ankle fracture six months after surgical intervention through the Y-Balance test. *Gait Posture* **2020**, *in press*. [CrossRef] [PubMed]
14. Day, G.A.; Swanson, C.E.; Hulcombe, B.G. Operative treatment of ankle fractures: A minimum ten-year follow-up. *Foot Ankle Int.* **2001**, *22*, 102–106. [CrossRef]
15. Nilsson, G.; Nyberg, P.; Ekdahl, C.; Eneroth, M. Performance after surgical treatment of patients with ankle fractures—14-month follow-up. *Physiother. Res. Int. J. Res. Clin. Phys. Ther.* **2003**, *8*, 69–82. [CrossRef]
16. Dean, D.M.; Ho, B.S.; Lin, A.; Fuchs, D.; Ochenjele, G.; Merk, B.; Kadakia, A.R. Predictors of Patient-Reported Function and Pain Outcomes in Operative Ankle Fractures. *Foot Ankle Int.* **2017**, *38*, 496–501. [CrossRef]
17. Kitaoka, H.B.; Alexander, I.J.; Adelaar, R.S.; Nunley, J.A.; Myerson, M.S.; Sanders, M. Clinical rating systems for the ankle-hindfoot, midfoot, hallux, and lesser toes. *Foot Ankle Int.* **1994**, *15*, 349–353. [CrossRef]

18. Olerud, C.; Molander, H. A scoring scale for symptom evaluation after ankle fracture. *Arch. Orthop. Trauma. Surg. Arch. Orthopadische Unf.-Chir.* **1984**, *103*, 190–194. [CrossRef]
19. Hsu, C.-Y.; Tsai, Y.-S.; Yau, C.-S.; Shie, H.-H.; Wu, C.-M. Differences in gait and trunk movement between patients after ankle fracture and healthy subjects. *Biomed. Eng. Online* **2019**, *18*, 26. [CrossRef]
20. Ng, R.; Broughton, N.; Williams, C. Measuring Recovery After Ankle Fractures: A Systematic Review of the Psychometric Properties of Scoring Systems. *J. Foot Ankle Surg.* **2018**, *57*, 149–154. [CrossRef]
21. Ekinci, M.; Birisik, F.; Ersin, M.; Şahinkaya, T.; Öztürk, İ. A prospective evaluation of strength and endurance of ankle dorsiflexors-plantar flexors after conservative management of lateral malleolar fractures. *Turk. J. Phys. Med. Rehabil.* **2021**, *67*, 300–307. [CrossRef]
22. Hollman, J.H.; McDade, E.M.; Petersen, R.C. Normative spatiotemporal gait parameters in older adults. *Gait Posture* **2011**, *34*, 111–118. [CrossRef]
23. McKay, M.J.; Baldwin, J.N.; Ferreira, P.; Simic, M.; Vanicek, N.; Wojciechowski, E.; Mudge, A.; Burns, J. 1000 Norms Project Consortium, Spatiotemporal and plantar pressure patterns of 1000 healthy individuals aged 3–101 years. *Gait Posture* **2017**, *58*, 78–87. [CrossRef]
24. Rosenbaum, D.; Macri, F.; Lupselo, F.S.; Preis, O.C. Gait and function as tools for the assessment of fracture repair—The role of movement analysis for the assessment of fracture healing. *Injury* **2014**, *45*, S39–S43. [CrossRef]
25. Chaparro-Cárdenas, S.L.; Lozano-Guzmán, A.A.; Ramirez-Bautista, J.A.; Hernández-Zavala, A. A review in gait rehabilitation devices and applied control techniques. *Disabil. Rehabil. Assist. Technol.* **2018**, *13*, 819–834. [CrossRef]
26. Muyor, J.M.; Arrabal-Campos, F.M.; Martínez-Aparicio, C.; Sánchez-Crespo, A.; Villa-Pérez, M. Test-retest reliability and validity of a motion capture (MOCAP) system for measuring thoracic and lumbar spinal curvatures and sacral inclination in the sagittal plane. *J. Back Musculoskelet. Rehabil.* **2017**, *30*, 1319–1325. [CrossRef]
27. Lee, M.M.; Song, C.H.; Lee, K.J.; Jung, S.W.; Shin, D.C.; Shin, S.H. Concurrent Validity and Test-retest Reliability of the OPTOGait Photoelectric Cell System for the Assessment of Spatio-temporal Parameters of the Gait of Young Adults. *J. Phys. Ther. Sci.* **2014**, *26*, 81–85. [CrossRef]
28. Bilney, B.; Morris, M.; Webster, K. Concurrent related validity of the GAITRite walkway system for quantification of the spatial and temporal parameters of gait. *Gait Posture* **2003**, *17*, 68–74. [CrossRef]
29. Washabaugh, E.P.; Kalyanaraman, T.; Adamczyk, P.G.; Claflin, E.S.; Krishnan, C. Validity and repeatability of inertial measurement units for measuring gait parameters. *Gait Posture* **2017**, *55*, 87–93. [CrossRef]
30. Kobsar, D.; Charlton, J.M.; Tse, C.T.F.; Esculier, J.-F.; Graffos, A.; Krowchuk, N.M.; Thatcher, D.; Hunt, M.A. Validity and reliability of wearable inertial sensors in healthy adult walking: A systematic review and meta-analysis. *J. Neuroeng. Rehabil.* **2020**, *17*, 62. [CrossRef]
31. Zijlstra, W.; Hof, A.L. Assessment of spatio-temporal gait parameters from trunk accelerations during human walking. *Gait Posture* **2003**, *18*, 1–10. [CrossRef]
32. Buganè, F.; Benedetti, M.G.; Casadio, G.; Attala, S.; Biagi, F.; Manca, M.; Leardini, A. Estimation of spatial-temporal gait parameters in level walking based on a single accelerometer: Validation on normal subjects by standard gait analysis. *Comput. Methods Programs Biomed.* **2012**, *108*, 129–137. [CrossRef] [PubMed]
33. Bravi, M.; Gallotta, E.; Morrone, M.; Maselli, M.; Santacaterina, F.; Toglia, R.; Foti, C.; Sterzi, S.; Bressi, F.; Miccinilli, S. Concurrent validity and inter trial reliability of a single inertial measurement unit for spatial-temporal gait parameter analysis in patients with recent total hip or total knee arthroplasty. *Gait Posture* **2020**, *76*, 175–181. [CrossRef] [PubMed]
34. Park, G.; Woo, Y. Comparison between a center of mass and a foot pressure sensor system for measuring gait parameters in healthy adults. *J. Phys. Ther. Sci.* **2015**, *27*, 3199–3202. [CrossRef]
35. De Ridder, R.; Lebleu, J.; Willems, T.; de Blaiser, C.; Detrembleur, C.; Roosen, P. Concurrent Validity of a Commercial Wireless Trunk Triaxial Accelerometer System for Gait Analysis. *J. Sport Rehabil.* **2019**, *28*, jsr.2018-0295. [CrossRef]
36. Nilsson, G.M.; Jonsson, K.; Ekdahl, C.S.; Eneroth, M. Effects of a training program after surgically treated ankle fracture: A prospective randomised controlled trial. *BMC Musculoskelet. Disord.* **2009**, *10*, 118. [CrossRef]
37. Suciu, O.; Onofrei, R.R.; Totorean, A.D.; Suciu, S.C.; Amaricai, E.C. Gait analysis and functional outcomes after twelve-week rehabilitation in patients with surgically treated ankle fractures. *Gait Posture* **2016**, *49*, 184–189. [CrossRef]
38. Van Hoeve, S.; Houben, M.; Verbruggen, J.P.A.M.; Willems, P.; Meijer, K.; Poeze, M. Gait analysis related to functional outcome in patients operated for ankle fractures. *J. Orthop. Res.* **2019**, *37*, 1658–1666. [CrossRef]
39. The American Orthopedic Foot and Ankle Score (AOFAS). Code Technol. We Collect Orthop. Patient Outcomes. 2017. Available online: https://www.codetechnology.com/american-orthopedic-foot-ankle-score-aofas/ (accessed on 23 February 2017).
40. Yang, S.; Li, Q. Inertial Sensor-Based Methods in Walking Speed Estimation: A Systematic Review. *Sensors* **2012**, *12*, 6102–6116. [CrossRef]
41. Vítečková, S.; Horáková, H.; Poláková, K.; Krupička, R.; Růžička, E.; Brožová, H. Agreement between the GAITRite®System and the Wearable Sensor BTS G-Walk®for measurement of gait parameters in healthy adults and Parkinson's disease patients. *PeerJ* **2020**, *8*, e8235. [CrossRef]
42. Cohen, J. *Statistical Power Analysis for the Behavioral Sciences*, 2nd ed.; L. Erlbaum Associates: Hillsdale, NJ, USA, 1988.
43. Weir, J.P. Quantifying test-retest reliability using the intraclass correlation coefficient and the SEM. *J. Strength Cond. Res.* **2005**, *19*, 231–240. [CrossRef]

44. Kottner, J.; Audige, L.; Brorson, S.; Donner, A.; Gajewski, B.J.; Hróbjartsson, A.; Roberts, C.; Shoukri, M.; Streiner, D.L. Guidelines for Reporting Reliability and Agreement Studies (GRRAS) were proposed. *Int. J. Nurs. Stud.* **2011**, *48*, 661–671. [CrossRef]
45. De Vet, H.C.W.; Terwee, C.B.; Knol, D.L.; Bouter, L.M. When to use agreement versus reliability measures. *J. Clin. Epidemiol.* **2006**, *59*, 1033–1039. [CrossRef]
46. Tyler, A.F.; Rose, T.; Day, S.; Kenia, J.; Horan, A.D.; Mehta, S.; Donegan, D.J. Comparison of Spatiotemporal Gait Parameters Following Operative Treatment of Trimalleolar Ankle Fractures vs Healthy Controls. *Foot Ankle Orthop.* **2020**, *5*, 247301142093105. [CrossRef]
47. Patel, S.; Park, H.; Bonato, P.; Chan, L.; Rodgers, M. A review of wearable sensors and systems with application in rehabilitation. *J. Neuroeng. Rehabil.* **2012**, *9*, 21. [CrossRef]
48. Lin, C.-W.C.; Donkers, N.A.J.; Refshauge, K.M.; Beckenkamp, P.R.; Khera, K.; Moseley, A.M. Rehabilitation for ankle fractures in adults. *Cochrane Database Syst. Rev.* **2012**, *11*, CD005595. [CrossRef]
49. Larsen, P.; Nielsen, H.B.; Lund, C.; Sørensen, D.S.; Larsen, B.T.; Matthews, M.; Vicenzino, B.; Elsoe, R. A novel tool for measuring ankle dorsiflexion: A study of its reliability in patients following ankle fractures. *Foot Ankle Surg.* **2016**, *22*, 274–277. [CrossRef]
50. Böpple, J.C.; Tanner, M.; Campos, S.; Fischer, C.; Müller, S.; Wolf, S.I.; Doll, J. Short-term results of gait analysis with the Heidelberg foot measurement method and functional outcome after operative treatment of ankle fractures. *J. Foot Ankle Res.* **2022**, *15*, 2. [CrossRef]
51. Stevens, J.E.; Walter, G.A.; Okereke, E.; Scarborough, M.T.; Esterhai, J.L.; George, S.Z.; Kelley, M.J.; Tillman, S.M.; Gibbs, J.D.; Elliott, M.A.; et al. Muscle adaptations with immobilization and rehabilitation after ankle fracture. *Med. Sci. Sports Exerc.* **2004**, *36*, 1695–1701. [CrossRef]
52. Stevens, J.E.; Pathare, N.C.; Tillman, S.M.; Scarborough, M.T.; Gibbs, C.P.; Shah, P.; Jayaraman, A.; Walter, G.A.; Vandenborne, K. Relative contributions of muscle activation and muscle size to plantarflexor torque during rehabilitation after immobilization. *J. Orthop. Res.* **2006**, *24*, 1729–1736. [CrossRef]
53. Hsiao, H.; Knarr, B.A.; Higginson, J.S.; Binder-Macleod, S.A. The relative contribution of ankle moment and trailing limb angle to propulsive force during gait. *Hum. Mov. Sci.* **2015**, *39*, 212–221. [CrossRef] [PubMed]
54. Egol, K.A.; Tejwani, N.C.; Walsh, M.G.; Capla, E.L.; Koval, K.J. Predictors of short-term functional outcome following ankle fracture surgery. *J. Bone Jt. Surg. Am.* **2006**, *88*, 974–979. [CrossRef]
55. Donisi, L.; Pagano, G.; Cesarelli, G.; Coccia, A.; Amitrano, F.; D'Addio, G. Benchmarking between two wearable inertial systems for gait analysis based on a different sensor placement using several statistical approaches. *Measurement* **2021**, *173*, 108642. [CrossRef]
56. Greene, B.R.; Foran, T.G.; McGrath, D.; Doheny, E.P.; Burns, A.; Caulfield, B. A Comparison of Algorithms for Body-Worn Sensor-Based Spatiotemporal Gait Parameters to the GAITRite Electronic Walkway. *J. Appl. Biomech.* **2012**, *28*, 349–355. [CrossRef]

Temporal Synergies Detection in Gait Cyclograms Using Wearable Technology

Marija M. Gavrilović * and Milica M. Janković

School of Electrical Engineering, University of Belgrade, Bulevar kralja Aleksandra 73, 11000 Belgrade, Serbia; piperski@etf.rs
* Correspondence: marijapetrovic48@yahoo.com

Abstract: The human gait can be described as the synergistic activity of all individual components of the sensory–motor system. The central nervous system (CNS) develops synergies to execute endpoint motion by coordinating muscle activity to reflect the global goals of the endpoint trajectory. This paper proposes a new method for assessing temporal dynamic synergies. Principal component analysis (PCA) has been applied on the signals acquired by wearable sensors (inertial measurement units, IMU and ground reaction force sensors, GRF mounted on feet) to detect temporal synergies in the space of two-dimensional PCA cyclograms. The temporal synergy results for different gait speeds in healthy subjects and stroke patients before and after the therapy were compared. The hypothesis of invariant temporal synergies at different gait velocities was statistically confirmed, without the need to record and analyze muscle activity. A significant difference in temporal synergies was noticed in hemiplegic gait compared to healthy gait. Finally, the proposed PCA-based cyclogram method provided the therapy follow-up information about paretic leg gait in stroke patients that was not available by observing conventional parameters, such as temporal and symmetry gait measures.

Keywords: gait; gait cycle; ground reaction force; inertial measurement unit; principal component analysis; stroke; synergy; wearable device

1. Introduction

The central nervous system (CNS) controls many degrees of freedom (DOFs) of the musculoskeletal system, coordinating many muscle activities on many joints. Human movements can have different trajectories, speeds, and accelerations even when they achieve the same goal. To control so many DOFs, it becomes necessary for the CNS to have a complex and delicate organizational structure [1]. Different mathematical approaches for modeling realistic multi-joint movements were suggested in the literature, based on the various optimization functions such as minimum jerk [2,3], minimum torque change [4], minimum effort [5], as well as more complex functions [6,7]. An organizational approach based on activities of functional groups (called synergies) was also suggested [8]. Synergies represent patterns of body segment coactivations. Researchers have hypothesized that the nervous system activates synergies by a neural signal and creates a set of temporal–spatial synergy modules. These modules represent a smaller dimensional space than the space formed by individual DOFs. Synergies can be found at various levels, such as joint coordinates or muscles [9,10]. Kinematic synergies may result from muscle synergies, i.e., as a consequence of muscle activity [11,12]. In addition, researchers have suggested that CNS develops synergies to execute endpoint motion [13,14]. Motor intra-limb coordination is the ability to coordinate segments in a sequence [15]. This coordination can be accomplished by controlling the endpoint trajectory.

The human gait can be described as a synergistic activity of all individual components of the human sensory–motor system. Different mathematical models of muscle synergies are known in the literature: invariant temporal ("temporal synergies"), spatial ("synchronous synergies"), and spatiotemporal ("time-varying synergies") [16]. All of these approaches reduce the dimensionality of the movements, but they are not equivalent to each other.

Temporal muscle synergies imply the existence of a set of temporal components common to different activation tasks [17,18]. Ivanenko et al. [19] showed that there is a basic set of five temporal components extracted from recorded electromyography (EMG) signals in controls and patients with a spinal cord injury (SCI). The consistent timing of motor patterns across various walking tasks was shown even with considerable variation of muscle coactivation. These temporal components represent the timings of the intersegmental coordination and may reflect a neural strategy for coordination in a low dimensional set of patterns that facilitate control of gait. Furthermore, these timings are argued to represent a control variable in central pattern generators [20]. Furthermore, it was reported that the nervous system's activation pattern during walking does not depend on walking speed, including running [21].

However, EMG analysis has certain limitations; for example, adipose tissue can affect EMG recordings. There is also the problem of muscle crosstalk and a lack of deep muscles reliability [22]. Furthermore, it was shown that the synergy structure is dependent on the number and choice of muscles [23]. On the other hand, the intermediate dynamic representation is a logical connection between highly variable muscle activity and whole-body mechanics [20].

The synergism in people without sensorimotor impairment differs from patients with sensorimotor disorders. Injury to the CNS, such as stroke, leads to changes in gait modality and synergism [24]. These differences can be observed concerning the parameters that characterize gait. Characteristics of gait in stroke hemiplegic patients are: decreased speed, decreased and asymmetrical step length, decreased stance and single support times on the affected side, changes in joint kinematics, and overall asymmetry in different metrics [25]. The rehabilitation process restores the gait, i.e., retrains the patient to stand and walk with reduced sensory–motor resources and to walk in the way most similar to the gait before the disorder. During rehabilitation, it is essential to objectively quantify the success of the applied protocols and therapies on gait performance.

The gold standard for quantitative gait analysis implies the usage of high cost, space, and time-consuming 3D motion capture systems and force platforms [26,27]. Recently, the development of wearable technology enabled the usage of alternative low-cost approaches for gait assessment based on inertial measurement units (IMU) and ground reaction force (GRF) sensors [28,29]. These portable, wireless systems are suitable for clinical and home monitoring [30]. They are easy to use, non-invasive, small, compact, and robust enough to provide valuable information for the objective evaluation of the gait performance of people with neurological disorders [31,32]. Conventionally, the prerequisite for quantitative gait analysis is gait segmentation. Several algorithms were developed to tackle this problem in IMU-based systems, such as zero-crossing and threshold methods [33,34]. However, these algorithms usually have lower accuracy in pathological gait [35]. The gold standard for gait phase partitioning is the measurement signal of the direct contact between the foot and the ground. For this reason, some wearable systems, in addition to the IMUs, also contain foot pressure insoles in shoes. However, gait phases' detection accuracy and reliability also depend on the location of the GRF sensors [36]. It is difficult to determine the heel-strike events automatically in the recordings of the person after a stroke, precisely because of the problem with the drop foot [37]. Thus, a gait analysis methodology that does not need the segmentation process is preferred.

The principal component analysis (PCA) has been widely used to discover "hidden" patterns in the high dimensional space of human gait signals in healthy and pathological gait [19,38,39]. Many researchers used PCA to identify muscle [21] and limb synergies [40], which are proposed to be building blocks for motor behavior [19]. Recently, it was shown that the space of two-dimensional PCA cyclograms allows simple assessment of gait performance in stroke hemiplegic patients [41].

This study aims to evaluate whether invariant (temporal) features of synergies can be extracted by analyzing foot (endpoint) dynamics (kinetics and kinematics) acquired by a wearable device, without the need for gait segmentation and need of EMG data acquisition. PCA was applied on the signals acquired by wearable sensors (IMU and GRF integrated into shoe insoles and mounted on feet) to detect temporal synergies in the space of two-dimensional PCA cyclograms. The idea of invariant temporal components "hidden" in motion dynamics signals was explored, as shown in the literature for EMG signals [19]. To test the hypothesis about invariant temporal dynamic synergies, the gait was analyzed at different speeds in healthy subjects. The gait of stroke hemiplegic patients before and after the rehabilitation therapy was also analyzed. The differences between healthy and pathological gait patterns were observed concerning the parameters which define the temporal dynamic synergies. Additionally, it was investigated whether the method for detecting temporal dynamic synergies from IMU and GRF signals has an additional practical value for the paretic side recovery follow-up of stroke patients compared to the conventional gait analysis results, such as symmetry and temporal gait parameters.

2. Materials and Methods

2.1. Subjects

Nineteen subjects took part in this study: 14 healthy persons (without sensory–motor deficiency) and five hemiplegic stroke patients in the subacute phase (4–6 months after stroke). Subject characteristics are shown in Table 1. The patients could follow instructions from clinicians. The patients could walk with or without cane support.

Table 1. Subject characteristics.

Variable	Mean ± SD	
	Healthy Subjects (n = 14)	Patients (n = 5)
Age (years)	34.8 ± 12.6	61 ± 5.1
Gender	8 male, 6 female	1 male, 4 female
Total body mass (kg)	73.3 ± 12.7	78.4 ± 9.2
Height (m)	1.78 ± 0.08	1.7 ± 0.05
BMI (kg/m^2)	23 ± 2.18	28.18 ± 3.6
Affected side	-	4 left, 1 right

The patients participated in functional electrical stimulation (FES)-based therapy. The effectiveness of FES therapy for the drop foot correction was assessed by observing the neuroplasticity changes using electroencephalography examination. Eight-channel MOTIMOVE electronic stimulator (3F—FIT FABRICANDO FABER, Belgrade, Serbia, [42]) was used for FES therapy, augmenting the patient's pedaling (OMEGO® Plus, Graz, Austria, [43]). The duration of the rehabilitation protocol was four weeks. The healthy subjects did not participate in the FES therapy.

The experimental design was approved by the ethical review board of the Rehabilitation Clinic "Dr Miroslav Zotović" in Belgrade. Participants were well-informed about the noninvasive protocol and they signed informed consent forms prior to gait assessment.

2.2. Instrumentation

The Gait Teacher (RehabShop, Belgrade, Serbia) [44] was used in the study. This system comprises 10 GRF sensors (five per foot insole) that measure vertical forces and two IMUs (MPU6050 module) with integrated three-axis accelerometers and gyroscopes into the insoles. Each foot insole has two piezoresistive GRF sensors in the heel zone (medial heel—HeelM, lateral heel—HeelL), two sensors in the metatarsal (medial metatarsal—MetaM, lateral metatarsal—MetaL), and one sensor in the toes zone (Toe). Each sensor can estimate pressure up to 3.5 MPa. The characteristics of GRF sensors are: linearity < ±0.25% FS, BFSL, repeatability < ±0.075% FS, hysteresis < ±0.05% FS, zero thermal error < 0.75% FS, @35 °C, span thermal error < 0.75% FS, @35 °C, and stability error < ±0.2% FS/year. The gyroscope and accelerometer specifications within IMU are: supply voltage 2.3–3.4 V, consumption 3.9 mA, calibration tolerance ±3%, I2C interface support, and operating temperature −40 °C to −85 °C. The IMU can measure the 3D acceleration (range of ±4 g) and the 3D angular velocity (range of ±500 deg/s). The 3D directions in the IMU are as follows: the z-axis directs up from the insole, the x-axis directs ahead, and the y-axis directs medially. The direction of angular velocity ω_x is from heel to toe. This angular rate is perpendicular to the insole (frontal plane). The rate ω_y is also orthogonal to the insole and directed laterally. The angular rate ω_z is in the plane of the insole pointing up. Each insole is wirelessly connected to the computer. Eleven signals from each insole are transferred at a sampling rate of 100 Hz. The acquisition software was built in LabView (National Instruments, Austin, TX, USA). The built-in software synchronizes IMU and GRF sensors. The system provides data with a time delay of 20 ms. Data are stored in text format (.txt) for further offline analysis (Figure 1). In conclusion, the data obtained with the Gait Teacher are a set of five GRF time series and six-time series of angular velocities and accelerations per insole. The output is a large matrix with 22 components [41].

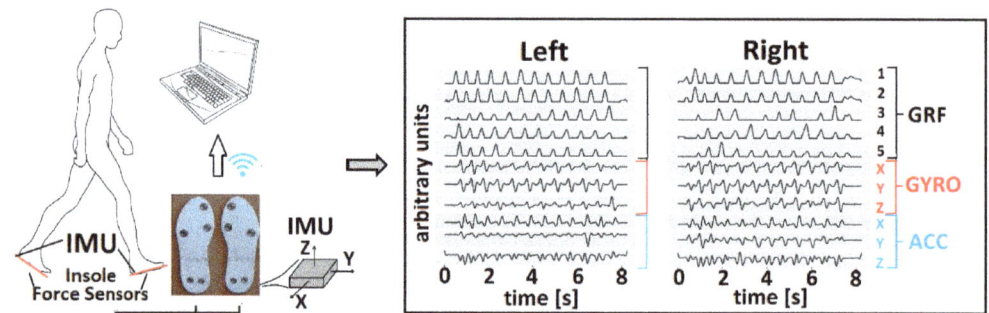

Figure 1. Gait Teacher instrumentation and output signals from both insoles.

2.3. Experiment Protocol

The Gait Teacher insoles were fitted to the subjects' shoes. First, the outputs from GRF sensors were zeroed: a participant raised the left foot and then the right and held it in the air for about 2 s (no load) while the clinician pressed the set button on the host computer. The IMU signals were zeroed while the participant stood on both feet for about 2 s.

Healthy subjects walked on a flat surface 10 m long. Before the recording, the respondent practiced walking for a few minutes. Signals from all sensors were recorded from three consecutive sessions. They walked at different speeds: 0.4 m/s, 0.8 m/s, 1 m/s, 1.6 m/s, and 2 m/s. The lowest speed was chosen to mimic the speed of the patients after stroke in the subacute phase ~0.4 m/s [45]. The highest speed was set to be the highest speed of the oldest participant. The oldest participant in the study was a healthy individual, 70 years old, and the maximal speed for this age is ~2 m/s [46]. Different speeds were recorded to address the diversity of different gaits and therefore generalize results from temporal synergies detection as much as possible, controlling for speed. To ensure a particular gait speed on the ground (avoiding the treadmill effect on the gait performance [47]), the subject followed the sound of the metronome, which signaled the cadence depending on the desired walking speed (Table 2). Markers were placed at one of the predefined distances: 0.5, 0.75, and 1 m, Figure 2. The markers were not moved between consecutive gait sessions of one participant for the same walking speed. This distance between markers was changed depending on the height or walking speed of the participant, so that the subject feels comfortable while walking. For higher subjects or higher speeds, markers were set at a greater distance. The metronome signaled the beginning of each stride, which occurred at specific markers on the floor. Table 2 shows the cadences required for different speeds, on a path of 10 m, for three possible stride lengths (the most suitable one for a particular respondent, heuristically chosen depending on the subject's height and the specified speed).

Table 2. Cadence for various speeds and stride lengths on a path of 10 m (SPM = strides per minute).

SPM	2 $\frac{m}{s}$	1.6 $\frac{m}{s}$	1 $\frac{m}{s}$	0.8 $\frac{m}{s}$	0.4 $\frac{m}{s}$
0.5 m	240	192	120	96	48
0.75 m	160	128	80	64	32
1 m	120	96	60	48	24

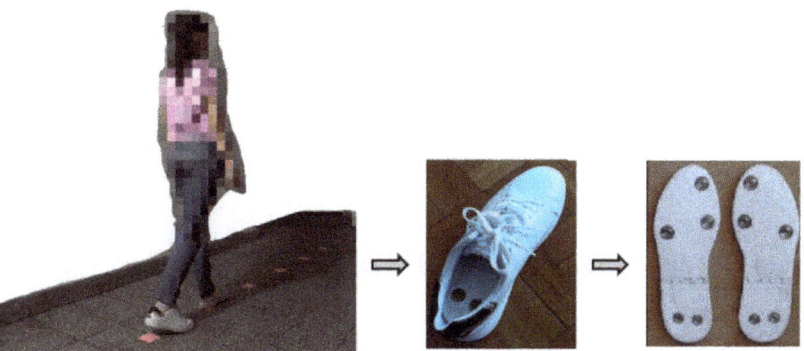

Figure 2. An example of the experimental setup.

The patients were asked to walk at a self-selected preferred speed. Signals from all sensors were recorded from three consecutive sessions. The rest between runs was about 1 min long. The clinician could monitor the signals on the computer screen during the recording. Signals recorded from sensors mounted on the paretic leg before therapy (p.b.), nonparetic leg before therapy (np.b.), paretic leg after therapy (p.a.), and nonparetic leg after therapy (np.a.) were separately analyzed. The number of strides performed by healthy subjects was 534, 534, 400, 366, and 300, respectively for speeds: 0.4 m/s, 0.8 m/s, 1 m/s, 1.6 m/s, and 2 m/s. The number of strides performed by patients was 110 before and 168 after therapy.

2.4. Data Preprocessing

The first and last strides were excluded from the gait analysis since the person needs to adapt the gait speed to the sound of a metronome. The signals were filtered by a low-pass Butterworth filter, third order, with a cut-off frequency of 5 Hz [48]. Signals obtained by sensors from different legs were analyzed separately. The input for PCA included five signals from five GRF sensors, angular velocity in the sagittal plane, Gyro_Y, and accelerations in the frontal plane, Acc_X, and transverse plane, Acc_Z, (in total, eight signals per leg, Figure 3). They are chosen heuristically because the gait is predominant in the profile plane. All PCA and statistical analyses were done in the R software environment, version 3.5.1.

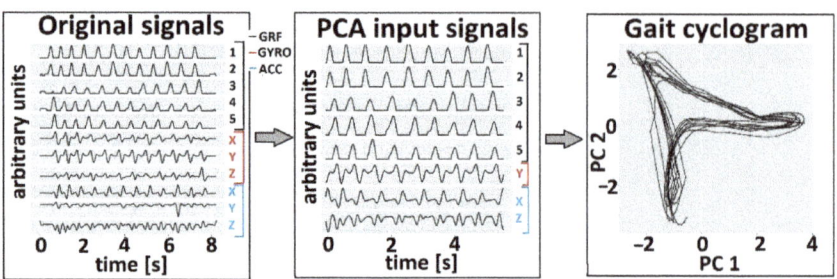

Figure 3. PCA cyclogram generation in the first two principal components space. Example data are from a person with no known sensory–motor impairment. The original signals were acquired by the Gait Teacher system (**left panel**). The subset of signals from the whole gait session (**middle panel**) was used to form a cyclogram (PC_2 vs. PC_1, **right panel**).

2.5. Detection of Temporal Synergies

PCA was used to find common temporal components hidden in the waveforms of dynamics' signals. The PCA input signals were normalized to have unit variance. Bartlett's sphericity test showed that the signals were suitable for PCA [49]. The PCA allowed the mapping of original data into the orthogonal space, where the principal axis is the direction of the data's maximal variance [50].

The analysis included calculating the correlation matrix, extracting the principal component of the varimax rotation, and calculating factor scores. These factor scores can be interpreted geometrically as the projections of the observations onto the principal components [49]. The whole preprocessed gait session (gait cyclogram) per subject was input for PCA. Therefore, the standardization across subjects with a different range of motions (subjects may engage in different walking strategies) was avoided [41]. After PCA, no stride segmentation was performed. Consequently, there was no need for the time interpolation of the signals for separate gait cycles.

The proposed method uses 2D gait cyclograms to represent recorded foot dynamics in the space of the first two principal components, PC_1 and PC_2 (Figure 3). The repetitive nature of near-cyclic events resulted in the overlapped cyclogram (cyclograms of gait cycles were overlapped) [41]. The calculation of principal components' quantitative parameter of cyclogram, introduced in [41], is shown in Equation (1) and expressed as an angle θ in each time point (observation).

$$\theta = arctg \frac{PC_2}{PC_1}, \qquad (1)$$

where PC_1 and PC_2 are the coordinates of the observations on the first two principal components (PC).

Figure 4a shows examples of specific time points where three temporal components exist during the single gait cycle by different colors (green, blue, yellow). These points correspond to the local extremums of PC_1 or PC_2. In Figure 4b the corresponding points of temporal synergy are presented in gait cyclogram using the same colors as in Figure 4a. The corresponding angles θ of observations that belong to each of three temporal components are marked by θ_1, θ_2, and θ_3.

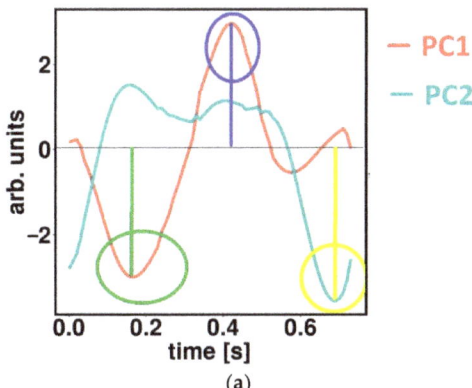 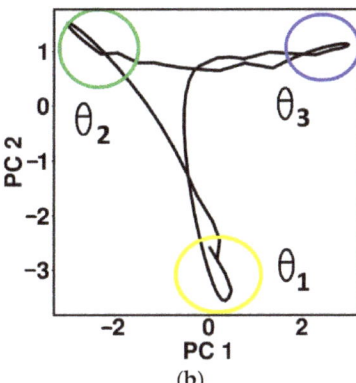

Figure 4. Representation of temporal synergies on the first two components on: (**a**) time PC signals; (**b**) PCA gait cyclograms. Time activations of temporal synergies are displayed using different colors (green, blue, yellow).

The overall schema of the performed methodology on the PCA gait cyclogram is shown in Figure 5, and it includes:

(1) Thresholding of gait cyclograms—Only observations (points in time) where principal components contribute significantly have been extracted and analyzed; namely, the threshold values for the squared cosine of the angle θ which was set heuristically to 0.8 ($cos^2_{PC_1} > 0.8$ and $cos^2_{PC_2} > 0.8$).

(2) Estimation of the distribution density applying nonparametric kernel density estimation (KDE) [51] on the angle θ (obtained after thresholding in the last stride)—KDE was obtained for nine groups of data separately: H_2, $H_{1.6}$, H_1, $H_{0.8}$, $H_{0.4}$ (both legs analyzed together for healthy subjects with the following walking speeds: 2 $\frac{m}{s}$, 1.6 $\frac{m}{s}$, 1 $\frac{m}{s}$, 0.8 $\frac{m}{s}$, 0.4 $\frac{m}{s}$, respectively), $P_{p.b}$ and $P_{p.a}$ (patients' paretic legs before and after therapy), $P_{np.b}$ and $P_{np.a}$ (patients' nonparetic legs before and after therapy). Shapiro–Wilk normality test [52] was used to check the (non)normality of the distributions.

(3) Clustering of distribution density to three clusters θ_1, θ_2, and θ_3 (related to three temporal components) for each of nine groups—distribution density was smoothed by the bandwidth parameter. The bandwidth of the kernel is a free parameter that exhibits a strong influence on the resulting estimate; it is the real positive number that defines the smoothness of the density plot. The formula used to calculate optimal bandwidth parameter bw for each group is shown in Equation (2) [53].

$$bw = \frac{0.9 * \min\left(\sqrt{Var(X)}, \frac{IQR(X)}{1.349}\right)}{\sqrt[5]{n}}, \tag{2}$$

where n is the number of observations of X, $Var(X)$ is its variance, and $IQR(X)$ is the interquartile range. Cluster limits were extracted as local minimums of the bandwidth smoothed distribution density.

(4) Statistical analysis—Mann–Whitney U nonparametric test was performed to determine whether the same clusters (detected temporal synergies) differ statistically between patients and healthy groups [54]. Wilcoxon test for partially matched two sample data (the combination of Wilcoxon signed-rank statistics for paired data and Mann–Whitney U statistics) was used to compare healthy groups for different speeds [55]. The same test was used to compare patients before and after therapy. Finally, it was analyzed whether the statistically significant results before and after therapy can be assessed based on temporal synergism and compared the effects to conventional parameters (Section 2.6). The significance level was $p = 0.001$ for estimating the statistically significant differences.

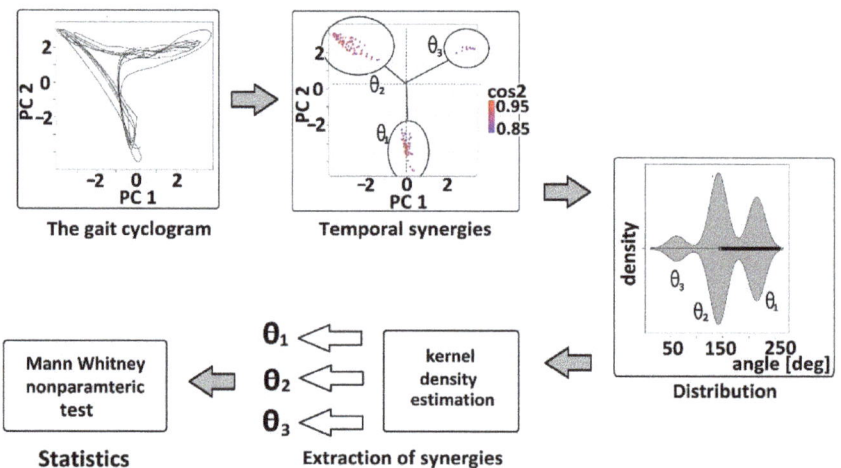

Figure 5. Temporal synergies detection from the PCA gait cyclograms.

2.6. Conventional Gait Analysis

The threshold method extracted the swing and stance phases for each gait session. The threshold was set to be 5% of the sum of all GRF signals in each insole divided by the number of force sensors, which was 5. The signals were filtered by a low-pass Butterworth filter, third order, with a cut-off frequency of 5 Hz. For each stride, stance and swing durations were calculated as a percentage of the gait cycle. In addition, since gait after stroke is characterized by high asymmetry, four symmetry measures were calculated for both the swing and stance phase, as in Equations (3)–(6). These measures were used to assess therapy impact on stroke patients [56,57].

$$\text{Symmetry ratio (SR)} : \frac{T_{left}}{T_{right}}, \tag{3}$$

$$\text{Symmetry index (SI)} : \left(\frac{|T_{left} - T_{right}|}{0.5 * (T_{left} + T_{right})} \right) * 100\%, \tag{4}$$

$$\text{Gait asymmetry (GA)} : \ln(\frac{T_{left}}{T_{right}}) * 100\%, \tag{5}$$

$$\text{Symmetry angle (SA)} : \frac{45° - \arctan\left(\frac{T_{left}}{T_{right}}\right)}{90°} * 100\%, \tag{6}$$

where T_{left} is the duration of the specific gait phase (stance or swing) for the left leg, and T_{right} is the duration of the specific gait phase (stance or swing) for the right leg.

Whether statistically significant results could be assessed before vs. after therapy was assessed using the Wilcoxon test for partially matched two-sample data. The significance level was $p = 0.001$ for estimating the statistically significant differences.

3. Results

3.1. PCA Cyclograms

Figure 6 (top) presents an example of overlapped cyclograms in a healthy subject for gait sessions with different gait speeds. For healthy subjects, the signals from sensors mounted on left and right feet were analyzed together. Figure 6 (bottom) shows thresholded cyclograms ($cos^2_{PC_1} > 0.8$ and $cos^2_{PC_2} > 0.8$, as explained in Section 2.5) that contain observations where temporal synergies are activated.

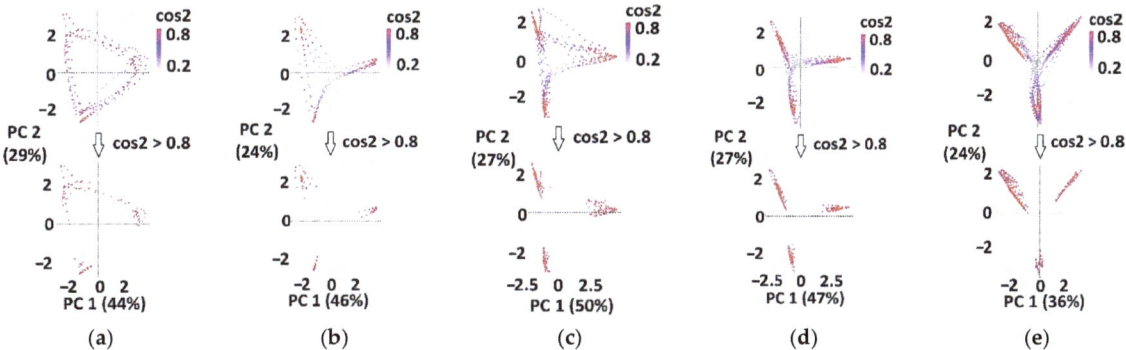

Figure 6. Examples of overlapped cyclograms for one healthy subject's gait session (**top**) and thresholded cyclograms (**bottom**). Extracted (red) observations on thresholded cyclograms correspond to temporal synergies in PCA space, for the following gait speeds: (**a**) 2 $\frac{m}{s}$; (**b**) 1.6 $\frac{m}{s}$; (**c**) 1 $\frac{m}{s}$; (**d**) 0.8 $\frac{m}{s}$; (**e**) 0.4 $\frac{m}{s}$. In brackets, the percentages of explained variance of the specific principal component (PC_1 or PC_2) are shown.

Cyclograms for patients' paretic and nonparetic sides, before and after therapy, were separately analyzed (Figure 7).

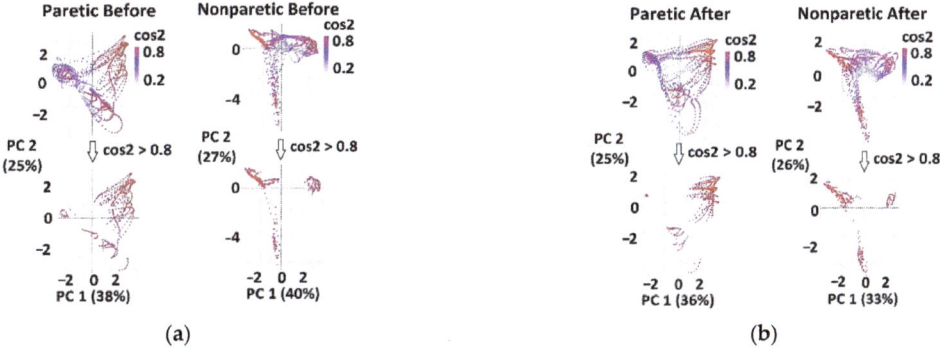

Figure 7. Examples of overlapped cyclograms for one patient (top) and thresholded cyclograms (bottom). Extracted (red) observations on thresholded cyclograms correspond to temporal synergies in PCA space: (**a**) before therapy (the paretic leg is in the left column, the nonparetic leg is in right column), and (**b**) after therapy (the paretic leg is in the left column and the nonparetic leg is in right column). In brackets, the percentages of explained variance of the specific principal component (PC_1 or PC_2) are shown.

Angles θ were calculated by Equation (1) for each observation on thresholded cyclograms (for red points in Figure 6 bottom and Figure 7 bottom). Arrays of angles' values for each of nine groups (H_2, $H_{1.6}$, H_1, $H_{0.8}$, $H_{0.4}$, $P_{p.b}$, $P_{np.b}$, $P_{p.a}$, $P_{np.a}$) were further used as an input for KDE.

3.2. Temporal Synergies Extracted by KDE

KDE was used to detect temporal synergies (clusters in time) for each of the nine groups. The cluster limits were estimated (Table 3) as local minimums in bandwidth-smoothed density distribution plots (red dots in Figures 8 and 9).

Table 3. Cluster limits (temporal components) in distribution density of angle values θ_1, θ_2, and θ_3, mean ± standard deviation, all expressed in degrees.

		Healthy Subjects					Patients before Therapy		Patients after Therapy	
		H_2	$H_{1.6}$	H_1	$H_{0.8}$	$H_{0.4}$	$P_{p.b}$	$P_{np.b}$	$P_{p.a}$	$P_{np.a}$
θ_1	cluster limits	[198–360]	[198–360]	[198–360]	[206–360]	[213–360]	[257–360]	[235–360]	[191–360]	[206–360]
	mean ± SD	265 ± 14.9	262 ± 15.7	266 ± 7.9	271 ± 15.8	276 ± 12.8	318 ± 24.4	295 ± 38.6	291 ± 40.3	272 ± 27.6
θ_2	cluster limits	[73–197]	[73–197]	[73–197]	[88–205]	[81–212]	[110–256]	[110–234]	[118–190]	[59–205]
	mean ± SD	138 ± 8.9	138 ± 7.5	140 ± 9.7	147 ± 14	147 ± 22.6	183 ± 26.1	172 ± 18.4	162 ± 4.3	152 ± 11.7
θ_3	cluster limits	[0–72]	[0–72]	[0–72]	[0–87]	[0–80]	[0–109]	[0–109]	[0–117]	[0–58]
	mean ± SD	16 ± 7	13 ± 5.2	13 ± 8.3	21 ± 12.9	23 ± 16.7	36 ± 18.9	39 ± 12.7	25 ± 12.7	12 ± 6.9

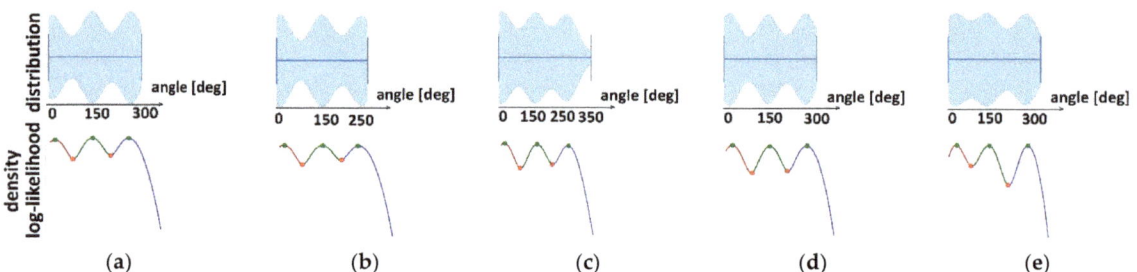

Figure 8. Clustering of temporal components in healthy subjects for the following gait speeds (red dots are cluster limits): (**a**) 2 $\frac{m}{s}$; (**b**) 1.6 $\frac{m}{s}$; (**c**) 1 $\frac{m}{s}$; (**d**) 0.8 $\frac{m}{s}$; (**e**) 0.4 $\frac{m}{s}$. Top graphics represent distribution densities, and bottom graphics represent bandwidth-smoothed distribution densities.

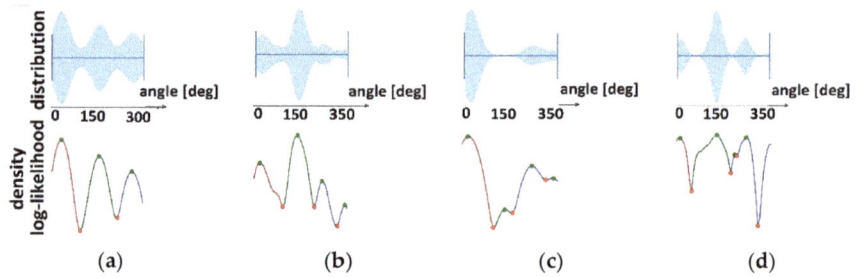

Figure 9. Clustering of temporal components (red dots are cluster limits) in patients for: (**a**) Paretic legs before therapy; (**b**) Nonparetic legs before therapy; (**c**) Paretic legs after therapy; (**d**) Nonparetic legs after therapy. Top graphics represent distribution densities, and bottom graphics represent bandwidth-smoothed distribution densities.

In Table 3, cluster limits in distribution density of angle values θ_1, θ_2, and θ_3 are shown in degrees for healthy subjects and patients before and after therapy.

Based on Equation (1), the mean values and standard deviations of the θ_1, θ_2, and θ_3 angles in cyclograms (i.e., the significant contribution of activation of the first two principal components) are shown in Table 3 for all patients and healthy subjects with different speeds. It could be noticed that the angles were shifted in time by approximately one-third of the walking cycle. These angles quantify temporal activations of gait synergies.

3.3. Comparison of Synergies between Different Speeds in Healthy Subjects

No significant differences were found between H_2, $H_{1.6}$, H_1, $H_{0.8}$, $H_{0.4}$ groups for θ_1, θ_2, and θ_3 ($p > 0.001$).

3.4. Comparison of Synergies between Patients and Healthy Subjects

Table 4 shows the results of statistic tests between healthy groups (H_2, $H_{1.6}$, H_1, $H_{0.8}$, $H_{0.4}$) and patients ($P_{p.b.}$, $P_{np.b.}$, $P_{p.a.}$, and $P_{np.a.}$). Significant differences were found in all angles (θ_1, θ_2, and θ_3) between all healthy groups and paretic leg gait before therapy ($P_{p.b.}$). After therapy, the shift in the angle towards a healthy angle can be found in some angles, specifically for the lowest gait speed (0.4 $\frac{m}{s}$), which is the most similar to the speed of the patient's gait after stroke [58].

Table 4. Statistical differences between healthy and patient groups (before and after therapy).

Healthy	Patients		$P_{p.b.}$	$P_{np.b.}$	$P_{p.a.}$	$P_{np.a.}$
H_2		θ_1	0 *	0 *	0 *	0 *
		θ_2	0 *	0 *	0 *	0 *
		θ_3	0 *	0 *	0 *	0.008
$H_{1.6}$		θ_1	0 *	0 *	0 *	0 *
		θ_2	0 *	0 *	0 *	0 *
		θ_3	0 *	0 *	0 *	0.332
H_1		θ_1	0 *	0 *	0.001	0.115
		θ_2	0 *	0 *	0 *	0 *
		θ_3	0 *	0 *	0 *	0.594
$H_{0.8}$		θ_1	0 *	0 *	0.022	0.045
		θ_2	0 *	0 *	0 *	0.004
		θ_3	0 *	0 *	0.024	0.002
$H_{0.4}$		θ_1	0 *	0.588	0.301	0.001
		θ_2	0 *	0 *	0.008	0.138
		θ_3	0 *	0.002	0.190	0.001

* $p < 0.001$.

3.5. Comparison of Synergies between Patients before and after Therapy

The significant differences in patients before and after therapy were found in all angles θ_1, θ_2, and θ_3 ($p < 0.001$). The boxplots for each angle θ_1, θ_2, and θ_3 for all nine groups are shown in Figure 10. The temporal synergies (angles) shift can be observed after therapy towards healthy synergies.

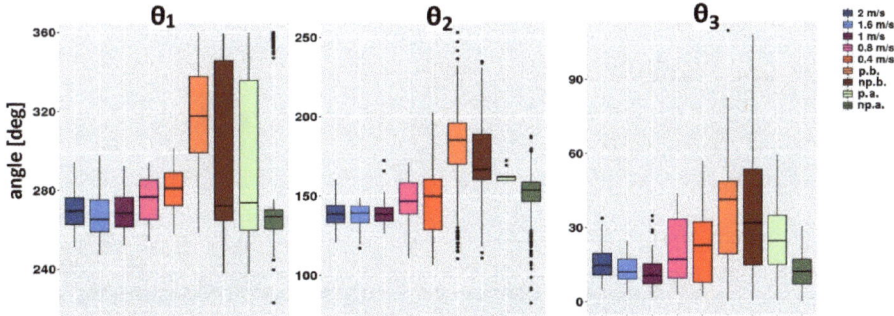

Figure 10. Temporal synergies (angles θ_1, θ_2, and θ_3) for all groups.

Additionally, it is important to consider the relative weight of each dynamic's signal, which is called loading. Loadings from the first two principal components are interpreted as the coefficients of the linear combination of the input variables from which the principal components are constructed. The relative strength of the effect of each factor on an input signal is given by this weighting coefficient. For each input signal, the mean weighting coefficients (loadings) of the first two components were obtained by averaging the values across all subjects for specific gait speed [19]. Figure 11 shows average weighting coefficients for all nine groups. Some input variables loaded highly on the specific component, such as angular velocity Gyro_Y on PC_2. Most of the input variables are loaded on both components. The noticeable gradual change of weightings with gait speed can be noticed in loadings on both PC_1 and PC_2. For patients, it could be noticed that loadings in PC_1 are approaching values from healthy subjects' gaits.

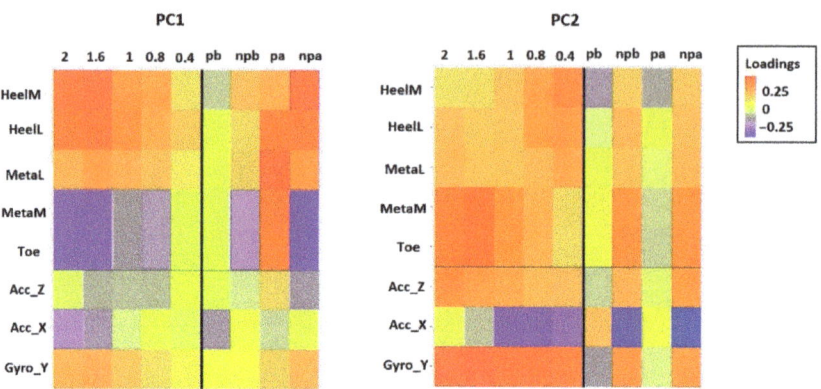

Figure 11. Weighting coefficients of the PC_1 and PC_2 for all groups. Coefficients are plotted on a color-coded scale.

3.6. Comparison with Conventional Methods

In Figure 12, boxplots for symmetry (SR, SI, GA, SA) and temporal (duration) parameters of stance and swing gait phases are shown.

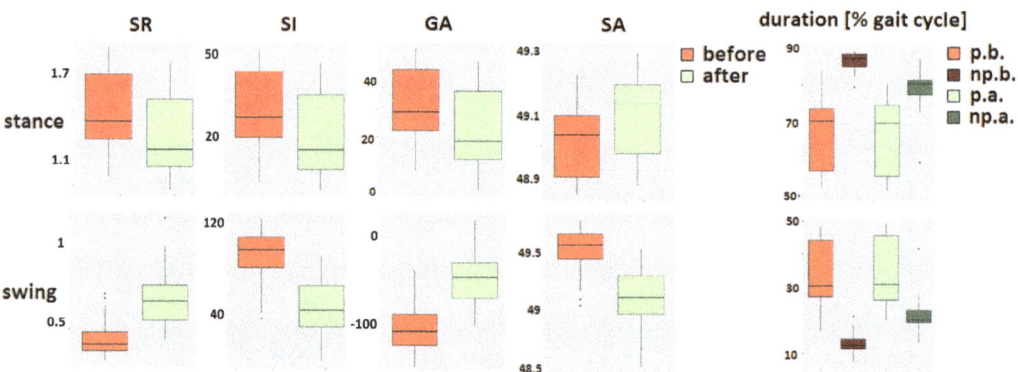

Figure 12. Boxplots of symmetry and temporal parameters for all patients' groups.

No significant differences between gait before and after therapy with the paretic leg could be found in swing or stance duration ($p = 0.94$). A significant difference has been found in swing and stance durations in nonparetic leg gait. Furthermore, this significant difference was reflected in swing symmetry parameters since it is proportional to the ratio of paretic and nonparetic leg parameters ($p < 0.001$) but not in the stance symmetry parameters ($p = 0.017$–0.019).

Unlike temporal parameters for the paretic leg, by observing the temporal synergies parameters (Equation (1)), the statistically significant differences for the paretic leg after therapy were found compared to before therapy ($p < 0.001$, Figure 10).

4. Discussion

This paper proposes a new method for detecting temporal gait synergies in dynamic space using PCA without recording muscle activity. The foot trajectory has been represented with respect to time in the PCA cyclogram space. The foot dynamics reflect the muscle activity but in a more straightforward way. Analyzing the dynamics of the endpoint—i.e., foot—is important since it is assumed that the control of limb dynamics, instead of muscle activity, would help ensure whole-body mechanical stability and energy [59]. The control of limb segment motion may happen by encoding the limb endpoint dynamics.

The inputs for PCA were GRF signals measured at the lateral and medial heel, lateral and medial metatarsal, and toe on each foot, as well as the accelerations and angular velocities measured at the rear part of each foot. The Gait Teacher system is easy to use, wearable, and relatively cheap compared to EMG-based and other gait analysis systems. It can be used in everyday life, not just in a hospital environment [60,61]. The clinician does not need the training to manage the system, unlike EMG equipment, where electrode montage and data acquisition are more time-consuming. The system's set-up comes down to putting on shoes with insoles and following the simple interface. Due to the high level of impairment of patients in the subacute phase of stroke [62], it is crucial to provide fast and straightforward screening to make the gait evaluation more comfortable and effortless for patients.

PCA used whole preprocessed gait session recordings as an input. There was no gait segmentation before or after PCA; therefore, there was no loss of information due to the interpolation to the specific time base or incorrect stride segmentation. The problem of gait phase detection accuracy and reliability was bypassed by observing the whole gait session and evaluating the sequence at once. Unlike when calculating symmetry and temporal parameters, valuable data were lost due to incorrect gait event detection.

In this paper, three temporal activations of synergies were extracted (three modules, related to angles θ_1, θ_2, and θ_3). Statistical tests proved the differences between healthy and patient gait before therapy and confirmed that the temporal synergies are invariant in healthy gait, regardless of different gait speeds, Table 4. These temporal activations are shifted 30% in time, which agrees with previous studies. Researchers have also claimed that three main temporal components from a set of five are also shifted by approximately 30% in time. Additionally, the existence of three synergies was statistically confirmed. The time shift of synergies was not significantly different in healthy gait for different speeds, which was not aligned with the observation from the literature [19].

The rehabilitation helps recovery of cortical neuronal networks controlling gait, and the re-emergence of healthy synergies can be noticed [63]. In this paper, synergies have been analyzed before and after therapy for stroke patients, and synergies were also compared to healthy subjects. Before the therapy, there were significant differences in all three temporal synergies compared to healthy gait. This can be explained by a change in double limb support and single limb support duration [64]. After therapy, the temporal activations 'moved' closer (i.e., cyclogram has rotated towards healthy cyclogram orientation) to the activations of lower speed healthy gait. The time-shift of specific synergies towards healthy values was statistically confirmed for synergies because of the FES therapy, Table 4. To the best of our knowledge, no prior studies have statistically compared temporal synergies from dynamics perspective between stroke hemiparetic gait before and after therapy with different healthy gait speeds.

On the other side, an observation can be reported about the second module related to the angle θ_2 in the paretic leg before and after therapy, indicating less complex locomotor control of the affected side (Figure 7). The reduction in observations for the second module could be noticed because the same amount of variance can be explained with fewer synergies. These results agree with previous findings of the relation between less complex control and poorer walking performance [17]. A decreased number of synergies ('disappearing' of the second module, from three to two synergies) in the paretic leg can be explained by the merging of synergies [17,65,66]. This decrease is explained by the greater cohesion between the parts of the body and the generally reduced complexity of movement due to injury. The merging of synergies was shown in paretic gait after the therapy, indicating the possible development of abnormal synergies [17,67].

The difference in the distribution of weightings reflects complex motor coordination, although the temporal synergies are consistent (Figure 11). This means that even though the input variables had a different contribution to each PC, the activations of PCs in time remained the same. It could be noticed that some weightings in the paretic leg after therapy became more exaggerated than in a healthy one, such as lateral metatarsal force weighting on PC_1 (Figure 11). This aligns with the possible development of abnormal synergies (merging of synergies) but needs further investigation.

By applying PCA, it was possible to characterize better the specific features of gait disorders in relation to commonly used techniques [40]. Therefore, the conventional temporal and symmetry parameters were also calculated. The proposed method was more advantageous than conventional gait analysis since the statistical test proved the significant difference in the paretic leg, which was not observed in temporal or symmetry parameters (Figure 12). After the therapy, symmetric gait may not be the only measure of therapy success and may not reveal the complete picture [68]. On the other hand, maximal gait variability was preserved by using PCA, and variability is a complementary way of quantifying locomotion and monitoring rehabilitation effects [69–71].

Other studies have examined the possibilities for follow-up of stroke patients based on the analysis of temporal muscle synergies [72]. Abnormal patterns of muscle synergies were used to provide additional measures for clinicians during various therapy sessions, such as robotic-assisted, conventional gait, or FES-cycling training [73,74]. Whether temporal synergies indicate the gait recovery of stroke patients is still arguable [65,73–75]. The present study showed significant changes in the temporal synergies during the rehabilitation from a dynamics perspective without considering muscle synergies.

The detection of temporal synergies from a dynamic perspective is helpful for gait assessment. Visually monitoring 2D cyclograms is a robust and straightforward qualitative measure for clinicians. The values of the proposed θ angles—i.e., temporal synergies—are quantitative measures of gait performance. The rotation of a 2D cyclogram (the change in temporal synergy) is a direct and simple measure that clinicians can use to assess gait performance by comparing values with healthy temporal synergies. As a result, clinicians will better understand and follow up with the therapy's effect on gait after a stroke. Whether the gait synergies represent an input or an output of neuromuscular control is still a point of debate [76,77]. Nevertheless, defining changes in gait from a dynamic systems perspective can be useful in rehabilitation for clinical gait assessments [41,78].

The performed study has several limitations. First, the COVID-19 pandemic restrictions caused a lack of participants following the rehabilitation protocol, and for that reason, a limited number of stroke patients were included in the study. Future studies will include a larger patient population. Additionally, for the therapy efficiency assessment, data could be acquired before and after different therapy protocols [73]. Second, the study was underpowered when comparing healthy subjects and patients since they were unmatched by confounding factors, such as age and gender. Future studies will also include matched healthy and patient groups by confounding factors. Third, the wearable device used in the study has lower accuracy and reliability than the gold standard optoelectronic systems with force platforms. However, the trade-off between good performance characteristics and high cost should also be considered [79]. Finally, the question may be asked whether data loss due to PCA affects the results. Even though the initial dataset of 11 signals per leg contains more information than two PCs, the valuable information about the gait variability is kept using PCs. This dimensionality reduction imitates the problem of neural control, where many input signals fire one control signal [41]. More synergies could be observed, and more data information could be kept by adding additional components and creating three-dimensional cyclograms. Nonetheless, observing cyclograms in 2D coordinate frames (and monitoring only θ angles) is more convenient for the clinician than monitoring the higher dimensionality graphs and parameters. The presented concept of 2D PCA-based temporal synergies assessment is suitable for near real-time monitoring purposes and can be used to improve the current clinical tools for gait assessment in the future.

5. Conclusions

In this paper, an innovative method for directly observing the limb's endpoint dynamics and detecting temporal synergies during walking with different speeds is proposed, without stride extraction, and without using EMG recordings. Furthermore, the hypothesis about invariant temporal dynamic synergies was statistically confirmed, and the potential use of this information in practical gait assessment during rehabilitation after stroke was highlighted.

Author Contributions: Conceptualization: M.M.G. and M.M.J.; Methodology: M.M.G.; Software: M.M.G.; Validation: M.M.G. and M.M.J.; Formal analysis: M.M.G.; Investigation: M.M.G.; Resources: M.M.G. and M.M.J.; Data curation: M.M.G.; Writing—original draft preparation: M.M.G. and M.M.J.; Writing—review and editing: M.M.G. and M.M.J.; Visualization: M.M.G. and M.M.J.; Supervision: M.M.J.; Project Administration: M.M.J. All authors have read and agreed to the published version of the manuscript.

Funding: This research was funded by the Ministry of Education, Science and Technological Development of the Republic of Serbia (No 175016).

Institutional Review Board Statement: The study was conducted according to the guidelines of the Declaration of Helsinki and approved by the ethics committee of the Rehabilitation Clinic "Dr Miroslav Zotović" in Belgrade, Serbia.

Informed Consent Statement: Informed consent was obtained from all subjects involved in the study.

Data Availability Statement: The data presented in this study are available on request from the corresponding author.

Acknowledgments: We would like to thank Dejan B. Popović for his initial advice in this research. We also thank Ljubica Konstantinović and Suzana Dedijer-Dujović, for providing gait data for patients who participated in the FES therapy (MOTIMOVE electronic stimulator, https://www.3-x-f.com/ (accessed on 20 February 2022)) augmenting the pedaling (OMEGO® Plus, https://tyromotion.com/en/products/omegoplus/ (accessed on 20 February 2022)).

Conflicts of Interest: The authors declare no conflict of interest.

References

1. Bernstein, N. *The Coordination and Regulation of Movements*; Pergamon: Oxford, UK, 1967.
2. Flash, T.; Hogan, N. The coordination of arm movements: An experimentally confirmed mathematical model. *J. Neurosci.* **1985**, *5*, 1688–1703. [CrossRef] [PubMed]
3. Embry, K.R.; Villarreal, D.J.; Macaluso, R.L.; Gregg, R.D. Modeling the Kinematics of Human Locomotion Over Continuously Varying Speeds and Inclines. *IEEE Trans. Neural Syst. Rehabil. Eng.* **2018**, *26*, 2342–2350. [CrossRef] [PubMed]
4. Uno, Y.; Kawato, M.; Suzuki, R. Formation and control of optimal trajectory in human multijoint arm movement. *Biol. Cybern.* **1989**, *61*, 89–101. [CrossRef]
5. Hasan, Z. Optimized movement trajectories and joint stiffness in unperturbed, inertially loaded movements. *Biol. Cybern.* **1986**, *53*, 373–382. [CrossRef] [PubMed]
6. Rosenbaum, D.A.; Meulenbroek, R.; Vaughan, J.; Jansen, C. Posture-based motion planning: Applications to grasping. *Psychol. Rev.* **2001**, *108*, 709–734. [CrossRef]
7. Oguz, O.S.; Zhou, Z.; Wollherr, D. A Hybrid Framework for Understanding and Predicting Human Reaching Motions. *Front. Robot. AI* **2018**, *5*, 27. [CrossRef] [PubMed]
8. d'Avella, A.; Saltiel, P.; Bizzi, E. Combinations of muscle synergies in the construction of a natural motor behavior. *Nat. Neurosci.* **2003**, *6*, 300–308. [CrossRef] [PubMed]
9. Oshima, H.; Aoi, S.; Funato, T.; Tsujiuchi, N.; Tsuchiya, K. Variant and Invariant Spatiotemporal Structures in Kinematic Coordination to Regulate Speed During Walking and Running. *Front. Comput. Neurosci.* **2019**, *13*, 63. [CrossRef] [PubMed]
10. Popovič, M.; Popovic, D. Cloning biological synergies improves control of elbow neuroprostheses. *IEEE Eng. Med. Biol.* **2001**, *20*, 74–81. [CrossRef] [PubMed]
11. Tagliabue, M.; Ciancio, A.L.; Brochier, T.; Eskiizmirliler, S.; Maier, M.A. Differences between kinematic synergies and muscle synergies during two-digit grasping. *Front. Hum. Neurosci.* **2015**, *9*, 165. [CrossRef] [PubMed]

12. Esmaeili, S.; Karami, H.; Baniasad, M.; Shojaeefard, M.; Farahmand, F. The association between motor modules and movement primitives of gait: A muscle and kinematic synergy study. *J. Biomech.* **2022**, *134*, 110997. [CrossRef]
13. Ivanenko, Y.P.; Cappellini, G.; Dominici, N.; Poppele, R.E.; Lacquaniti, F. Modular Control of Limb Movements during Human Locomotion. *J. Neurosci.* **2007**, *27*, 11149–11161. [CrossRef] [PubMed]
14. Huang, B.; Xiong, C.; Chen, W.; Liang, J.; Sun, B.-Y.; Gong, X. Common kinematic synergies of various human locomotor behaviours. *R. Soc. Open Sci.* **2021**, *8*, 210161. [CrossRef] [PubMed]
15. Cech, D.; Martin, S. *Functional Movement Development Across the Life Span*, 3rd ed.; Elsevier: Amsterdam, The Netherlands, 2012.
16. Chiovetto, E.; Berret, B.; Delis, I.; Panzeri, S.; Pozzo, T. Investigating reduction of dimensionality during single-joint elbow movements: A case study on muscle synergies. *Front. Comput. Neurosci.* **2013**, *7*, 11. [CrossRef]
17. Clark, D.J.; Ting, L.H.; Zajac, F.E.; Neptune, R.R.; Kautz, S.A. Merging of Healthy Motor Modules Predicts Reduced Locomotor Performance and Muscle Coordination Complexity Post-Stroke. *J. Neurophysiol.* **2010**, *103*, 844–857. [CrossRef]
18. Chvatal, S.A.P.; Ting, L.H.P. Common muscle synergies for balance and walking. *Front. Comput. Neurosci.* **2013**, *7*, 48. [CrossRef] [PubMed]
19. Ivanenko, Y.P.; Grasso, R.; Zago, M.; Molinari, M.; Scivoletto, G.; Castellano, V.; Macellari, V.; Lacquaniti, F. Temporal Components of the Motor Patterns Expressed by the Human Spinal Cord Reflect Foot Kinematics. *J. Neurophysiol.* **2003**, *90*, 3555–3565. [CrossRef] [PubMed]
20. Lacquaniti, F.; Grasso, R.; Zago, M. Motor patterns in walking. *Physiology* **1999**, *14*, 168–174. [CrossRef]
21. Ivanenko, Y.P.; Poppele, R.E.; Lacquaniti, F. Five basic muscle activation patterns account for muscle activity during human locomotion. *J. Physiol.* **2004**, *556*, 267–282. [CrossRef] [PubMed]
22. Kuiken, T.A.; Lowery, M.; Stoykov, N.S. The effect of subcutaneous fat on myoelectric signal amplitude and cross-talk. *Prosthetics Orthot. Int.* **2003**, *27*, 48–54. [CrossRef] [PubMed]
23. Steele, K.M.; Tresch, M.C.; Perreault, E.J. The number and choice of muscles impact the results of muscle synergy analyses. *Front. Comput. Neurosci.* **2013**, *7*, 105. [CrossRef] [PubMed]
24. Fox, E.J.; Tester, N.; Kautz, S.; Howland, D.R.; Clark, D.J.; Garvan, C.; Behrman, A.L. Modular control of varied locomotor tasks in children with incomplete spinal cord injuries. *J. Neurophysiol.* **2013**, *110*, 1415–1425. [CrossRef] [PubMed]
25. Woolley, S.M. Characteristics of Gait in Hemiplegia. *Top. Stroke Rehabil.* **2001**, *7*, 1–18. [CrossRef] [PubMed]
26. Akhtaruzzaman, M.D.; Shafie, A.A.; Khan, M.R. Gait analysis: Systems, technologies, and importance. *J. Mech. Med. Biol.* **2016**, *16*, 1630003. [CrossRef]
27. do Carmo Vilas-Boas, M.; Choupina, H.M.; Rocha, A.P.; Fernandes, J.M.; Cunha, J.P. Full-body motion assessment: Concurrent validation of two body tracking depth sensors versus a gold standard system during gait. *J. Biomech.* **2019**, *87*, 189–196. [CrossRef] [PubMed]
28. Benson, L.C.; Clermont, C.A.; Bošnjak, E.; Ferber, R. The use of wearable devices for walking and running gait analysis outside of the lab: A systematic review. *Gait Posture* **2018**, *63*, 124–138. [CrossRef] [PubMed]
29. Kokolevich, Z.M.; Biros, E.; Tirosh, O.; Reznik, J.E. Distinct Ground Reaction Forces in Gait between the Paretic and Non-Paretic Leg of Stroke Patients: A Paradigm for Innovative Physiotherapy Intervention. *Healthcare* **2021**, *9*, 1542. [CrossRef] [PubMed]
30. Petraglia, F.; Scarcella, L.; Pedrazzi, G.; Brancato, L.; Puers, R.; Costantino, C. Inertial sensors versus standard systems in gait analysis: A systematic review and meta-analysis. *Eur. J. Phys. Rehabil. Med.* **2019**, *55*, 265–280. [CrossRef] [PubMed]
31. Panero, E.; Digo, E.; Dimanico, U.; Alberto Artusi, C.; Zibetti, M.; Gastaldi, L. Effect of Deep Brain Stimulation Frequency on Gait Symmetry, Smoothness and Variability using IMU. In Proceedings of the 2021 IEEE International Symposium on Medical Measurements and Applications (MeMeA), Lausanne, Switzerland, 23–25 June 2021.
32. Vienne, A.; Barrois, R.P.; Buffat, S.; Ricard, D.; Vidal, P.-P. Inertial Sensors to Assess Gait Quality in Patients with Neurological Disorders: A Systematic Review of Technical and Analytical Challenges. *Front. Psychol.* **2017**, *8*, 817. [CrossRef] [PubMed]
33. Gouwanda, D.; Gopalai, A.A.; Khoo, B.H. A Low Cost Alternative to Monitor Human Gait Temporal Parameters–Wearable Wireless Gyroscope. *IEEE Sens. J.* **2016**, *16*, 9029–9035. [CrossRef]
34. Mei, C.; Gao, F.; Li, Y. A Determination Method for Gait Event Based on Acceleration Sensors. *Sensors* **2019**, *19*, 5499. [CrossRef] [PubMed]
35. Pérez-Ibarra, J.C.; Williams, H.; Siqueira, A.A.; Krebs, H.I. Real-time identification of impaired gait phases using a single foot-mounted inertial sensor: Review and feasibility study. In Proceedings of the 2018 7th IEEE International Conference on Biomedical Robotics and Biomechatronics (Biorob), Enschede, The Netherlands, 26–29 August 2018; pp. 1157–1162.
36. Lyons, G.; Sinkjaer, T.; Burridge, J.; Wilcox, D. A review of portable FES-based neural orthoses for the correction of drop foot. *IEEE Trans. Neural Syst. Rehabil. Eng.* **2002**, *10*, 260–279. [CrossRef]
37. Beckerman, H.; Becher, J.; Lankhorst, G.J.; Verbeek, A. Walking ability of stroke patients: Efficacy of tibial nerve blocking and a polypropylene ankle-foot orthosis. *Arch. Phys. Med. Rehabil.* **1996**, *77*, 1144–1151. [CrossRef]
38. Chau, T. A review of analytical techniques for gait data. Part 1: Fuzzy, statistical and fractal methods. *Gait Posture* **2001**, *13*, 49–66. [CrossRef]
39. Daffertshofer, A.; Lamoth, C.J.; Meijer, O.G.; Beek, P.J. PCA in studying coordination and variability: A tutorial. *Clin. Biomech.* **2004**, *19*, 415–428. [CrossRef] [PubMed]
40. Milovanović, I.; Popovic, D.B. Principal Component Analysis of Gait Kinematics Data in Acute and Chronic Stroke Patients. *Comput. Math. Methods Med.* **2012**, *2012*, 649743. [CrossRef] [PubMed]

41. Gavrilović, M.; Popović, D.B. A principal component analysis (PCA) based assessment of the gait performance. *Biomed. Tech.* **2021**, *66*, 449–457. [CrossRef] [PubMed]
42. 3F-FIT FABRICANDO FABER. Available online: https://www.3-x-f.com/ (accessed on 20 February 2022).
43. Robotic Gait Therapy I OMEGO®Plus I Tyromotion. Available online: https://tyromotion.com/en/products/omegoplus/ (accessed on 20 February 2022).
44. REHAB SHOP. Available online: https://www.rehabshop.rs (accessed on 20 February 2022).
45. Fulk, G.D.; Echternach, J.L. Test-Retest Reliability and Minimal Detectable Change of Gait Speed in Individuals Undergoing Rehabilitation after Stroke. *J. Neurol. Phys. Ther.* **2008**, *32*, 8–13. [CrossRef]
46. Bohannon, R.W. Comfortable and maximum walking speed of adults aged 20–79 years: Reference values and determinants. *Age Ageing* **1997**, *26*, 15–19. [CrossRef] [PubMed]
47. Asmussen, M.J.; Kaltenbach, C.; Hashlamoun, K.; Shen, H.; Federico, S.; Nigg, B.M. Force measurements during running on different instrumented treadmills. *J. Biomech.* **2018**, *84*, 263–268. [CrossRef] [PubMed]
48. Crenna, F.; Rossi, G.; Berardengo, M. Filtering Biomechanical Signals in Movement Analysis. *Sensors* **2021**, *21*, 4580. [CrossRef] [PubMed]
49. Bartlett, M.S. Properties of sufficiency and statistical tests. In *Proceedings of the Royal Society of London*; Series A-Mathematical and Physical Sciences; Royal Society: London, UK, 1937; Volume 160, pp. 268–282.
50. Milovanović, I. Synergy Patterns of Stroke Subjects While Walking: Implications for Control of FES Assistive Devices. Ph.D. Thesis, Faculty of Electrical Engineering University of Belgrade, Belgrade, Serbia, 2013.
51. Rosenblatt, M. Remarks on Some Nonparametric Estimates of a Density Function. *Ann. Math. Stat.* **1956**, *27*, 832–837. [CrossRef]
52. Shapiro, S.S.; Wilk, M.B. An analysis of variance test for normality (complete samples). *Biometrika* **1965**, *52*, 591–611. [CrossRef]
53. Silverman, B.W. *Density Estimation for Statistics and Data Analysis*; Chapman and Hall: London, UK, 1986.
54. Mann, H.B.; Whitney, D.R. On a Test of Whether one of Two Random Variables is Stochastically Larger than the Other. *Ann. Math. Stat.* **1947**, *18*, 50–60. [CrossRef]
55. Fong, Y.; Huang, Y.; Lemos, M.P.; McElrath, M.J. Rank-based two-sample tests for paired data with missing values. *Biostatistics* **2017**, *19*, 281–294. [CrossRef]
56. Gavrilović, M. Gyroscope based method for evaluation of gait symmetry. In Proceedings of the 5th IcETRAN, Palić, Serbia, 11–14 June 2018.
57. Błażkiewicz, M.; Wiszomirska, I.; Wit, A. Comparison of four methods of calculating the symmetry of spatial-temporal parameters of gait. *Acta Bioeng. Biomech.* **2014**, *16*, 29–35. [CrossRef]
58. Wing, K.; Lynskey, J.V.; Bosch, P.R. Walking speed in stroke survivors: Considerations for clinical practice. *Top. Geriatr. Rehab.* **2012**, *28*, 113–121. [CrossRef]
59. Pearson, K.G. Common Principles of Motor Control in Vertebrates and Invertebrates. *Annu. Rev. Neurosci.* **1993**, *16*, 265–297. [CrossRef] [PubMed]
60. Rinehart, N.J.; Tonge, B.J.; Iansek, R.; McGinley, J.; Brereton, A.V.; Enticott, P.G.; Bradshaw, J.L. Gait function in newly diagnosed children with autism: Cerebellar and basal ganglia related motor disorder. *Dev. Med. Child Neurol.* **2006**, *48*, 819–824. [CrossRef]
61. Winter, D.A. Chapter 9: Kinesiological Electromyography. In *Biomechanics and Motor Control of Human Movement*, 3rd ed.; Winter, D.A., Ed.; John Wiley & Sons, Inc.: Hoboken, NJ, USA, 2005.
62. Frenkel-Toledo, S.; Ofir-Geva, S.; Mansano, L.; Granot, O.; Soroker, N. Stroke Lesion Impact on Lower Limb Function. *Front. Hum. Neurosci.* **2021**, *15*, 27. [CrossRef]
63. Maguire, C.C.; Sieben, J.M.; De Bie, R.A. Movement goals encoded within the cortex and muscle synergies to reduce redundancy pre and post-stroke. The relevance for gait rehabilitation and the prescription of walking-aids. A literature review and scholarly discussion. *Physiother. Theory Pract.* **2018**, *35*, 1–14. [CrossRef] [PubMed]
64. Goldie, P.A.; Matyas, T.A.; Evans, O.M. Gait after stroke: Initial deficit and changes in temporal patterns for each gait phase. *Arch. Phys. Med. Rehabil.* **2001**, *82*, 1057–1065. [CrossRef] [PubMed]
65. Gizzi, L.; Nielsen, J.F.; Felici, F.; Ivanenko, Y.; Farina, D. Impulses of activation but not motor modules are preserved in the locomotion of subacute stroke patients. *J. Neurophysiol.* **2011**, *106*, 202–210. [CrossRef] [PubMed]
66. Bowden, M.G.; Clark, D.J.; Kautz, S.A. Evaluation of Abnormal Synergy Patterns Poststroke: Relationship of the Fugl-Meyer Assessment to Hemiparetic Locomotion. *Neurorehabil. Neural Repair* **2009**, *24*, 328–337. [CrossRef] [PubMed]
67. Van Criekinge, T.; Vermeulen, J.; Wagemans, K.; Schröder, J.; Embrechts, E.; Truijen, S.; Hallemans, A.; Saeys, W. Lower limb muscle synergies during walking after stroke: A systematic review. *Disabil. Rehabil.* **2020**, *42*, 2836–2845. [CrossRef]
68. Krasovsky, T.; Levin, M.F. Review: Toward a Better Understanding of Coordination in Healthy and Poststroke Gait. *Neurorehabil. Neural Repair* **2009**, *24*, 213–224. [CrossRef] [PubMed]
69. Hausdorff, J.M. Gait variability: Methods, modeling and modeling meaning. *J. Neuroeng. Rehab.* **2005**, *2*, 19. [CrossRef] [PubMed]
70. Keklicek, H.; Kirdi, E.; Yalcin, A.; Topuz, S.; Ulger, O.; Erbahceci, F.; Sener, G. Comparison of gait variability and symmetry in trained individuals with transtibial and transfemoral limb loss. *J. Orthop. Surg.* **2019**, *27*. [CrossRef]
71. Kim, W.-S.; Choi, H.; Jung, J.-W.; Yoon, J.S.; Jeoung, J.H. Asymmetry and Variability Should Be Included in the Assessment of Gait Function in Poststroke Hemiplegia with Independent Ambulation During Early Rehabilitation. *Arch. Phys. Med. Rehabil.* **2020**, *102*, 611–618. [CrossRef]

72. Rosa, M.C.N.; Marques, A.; Demain, S.; Metcalf, C.D. Lower limb co-contraction during walking in subjects with stroke: A systematic review. *J. Electromyogr. Kinesiol.* **2014**, *24*, 1–10. [CrossRef]
73. Tan, C.K.; Kadone, H.; Watanabe, H.; Marushima, A.; Hada, Y.; Yamazaki, M.; Sankai, Y.; Matsumura, A.; Suzuki, K. Differences in Muscle Synergy Symmetry Between Subacute Post-stroke Patients With Bioelectrically-Controlled Exoskeleton Gait Training and Conventional Gait Training. *Front. Bioeng. Biotechnol.* **2020**, *8*, 770. [CrossRef]
74. Ambrosini, E.; Parati, M.; Peri, E.; De Marchis, C.; Nava, C.; Pedrocchi, A.; Ferriero, G.; Ferrante, S. Changes in leg cycling muscle synergies after training augmented by functional electrical stimulation in subacute stroke survivors: A pilot study. *J. Neuroeng. Rehabil.* **2020**, *17*, 35. [CrossRef] [PubMed]
75. Den Otter, A.R.; Geurts, A.C.H.; Mulder, T.H.; Duysens, J. Gait recovery is not associated with changes in the temporal patterning of muscle activity during treadmill walking in patients with post-stroke hemiparesis. *Clin. Neurophysiol.* **2006**, *117*, 4–15. [CrossRef] [PubMed]
76. Tresch, M.C.; Jarc, A. The case for and against muscle synergies. *Curr. Opin. Neurobiol.* **2009**, *19*, 601–607. [CrossRef] [PubMed]
77. Cheung, V.C.K.; Seki, K. Approaches to revealing the neural basis of muscle synergies: A review and a critique. *J. Neurophysiol.* **2021**, *125*, 1580–1597. [CrossRef]
78. Singh, R.E.; Iqbal, K.; White, G.; Hutchinson, T.E. A Systematic Review on Muscle Synergies: From Building Blocks of Motor Behavior to a Neurorehabilitation Tool. *Appl. Bionics Biomech.* **2018**, *2018*, 3615368. [CrossRef] [PubMed]
79. Zhou, L.; Fischer, E.; Tunca, C.; Brahms, C.M.; Ersoy, C.; Granacher, U.; Arnrich, B. How We Found Our IMU: Guidelines to IMU Selection and a Comparison of Seven IMUs for Pervasive Healthcare Applications. *Sensors* **2020**, *20*, 4090. [CrossRef] [PubMed]

Article

Step Length Estimation Using the RSSI Method in Walking and Jogging Scenarios

Zanru Yang *, Le Chung Tran and Farzad Safaei

School of Electrical, Computer and Telecommunications Engineering, University of Wollongong, Wollongong, NSW 2522, Australia; lctran@uow.edu.au (L.C.T.); farzad@uow.edu.au (F.S.)
* Correspondence: zy482@uowmail.edu.au

Abstract: In this paper, human step length was estimated based on wireless channel properties and the received signal strength indicator (RSSI) method. Path loss between two ankles of the person under test was converted from the RSSI, which was measured using our developed wearable transceivers with embedded micro-controllers in four scenarios, namely indoor walking, outdoor walking, indoor jogging, and outdoor jogging. For brevity, we call it on-ankle path loss. The histogram of the on-ankle path loss showed clearly that there were two humps, where the second hump was closely related to the maximum path loss, which, in turn, corresponded to the step length. This histogram can be well approximated by a two-term Gaussian fitting curve model. Based on the histogram of the experimental data and the two-term Gaussian fitting curve, we propose a novel filtering technique to filter out the path loss outliers, which helps set up the upper and lower thresholds of the path loss values used for the step length estimation. In particular, the upper threshold was found to be on the right side of the second Gaussian hump, and its value was a function of the mean value and the standard deviation of the second Gaussian hump. Meanwhile, the lower threshold lied on the left side of the second hump and was determined at the point where the survival rate of the measured data fell to 0.68, i.e., the cumulative distribution function (CDF) approached 0.32. The experimental data showed that the proposed filtering technique resulted in high accuracy in step length estimation with errors of only 10.15 mm for the indoor walking, 4.40 mm for the indoor jogging, 4.81 mm for the outdoor walking, and 10.84 mm for the outdoor jogging scenarios, respectively.

Keywords: data histogram; distance estimation; gait speed; on-ankle path loss; RSSI; step length estimation; strike length estimation; two-term Gaussian distribution

1. Introduction

Step length (or stride length) plays an important role in addressing the issue of human health conditions, especially for seniors. It is an indicator that predicts accidental falls and fall-related injury in the elderly [1], which may cause fatality [2]. A reduced step length has been found to be associated with the increased dependence, mortality, and institutionalization of older people [3]. The variability of the step length also indicates the integrity of gray matter, which is closely related to personal memory and executive functions [4]. Furthermore, step length is one of the significant components in gait patterns. It can be converted to gait speed, which is useful in predicting life expectancy [5]. Therefore, monitoring the human step length is a vital topic that is worthy of investigating.

The estimation of the step length can be traced back to the problem of distance estimation. Although distance estimation has been intensively researched for general communication systems, there are few papers explicitly researching the human step length in daily activities, such as walking and jogging, in both indoor and outdoor environments. Moreover, as mentioned in more detail in the next section of this paper, the existing publications that address the estimation of step length either have modest accuracy or follow privacy-invasive, health-concerning, and strictly space-confined approaches. Specifically, camera-based technologies [6,7] are privacy-invasive and prone to error as they may record images or video footage of the participants. The camera-based methods also require a specific experimental setting because any obstacle appearing between the camera and the person under test can cause measurement errors. Meanwhile, laser-based methods [8] may arouse health concerns because a long-time exposure to lasers in these methods may cause some health hazards. On the other hand, sensing mats [9–11] have been well adopted to improve the safety of patients, especially the disabled and those with disorders. However, the sensing mat approach is confined to particular spaces, such as clinics, hospitals, or a specific laboratory setting where the sensing mat is laid, because the person under test must walk or run on this mat. Therefore, a more-accurate, less-invasive, less-health-concerning, and less-space-confined, but also cost-efficient technique for step length estimations in daily activities is still missing.

Thus, this paper aimed to estimate the step length based on the received signal strength indicator (RSSI) method in both walking and jogging activities in indoor and outdoor scenarios. The RSSI has been widely employed in distance estimation, and it might provide reliable performance [12–17], especially for measurements in line-of-sight (LOS) paths over short distances, such as the step length measurements in this paper. The step length in this paper refers to the average distance between two ankles of the person under test when the person is walking or jogging at a normal and equal pace. Unlike our previous work in [18], which only considered a static environment, this paper undertook experiments in actual moving activities. In particular, in this paper, we propose a novel filtering technique to be applied along with the empirical path loss model proposed in [18] to estimate the step length in walking and jogging situations.

The main contributions of this paper are summarized as follows:

- A novel filtering technique is proposed to eliminate on-ankle path loss outliers and keep the remaining as a reliable range with a pair of upper and lower thresholds. This range of path loss values was used to estimate the human step length in daily activities, such as walking and jogging;
- The distribution of the on-ankle path loss was revealed to follow a two-term Gaussian distribution, and the two thresholds lied on each side of its second hump;
- The thresholds can be determined mathematically. The upper threshold relates to the fitting equation of the second hump of the two-term Gaussian distribution, which was found as $\mu + 0.5\sigma$ for an outdoor and $\mu + \sigma$ for an indoor environment. The lower threshold relates to the survival rate, which is located at the point where the survival rate of the measured data is 0.68;
- The proposed filtering technique resulted in an accurate estimation of the step length, with errors of only 10.15 mm and 4.40 mm for walking and jogging in an indoor environment, respectively, and only 4.81 mm and 10.84 mm for the same activities in an outdoor environment.

The rest of the paper is organized as follows. Section 2 reviews the related works. Section 3 describes the proposed system model. In Section 4, the experimental procedures are detailed. Section 5 presents the experimental results and analyses of the step length estimation accuracy in the indoor walking, indoor jogging, outdoor walking, and outdoor jogging situations. Section 6 concludes the paper. Finally, Section 7 states the limitations and the future works.

2. Related Works

Accurate estimation of the human step length is a challenging task, especially in human daily activities, due to the randomness of these activities. As a result, there are few research papers that explicitly address the problem of step length estimation, although the overarching topic of distance measurements has been intensively researched for general communication systems. These research papers are briefly reviewed as follows.

The researchers in [6] used cameras as additional sensors in pedestrian dead reckoning (PDR) to analyze step length and step frequency. Currently, PDR is a popular indoor localization method [19,20] due to the wide availability of smart devices. Cameras were also employed in [7] to track the motions of the person under test. The stride length can be estimated by detecting and extracting several pieces of perspective information related to predefined markers and edges. The experiment results implied that the camera-based method was a promising way to detect all steps when the user was moving slowly, especially in an indoor environment. Recently, the researchers in [21] proposed a machine-learning-based step length estimation algorithm with the use of cameras and smartphones. This research considered a systematic feature selection algorithm to determine the choice of user-specific parameters from a large collection. The mean absolute errors of the step length estimations were 3.48 cm and 4.19 cm for a known test person and an unknown test person, respectively. However, the above camera-based techniques are flexibility-constrained because the camera must be arranged at a certain place and has a limited horizon. Moreover, its accuracy may be reduced in fast-moving situations or by obstacles appearing between the cameras and the person under test.

The gait patterns can also be detected by infrared thermography, such as in [8], where the best accuracy was found to be 91%. However, the drawback is that lasers are not common in daily usage because of the training requirements, costly equipment, and the potential health concern for long-term exposure.

An inertial sensor can be utilized in an inertial measurement unit (IMU) to collect gait-related parameters, which then help to estimate the human step length. An IMU generally consists of an accelerometer, a compass, and a gyroscope. Currently, most smart devices have built-in inertial sensors. The smart device can be held in hand [22] or attached to the body, such as the pelvis [23], which provides useful information and helps position the point of interest. References [19,20] estimated the human stride length based on the data collected from inertial sensor measurements from a smartphone. The experimental results demonstrated that the step length can be estimated with an error rate of 4.63% for indoor scenarios. Considering a general step length of 0.7 m, the corresponding absolute error would be 3.24 cm. The error of step length estimation was reduced to 2% in [24] based on a back-propagation artificial neural network using an IMU that was placed on the foot. The research in [25] compared the accuracy of estimation between different placements of the IMUs. Firstly, this paper utilized only one inertial sensor on each shank, called the integrator-based method, providing an average accuracy of 91.21%. The accuracy was improved to 95.37% if two sensors were employed on each leg, namely the angle-based method. As a result, the maximum error was 11.26 cm and 5.51 cm for the integration and angle mode, respectively. Although the integrator-based method was simpler, the angle-based method achieved better accuracy in terms of step length estimation since it was not sensitive to the initial conditions and errors caused by double integration. However, experiments and analyses in the outdoors are still missing. Moreover, a major disadvantage of using IMUs is that they typically suffer from an accumulated error, which means the accuracy will be degraded over time.

Deep learning has been adopted to estimate human step length because it can learn the features of the data automatically and has shown excellent performance in different application domains with the cost of powerful computing facilities. The proposed deep-learning-based algorithm in [26] can adapt to different phone carrying ways and does not require individual stature information and spatial constraints. The average error of this method was 3.01%, which means if the actual step length was 0.7 m, then the corresponding error range was within 2.1 cm. Paper [27] defined a deep-learning-based framework with an activity recognition model to regress the user change in distance and step length. The average error of the proposed method was 2.1%, which was about 1.47 cm if the step length was 0.7 m. It is worth noting that the positions (e.g., handheld position or pocket position) of the smartphone also had a huge influence on the estimation by around 5% [28]. The researchers in [29] investigated human step length and step width using wearable sensors in a computer-assisted rehabilitation environment. The results showed that in a specific experimental environment, gait patterns could be detected and the mean absolute errors were 0.2396 cm and 1.92 cm, respectively. However, the data in this paper were collected using specific equipment under a specific environment, rather than normal indoor and outdoor propagation environments in daily human activities.

Therefore, in this paper, we aimed to propose a step length estimation technique that has high accuracy and is less-privacy-invasive, less-health-concerning, and less-space-confined than the aforementioned techniques, without requiring powerful computing facilities as the deep-learning-based ones.

Our previous work presented in [18] proposed an empirical path loss model to estimate the human step length in both indoor and outdoor scenarios under a static context rather than in a dynamic one. Therefore, this paper aimed to estimate human step length in daily activities. In particular, a novel filtering technique is proposed in this paper, which was used along with the hardware transceivers and the empirical path loss model developed in our previous work [18] to estimate human step length correctly in both walking and jogging activities in both indoor and outdoor environments.

3. System Model

In this paper, we adopted the transceivers and the experimental path loss model between two human ankles developed in [18]. The experimental path loss PL_{OA} between two transceivers attached to the ankles of the person under test can be described as a modified free-space path loss model with a correction factor ΔPL (cf. (1) in [18]):

$$PL_{OA}(\text{dB}) = PL_{FS} + \Delta PL, \tag{1}$$

where PL_{FS} (dB) is the free-space path loss and ΔPL (dB) is the correction factor, which accounts for the hardware non-linearity, multipath propagation, insertion, and mismatch losses. For the transceivers considered, the correction factor was empirically found as 10 dB [18]. Therefore, (1) can be written as:

$$PL_{OA}(\text{dB}) = PL_{FS} + 10. \tag{2}$$

It is noted that the free-space path loss [30] is defined as:

$$PL_{FS}(\text{dB}) = 20 \log_{10}\left(\frac{4\pi d}{\lambda}\right), \tag{3}$$

where d (m) is the distance between the two antennas and λ (m) is the signal wavelength. From (2) and (3), this distance could be estimated as:

$$d = \frac{\lambda}{4\pi} 10^{\left(\frac{PL_{OA}(\text{dB})-10}{20}\right)}. \tag{4}$$

In the later analysis, we used this equation to calculate the human step length.

4. Experiment Setups

In this section, we detail our experimental settings. Similar to our previous work in [18], the Arduino Integrated Development Environment (IDE), XBee Configuration & Test Unit (X-CTU), Arduino UNO microprocessors, and XBee-PRO S2C wireless transceivers were employed in this experiment. The core communication technology used in the XBee-PRO S2C modules is the spreading spectrum technique regulated by the IEEE 802.15.4 standard for low-rate wireless personal area networks (LR-WPANs) [31]. In particular, each group of four data bits is mapped into one of 16 nearly orthogonal spreading sequences, each of which is 32 chips long. The resulting chip sequence is modulated on the radio-frequency carrier in the 2.4 GHz band by the offset quadrature phase shift keying (O-QPSK) modulation scheme. The components of the transceivers are depicted in Figure 1. The parameters were configured as follows: transmission power $P_0 = 0$ dBm and data rate

9600 bps. This is the most proper configuration of the developed transceivers for measuring the distance between two ankles, as discovered from our previous experiments in [18].

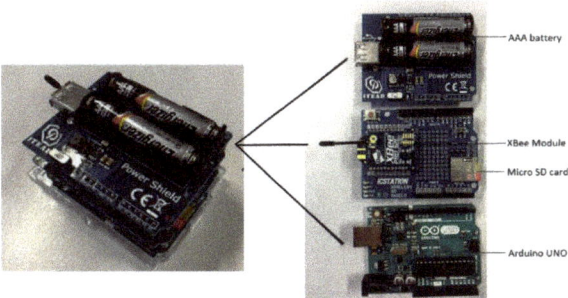

Figure 1. Components of the transceivers.

The transceivers were attached to the inner side of human ankles at the same height h, as shown in Figure 2. The distance between two antennas was regarded as the real step length d_0 (m). In our experiments, the transmitter and the receiver were placed on the medial side of the ankles of the subject under test in a way that the antennas faced each other, as shown in Figure 2b. This means that there existed an LOS path between the transceivers, even when the person under test was walking or jogging, and that there was no human body part appearing between them. As a result, this placement of equipment can eliminate the shadowing effect caused by any body parts. This intuitive prediction was confirmed in our previous work [18], where experiments were performed both off-body and on ankles to compare the shadowing effect. The results in [18] showed that the shadowing effect caused by the human body was negligible in our experiments.

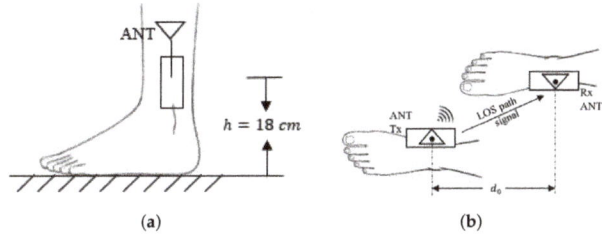

Figure 2. Schematic diagrams of the on-ankle transceivers. (**a**) Side view; (**b**) top view.

The main purpose of this system was to transmit and receive continuous data packets to/from each other, and the assembled micro SD card in the receiver recorded the RSSI values continuously. From the RSSI values, the on-ankle path loss can be calculated as (cf. (5) in [18]):

$$PL_{OA}(\text{dB}) = P_t + RSSI, \tag{5}$$

where P_t (dB) is the transmitted power. From (4) and (5), the distance between the two transceivers is:

$$d = \frac{\lambda}{4\pi} 10^{\left(\frac{P_t(\text{dB}) + RSSI(\text{dB}) - 10}{20}\right)}. \tag{6}$$

Following is a trial experiment of the indoor walking situation to explore the relationship between the measured path loss values and the positions of the two ankles. Figure 3a plots the on-ankle path loss over time. During the first 0.64 s, the transmitter and the receiver initialize themselves and synchronize with each other. Once the transmitter and the receiver are synchronized, it takes around 0.02 s for the hardware to measure and record each RSSI value into the micro-SD card, as shown in Figure 3b.

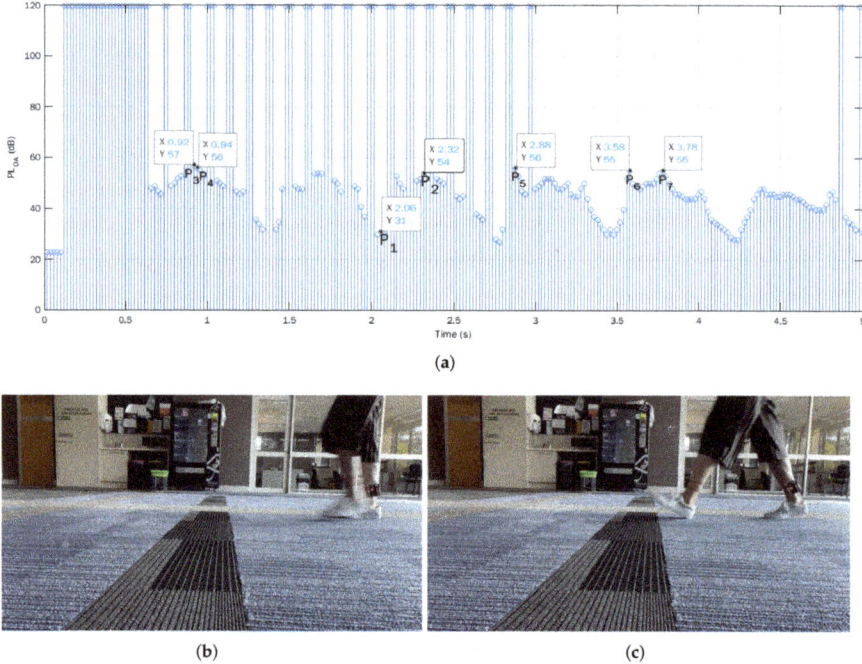

Figure 3. Trial indoor walking experiment. (**a**) On-ankle path loss at different time; (**b**) feet positions at P_1 (t = 2.08 s); (**c**) feet positions at P_2 (t = 2.32 s).

After the initial synchronization phase, the Arduino may encounter erroneous transmissions from time to time due to temporarily being out-of-synchronization. To cope with this, in our experiments, the Arduino UNO hardware was programmed in a way that, if an erroneous transmission occurs (i.e., the receiver does not receive the packet successfully), a very big value of path loss (120 dB was chosen in our experiments) would be recorded to the data file in the micro-SD card to flag this erroneous transmission. Thereby, in the later analysis, any erroneous transmission would be easily detected and omitted. As shown in Figure 3a, the temporary out-of-synchronization status was normally very short, and the Arduino UNOs could quickly synchronize again with each other. Hence, in general, the Arduino UNO transceivers were relatively stable and reliable.

Because of the modest computation capability of the Arduino UNO, the transceivers in our experiments were programmed to only transmit and receive data packets to record the RSSI values in order to avoid any unnecessary delay. Processing of the raw data was performed offline on a computer instead. It is also noted that we aimed to estimate the average step length over a certain period, rather than outputting the instant estimated step length values, to mitigate the randomness in the measurement process. As a result, the processing time of our algorithm had a negligible effect on the RSSI calculations.

It was observed that the measured path losses had a periodical pattern. To explore the meaning of the peaks and troughs of the path loss, let us consider two points P_1(2.08 s, 30 dB) and P_2(2.32 s, 54 dB) from the plot, where P_1 is at a trough and P_2 is the following peak. A video of the footage was captured in tandem with the path loss measurements. Based on the time stamps, we obtained the corresponding video frames, which corresponded to P_1 and P_2, as shown in Figure 3b,c. In Figure 3b, two feet are aligned with each other. In other words, at P_1, the distance between two ankles is the shortest, which indicates the pedestrian has moved the left leg from behind to the middle position and is about to step forward. Hence, a step is half-finished at the bottom points of Figure 3a. The step is fully finished in Figure 3c. The ankles are at the largest distance from each other, where P_2 is located. This means the peak path loss value at P_2 in the time duration [2.08 s, 2.32 s] coincidentally corresponds to the step length. Note that $PL_{OA} = 54$ dB is not the global largest value of path loss in Figure 3a. For example, the peak path loss values at the points P_3–P_7 at the time instants 0.92 s, 0.94 s, 2.88 s, 3.58 s, and 3.78 s were even bigger than 54 dB. In other words, the path loss corresponding to the step length is expected to be in a high range of the path loss values, but not necessarily the largest value. Hence, to find the step length, it was necessary to examine the histogram of the experimental data.

The bar chart in Figure 4 depicts the probability histogram of the on-ankle path loss in this trial experiment. Clearly, the histogram shows a two-hump shape with the most likely path loss occurring at the peak density $PL_{OA} \approx 46$ dB. The first, smaller hump corresponds to the half-finished steps, i.e., when the two feet are about to cross each other. The second, bigger hump corresponds to the events when the two feet are likely most separated from each other. The step length (i.e., the maximum distance between the two transceivers) may occur somewhere around the peak density rather than always at the peak density in the histogram. To demonstrate this point, let us consider the two different moments $t = 2.22$ s and $t = 2.80$ s when the path loss of 46 dB took place (cf. Figure 5a,b). These two figures suggest that, although the on-ankle path losses at these time instants were the same and both corresponded to the peak density in the histogram, the feet of the person under test were not in the identical posture. This means that the path loss corresponding to the peak density did not always correspond to the step length due to the randomness of the propagation channel. This observation is confirmed again in Figure 5c,d, where we show the two maximum distance events at the time instants $t = 3.12$ s and $t = 3.72$ s when $PL_{OA} \approx 50$ dB. The path loss $PL_{OA} \approx 50$ dB corresponds to the second maximum density, rather than the peak one in Figure 4.

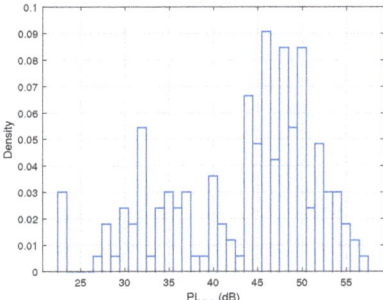

Figure 4. The probability histogram of the trial indoor walking experiment.

From the aforementioned observations, we conjectured that the human step length can be estimated within a certain range around the peak density of the histogram. This is because the actual step length may occur before or after the peak density due to the randomness of the propagation channel caused by the dynamic motions of the person under test. Therefore, in the following experiments, we propose a filtering technique to discard outlier data to form a range of reliable path loss values for estimating the step length. The accuracy analyses are also mentioned in the next section.

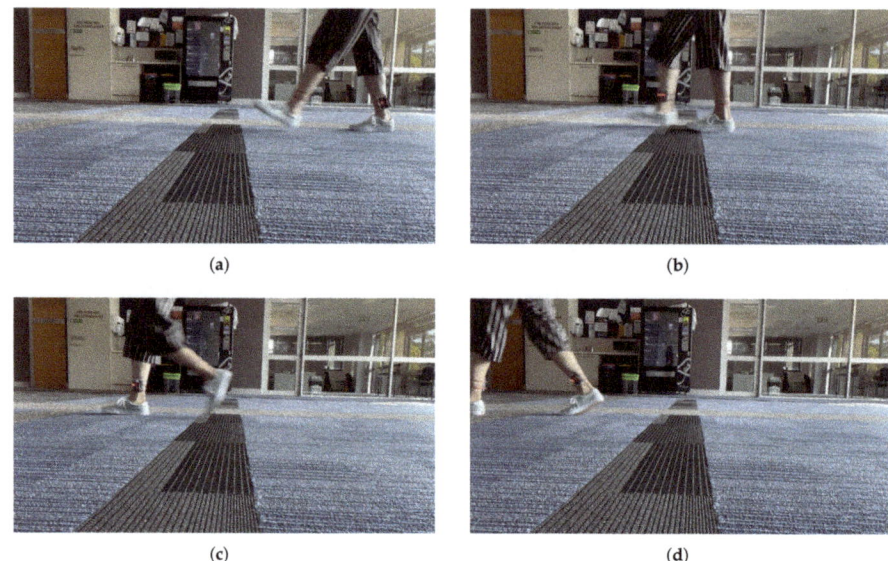

Figure 5. Feet positions at different time stamps of the indoor walking experiment. (**a**) t = 2.22 s (PL_{OA} = 46 dB); (**b**) t = 2.80 s (PL_{OA} = 46 dB); (**c**) t = 3.12 s (PL_{OA} = 50 dB); (**d**) t = 3.72 s (PL_{OA} = 50 dB).

5. Experimental Results and Analysis

In this section, experiments were conducted in four dynamic scenarios, including indoor walking, outdoor walking, indoor jogging, and outdoor jogging. The indoor experiments were carried out in a corridor of a building, while the outdoor ones were conducted along some pavement, which can be seen as an open area in Figure 6. The participant walked or jogged along a straight path with a length of 35.7 m. There were 50 steps and 38 steps in the walking and jogging scenarios, respectively. Therefore, the real average step length for walking was $d_{0w} = 35.7 \div 50 = 0.7140$ m, while for jogging, it was $d_{0j} = 35.7 \div 38 = 0.9395$ m. In each scenario, the experiments were carried out 10 times with over 1500 data in each dataset. Altogether, there were more than 15,000 data for each scenario. In our previous work [18], we derived the empirical path loss model for the wireless channel between the two ankles in a static situation, as shown in (1). As mentioned above, there existed randomness of the path loss in dynamic situations where the person under test was walking or jogging. Thus, we propose a filtering technique to apply along with the empirical model in (1) in order to eliminate the on-ankle path loss outliers. The resulting ranges of on-ankle path loss were then used to estimate the step length in the four motion scenarios. The following subsections are the experiment results and analyses for the four motion circumstances.

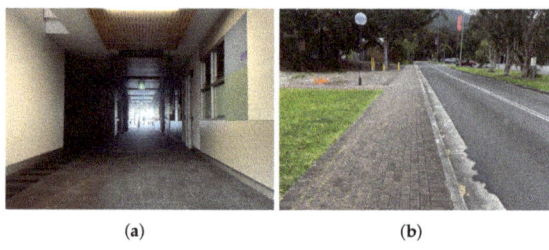

Figure 6. Experimental environments. (**a**) Indoors; (**b**) outdoors.

5.1. Empirical Threshold Pair

We propose a novel filtering technique to filter out the path loss outliers by setting a threshold pair, which consisted of an upper threshold and a lower threshold. As these two thresholds work together, we found both thresholds simultaneously. As shown in Figures 3 and 5, the path loss for the step length could be neither the maximum path loss value nor the path loss value corresponding to the peak density of the histogram. This was because the randomness of the propagation channel was caused by the dynamic movements of the person under test. Thus, it is important to consider a suitable range of the path loss values that might possibly correspond to the maximum distance between two ankles. To this end, based on the collected datasets, we first examined different combinations of the lower bound and the upper bound of this range to find the pair of boundaries that minimized the error between the average estimated step length and the true step length. The path loss values higher than the upper threshold or lower than the lower threshold were considered as outlier values. Figure 7 demonstrates the normalized errors of the step length estimations in the indoor walking and indoor jogging scenarios for different lower and upper thresholds. The relative (or normalized) error ϵ in percentage is defined as:

$$\epsilon = \frac{|\bar{d} - d_{0i}|}{d_{0i}} \times 100\%, \quad (7)$$

where $\bar{d}$ is the average estimated distance between two ankles under a certain experimental scenario, which involves 10 datasets, d_{0i} is the real step length, and i is either w for the walking scenario or j for the jogging scenario. Figure 7 shows that the (lower, upper) threshold pairs of (40 dB, 52 dB) and (40 dB, 56 dB) resulted in the average estimated step lengths being the closest to the true step lengths (i.e., the smallest normalized error ϵ) in the indoor walking and indoor jogging scenarios, respectively. Along with Figure 7, Tables 1 and 2 show in more detail the estimated step length (cf. (4)), averaged over all ten datasets for some different pairs of the (lower, upper) thresholds for the indoor walking and indoor jogging scenarios. In each cell of the table, there are three numbers. The average estimated step length in meters, which is the average result based on 10 experimental datasets, is located outside of the brackets. Following in the brackets are the average absolute error in millimeters and the average relative error in percentage, respectively.

The average absolute error was calculated as $|\bar{d} - d_{0i}|$. Tables 1 and 2 confirm further the observation gained from Figure 7 that the best pairs of (lower, upper) thresholds of the path losses were (40 dB, 52 dB) and (40 dB, 56 dB) for the indoor walking and indoor jogging cases, respectively. The average absolute and normalized estimation errors were just 10.15 mm and 1.42% for the indoor walking case, while these numbers were 4.40 mm and 0.47% for the indoor jogging case.

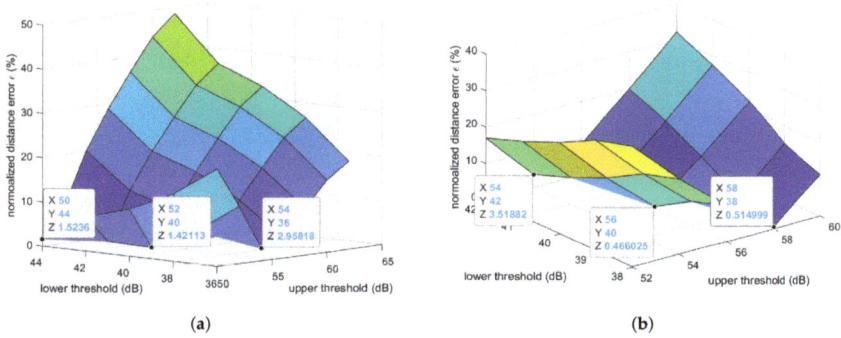

Figure 7. Normalized step length estimation errors of the indoor experiments. (**a**) Indoor walking; (**b**) indoor jogging.

Table 1. Estimation of the step length (m) in the indoor walking scenario for different pairs of upper threshold PL_u (dB) and lower threshold PL_l (dB). Two values in the brackets of each table cell are the corresponding absolute estimation error (mm) and relative estimation error (%), respectively.

PL_l (dB) \ PL_u (dB)	50	52	54	56	58
36	0.5556 (158.39, 22.18)	0.6206 (93.41, 13.08)	0.6929 (21.12, 2.96)	0.7452 (31.21, 4.40)	0.7896 (75.55, 10.58)
38	0.6040 (109.96, 15.40)	0.6701 (43.86, 6.14)	0.7448 (30.83, 4.32)	0.7997 (85.65, 12.00)	0.8466 (132.56, 18.57)
40	0.6372 (76.83, 10.76)	**0.7039 (10.15, 1.42)**	0.7802 (66.19, 9.27)	0.8368 (122.82, 17.20)	0.8856 (171.60, 24.03)
42	0.6577 (56.30, 7.88)	0.7251 (11.14, 1.56)	0.8029 (88.92, 12.45)	0.8610 (146.98, 20.59)	0.9112 (197.21, 27.62)
44	0.7031 (10.88, 1.52)	0.7746 (60.60, 8.49)	0.8578 (143.82, 20.14)	0.9207 (206.66, 28.94)	0.9755 (261.53, 36.63)

Table 2. Estimation of the step length (m), absolute estimation error (mm), and relative error (%) in the indoor jogging scenario for different pairs of upper threshold PL_u (dB) and lower threshold PL_l (dB).

PL_l (dB) \ PL_u (dB)	52	54	56	58	60
38	0.6282 (311.28, 33.13)	0.7458 (193.70, 20.62)	0.8461 (93.37, 9.94)	0.9443 (4.81, 0.51)	1.0450 (105.55, 11.23)
39	0.6557 (283.77, 30.20)	0.7758 (163.66, 17.42)	0.8785 (61.03, 6.50)	0.9791 (39.59, 4.21)	1.0825 (143.03, 15.22)
40	0.7050 (234.47, 24.96)	0.8288 (110.70, 11.78)	**0.9351 (4.40, 0.47)**	1.0397 (100.21, 10.67)	1.1477 (208.21, 22.16)
41	0.7450 (194.48, 20.70)	0.8708 (68.73, 7.32)	0.9795 (40.01, 4.26)	1.0870 (147.48, 15.70)	1.1984 (258.86, 27.55)
42	0.7795 (160.00, 17.03)	0.9064 (33.09, 3.52)	1.0170 (77.51, 8.25)	1.1268 (187.30, 19.94)	1.2410 (301.49, 32.09)

Similarly, Figure 8 and Tables 3 and 4 clearly show that the best (lower, upper) thresholds of the path losses used for estimating the average step length in the outdoor walking and jogging scenarios were (39 dB, 51 dB) and (42 dB, 54 dB), respectively. The average absolute and relative estimation errors for the former case were just 4.81 mm and 0.67%, while they were 10.84 mm and 1.15% for the latter one.

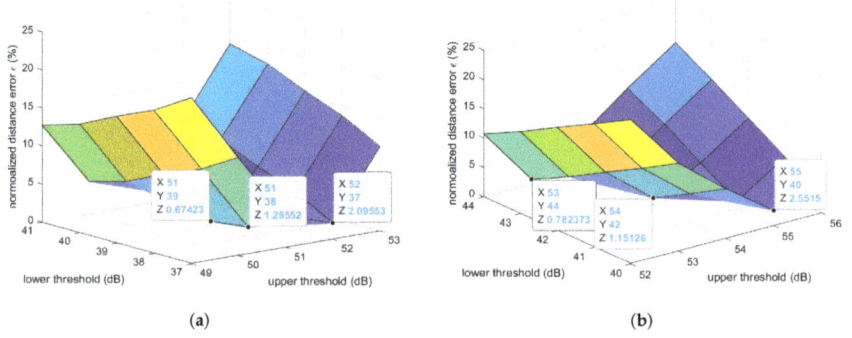

Figure 8. Normalized step length estimation errors of the outdoor experiments. (**a**) Outdoor walking; (**b**) Outdoor jogging.

Table 3. Estimation of the step length (m), absolute estimation error (mm), and relative error (%) in the outdoor walking scenario for different pairs of upper threshold PL_u (dB) and lower threshold PL_l (dB).

PL_l (dB) \ PL_u (dB)	49	50	51	52	53
37	0.5584 (155.56, 21.79)	0.6225 (91.54, 12.82)	0.6851 (28.93, 4.05)	0.7290 (14.96, 2.10)	0.7925 (78.54, 11.00)
38	0.5798 (134.16, 18.79)	0.6430 (71.02, 9.95)	0.7048 (9.18, 1.29)	0.7484 (34.40, 4.82)	0.8118 (97.79, 13.70)
39	0.5952 (118.81, 16.64)	0.6576 (56.41, 7.90)	**0.7188 (4.81, 0.67)**	0.7622 (48.15, 6.74)	0.8254 (111.38, 15.60)
40	0.6125 (101.55, 14.22)	0.6740 (40.05, 5.61)	0.7345 (20.46, 2.87)	0.7775 (63.52, 8.90)	0.8406 (126.59, 17.73)
41	0.6229 (91.06, 12.75)	0.6839 (30.07, 4.21)	0.7440 (30.02, 4.21)	0.7869 (72.94, 10.22)	0.8499 (135.95, 19.04)

Table 4. Estimation of the step length (m), absolute estimation error (mm), and relative error (%) in the outdoor jogging scenario for different pairs of upper threshold PL_u (dB) and lower threshold PL_l (dB).

PL_l (dB) \ PL_u (dB)	52	53	54	55	56
40	0.7082 (231.29, 24.62)	0.7990 (140.54, 14.96)	0.8599 (79.64, 8.48)	0.9155 (24.00, 2.55)	0.9651 (25.58, 2.72)
41	0.7420 (197.45, 21.02)	0.8338 (105.70, 11.25)	0.8952 (44.30, 4.72)	0.9515 (11.98, 1.28)	1.0018 (62.32, 6.63)
42	0.7745 (164.97, 17.56)	0.8669 (72.56, 7.72)	**0.9287 (10.84, 1.15)**	0.9855 (45.95, 4.89)	1.0365 (96.96, 10.32)
43	0.8085 (130.98, 13.94)	0.9013 (38.16, 4.06)	0.9632 (23.74, 2.53)	1.0205 (80.98, 8.62)	1.0721 (132.64, 14.12)
44	0.8391 (100.41, 10.69)	0.9321 (7.38, 0.79)	0.9941 (54.60, 5.81)	1.0517 (112.21, 11.94)	1.1040 (164.46, 17.51)

It is noted that the estimation error in the indoor walking scenario was higher than that in the indoor jogging one. This can be explained as follows. In general, one might expect that the error of the walking scenarios is smaller than that of the jogging ones as walking is a slower and more stable activity than jogging. This expectation was confirmed from the experimental results of the outdoor scenarios, where the errors for outdoor walking and jogging were 4.81 mm and 10.84 mm, respectively. However, this expectation may not always be the case for an indoor environment since there are more multipaths indoors than outdoors. Because walking takes a longer time than jogging to complete a step, when multipath propagation occurred, more affected RSSI (thus path loss) values during that step were recorded to the dataset in the walking scenario than in the jogging one. As a result, the histogram of the path loss dataset collected for the indoor walking scenario may have some (local) peaks that were far more distinct from the remaining non-peak values, compared to the indoor jogging case. This phenomenon can be observed in Figure 9a (mentioned later in Section 5.2), where the density of the path loss value of 46 dB was much more prominent than other non-peak values, while the local peaks in Figure 9b are less prominent compared to their surrounding values. This led to a slightly worse accuracy in average step length estimation in the indoor walking compared to the indoor jogging.

5.2. Upper Threshold Analysis

The data analyses mentioned in Section 5.1 are critical as they allowed us to devise the novel filtering technique, which is detailed below.

In order to formulate the thresholds mathematically, we firstly depict the probability histogram for all the datasets (around 15,000 data) collected in each experimental scenario, as shown in Figure 9. The probability histogram of the measured on-ankle path loss is represented by blue bars. It is noted that the plotted histogram has two humps, which correspond to the half-finished step, where the two feet are about to pass each other, and the fully finished step, when the two feet are most apart from each other, respectively. The plotted histogram can be well approximated by the probability density function (PDF) of a two-term Gaussian distribution model via the curve-fitting process indicated by the solid green curve in Figure 9 with the general PDF equation:

$$f(x) = f_1(x) + f_2(x)$$
$$= a_1 e^{-(\frac{x-b_1}{c_1})^2} + a_2 e^{-(\frac{x-b_2}{c_2})^2}, \tag{8}$$

where $f_k(x) = a_k e^{-(\frac{x-b_k}{c_k})^2}$, a_k is the amplitude, b_k is the centroid, and c_k relates to the peak width of this Gaussian distribution ($k = 1, 2$). These coefficients can be found from the curve fitting of the two-term Gaussian distribution model. Ideally, the step length is related to the maximum on-ankle path loss. However, due to the randomness of the propagation channel, the actual step length may correspond to a non-peak path loss around the peak of the second hump. This means that the pair of the (lower, upper) thresholds should capture a suitable range of the path loss values around the peak of the second hump. The values bigger than the upper threshold or smaller than the lower threshold were considered as outliers for estimating the path loss that corresponds to the step length. To capture the suitable window of the possible path loss values for estimating the step length, intuitively, the upper threshold should be located somewhere at the right slope of the second hump, while the lower threshold lies somewhere at the left slope of the second hump, i.e., in between the first hump and the second hump.

From Figure 9, it is observed that the impact of the first hump on the right slope of the second hump was negligible. Thus, we can extract the second hump and approximate its right slope by the Gaussian distribution:

$$f_2(x) = a_2 e^{-(\frac{x-b_2}{c_2})^2}. \tag{9}$$

This observation is confirmed in Figure 9a, where the bell-shaped red dashed curve representing the Gaussian distribution in (9) coincides with the right slope of the second hump of the two-term Gaussian distribution. As a result, we can obtain the mean μ and the standard deviation σ of the second hump based on the above Gaussian distribution in (9) as:

$$\mu = b_2, \tag{10}$$

$$\sigma = \frac{c_2}{\sqrt{2}}. \tag{11}$$

The above observations and analyses hold for all indoor/outdoor walking and indoor/outdoor jogging cases, as shown in Figure 9a–d.

The curve fitting parameters a_2, b_2, c_2, μ, and σ for the second hump in the four scenarios can be found in Table 5. Since the path loss, which corresponds to the step length, is a random variable, its upper threshold should be determined as a function of both the mean value μ and the standard deviation value σ of the second term of the two-term Gaussian distribution in (9). This philosophy is similar to the well-known concept of calculating the retransmission timeout (RTO) on the Internet where the RTO is the function of both the mean value of the round-trip time (RTT) and its deviation value.

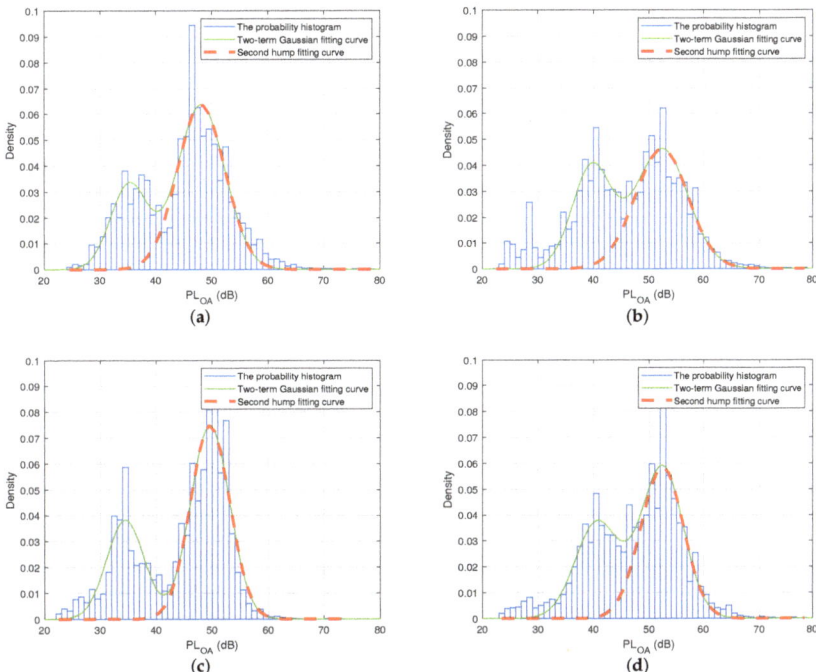

Figure 9. The probability histogram, the two-term Gaussian distribution, and the fitting curve of the second hump for the indoor and outdoor experiments. (**a**) Indoor walking; (**b**) indoor jogging; (**c**) outdoor walking; (**d**) outdoor jogging.

Table 5. Coefficients for the second hump-fitting equation.

	Indoor Walking	Indoor Jogging	Outdoor Walking	Outdoor Jogging
a_2	0.06369	0.04639	0.07489	0.05866
b_2	48.0900	52.3400	49.6100	52.3900
c_2	5.9990	6.7870	4.9330	5.4610
μ	48.0900	52.3400	49.6100	52.3900
σ	4.2419	4.7991	3.4882	3.8615

Table 6 presents the values of function $\mu + k\sigma$ ($k = 0, 0.5, 1, 1.5, 2$), and the corresponding difference, denoted as Δ (dB), between these values and the upper thresholds, which were worked out empirically from the actual measured data in Section 5.1. Table 6 clearly shows that the empirical upper thresholds in the indoor walking and jogging scenarios were both very well approximated by $\mu + \sigma$ with the differences Δ of only 0.3319 dB and 1.1391 dB, respectively. This finding makes sense because the upper threshold is equal to the mean path loss value μ plus a margin, which is equal to the standard deviation σ in this case.

Similarly, the empirical upper thresholds in the outdoor walking and jogging scenarios were both very close to $\mu + 0.5\sigma$ with the difference Δ of merely 0.3541 dB and 0.3208 dB, respectively. The upper thresholds in the two indoor cases were higher than those in the outdoor scenarios due to the fact that there were more multipaths indoors than outdoors; thus, the actual path loss that corresponds to the step lengths might vary more widely around its mean value.

Table 6. Absolute difference Δ (dB) between the function $\mu + k\sigma$ and the empirical upper threshold (indoor walking: 52 dB; indoor jogging: 56 dB; outdoor walking: 51 dB; outdoor jogging: 54 dB).

	Indoor Walking	Indoor Jogging	Outdoor Walking	Outdoor Jogging
$\mu(\Delta)$	48.0900 (3.9100)	52.3400 (3.6600)	49.6100 (1.3900)	52.3900 (1.6100)
$\mu + 0.5\sigma(\Delta)$	50.2110 (1.7890)	54.7396 (1.2604)	**51.3541 (0.3541)**	**54.3208 (0.3208)**
$\mu + \sigma(\Delta)$	**52.3319 (0.3319)**	**57.1391 (1.1391)**	53.0982 (2.0982)	56.2515 (2.2515)
$\mu + 1.5\sigma(\Delta)$	54.4529 (2.4529)	59.5387 (3.5387)	54.8422 (3.8422)	58.1823 (4.1823)
$\mu + 2\sigma(\Delta)$	56.5738 (4.5738)	61.9383 (5.9383)	56.5863 (5.5863)	60.1130 (6.1130)

5.3. Lower Threshold Analysis

As mentioned in Section 5.2, the lower threshold was located between the first hump and the second hump of the two-term Gaussian distribution, which means its value would be affected by both humps. Therefore, it was impossible to analyze the lower threshold based on a single hump as for the upper bound mentioned above. Thus, other techniques should be used to analyze the lower threshold. One of the possible techniques is based on the cumulative distribution function (CDF) or the survival function. The survival function is complementary to the CDF. It indicates the probability of the path loss value greater than or equal to a certain value. Figure 10 depicts the probability histogram, the CDF (the red curves), and the survival function (the bold green curves) of the measured path loss data for all four scenarios together with the lower thresholds (the black dashed lines), which were empirically found to be 39 dB and 42 dB in the outdoor walking and jogging cases, respectively, and 40 dB in the indoor cases, as detailed in Section 5.1.

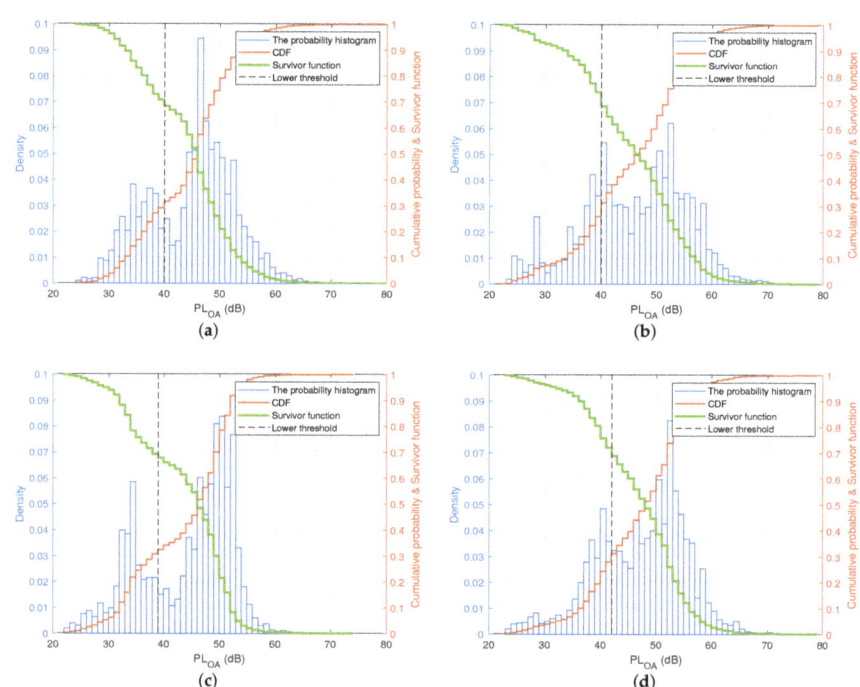

Figure 10. The probability histogram, the CDF, and the survivor function with respect to the lower threshold for the indoor and outdoor experiments. (**a**) Indoor walking (lower threshold = 40 dB); (**b**) indoor jogging (lower threshold = 40 dB); (**c**) outdoor walking (lower threshold = 39 dB); (**d**) outdoor jogging (lower threshold = 42 dB).

Figure 10 reveals an interesting fact that the intersections between the empirical lower thresholds and the survival curves were around 0.68 in all four cases. In other words, the measured path loss value was bigger than or at least equal to the value of the lower threshold 68% of the time in all four scenarios. Path loss values between the lower threshold and the upper one should be considered as the potential path losses corresponding to the step lengths. Based on the above empirical measurements and statistical analyses, we deduced that the lower threshold can be numerically found as the corresponding path loss value when the survival rate reaches 0.68.

6. Conclusions

This paper estimated the human step length in daily activities based on our developed wearable transceivers and the RSSI method. We conducted experiments for both walking and jogging activities in both indoor and outdoor environments. By analyzing the statistical properties of the collected datasets, for the first time, we proposed a filtering method to set up the lower and upper thresholds in order to eliminate the path loss outliers. The resulting range of path loss values between the two thresholds was used to estimate the step length. Mathematically, the upper threshold for an indoor environment was $\mu + \sigma$, while this value for an outdoor scenario was $\mu + 0.5\sigma$. The lower threshold relates to the survival function of the experimental datasets. This threshold was found numerically to be the path loss value where the survival rate was around 0.68 for both the indoor and outdoor environments and for both the walking and jogging activities. Our experiments showed that the step length can be accurately estimated with errors of only 10.15 mm and 4.40 mm for the indoor walking and jogging activities and errors of 4.81 mm and 10.84 mm for the outdoor walking and jogging activities, respectively.

7. Limitations and Future Works

The experimental results showed that the proposed system along with the proposed technique can estimate the average human step length with a sub-centimeter error. However, a limitation of this project is that we need to collect the dataset for the whole intended period of time, then proceed to the offline data processing phase, rather than processing data to estimate the step length and updating this estimation in a continuous manner while the person under test is moving. Overcoming this limitation is the motivation for our future work. More specifically, to guarantee both accuracy and efficiency, instead of waiting for the whole dataset to be collected, we may apply the weighted moving average algorithm to continuously estimate the average step length and keep updating this estimation over a shorter period of time. In this way, the dynamic essence of human activities will be captured more accurately than the simple averaging technique. In addition, we may consider a hybrid RSSI-based technology [32], such as adopting an IMU in the existing RSSI-measuring system along with an RSSI/IMU data fusion approach, to further improve the precision and robustness of the step length estimation.

Author Contributions: Conceptualization, Z.Y., L.C.T. and F.S.; data curation, Z.Y.; methodology, Z.Y., L.C.T. and F.S.; software, Z.Y.; validation, Z.Y., L.C.T. and F.S.; formal analysis, Z.Y. and L.C.T.; investigation, Z.Y.; writing—original draft preparation, Z.Y.; writing—review and editing, Z.Y., L.C.T. and F.S.; visualization, Z.Y.; supervision, L.C.T. and F.S.; and project administration, L.C.T. and F.S. All authors have read and agreed to the published version of the manuscript.

Funding: This research received no external funding.

Institutional Review Board Statement: Ethical review and approval were waived for this study because the experiments were not performed on any patients or on any individual other than the authors of this paper. The collected data are not sensitive information and contain no private information.

Informed Consent Statement: Patient consent was waived for this study because the experiments were not performed on any patients.

Data Availability Statement: The data presented in this study are available upon request from the corresponding author.

Conflicts of Interest: The authors declare no conflict of interest.

Abbreviations

The following abbreviations are used in this manuscript:

CDF	Cumulative distribution function
IDE	Integrated Development Environment
IMU	Inertial measurement unit
LOS	Line-of-sight
LR-WPAN	Low-rate wireless personal area network
O-QPSK	Offset quadrature phase shift keying
PDR	Pedestrian dead reckoning
RF	Radio frequency
RSSI	Received signal strength indicator
X-CTU	XBee Configuration & Test Unit

References

1. Allet, L.; Kim, H.; Ashton-Miller, J.; Mott, T.D.; Richardson, J.K. Step length after discrete perturbation predicts accidental falls and fall-related injury in elderly people with a range of peripheral neuropathy. *J. Diabetes Its Complicat.* **2014**, *28*, 79–84. [CrossRef] [PubMed]
2. Moyer, B.E.; Chambers, A.J.; Redfern, M.S.; Cham, R. Gait parameters as predictors of slip severity in younger and older adults. *Ergonomics* **2006**, *49*, 329–343. [CrossRef] [PubMed]
3. Woo, J.; Ho, S.C.; Yu, A.L. Walking speed and stride length predicts 36 months dependency, mortality, and institutionalization in Chinese aged 70 and older. *J. Am. Geriatr. Soc.* **1999**, *47*, 1257–1260. [CrossRef] [PubMed]
4. Rosso, A.L.; Hunt, M.J.O.; Yang, M.; Brach, J.S.; Harris, T.B.; Newman, A.B.; Satterfield, S.; Studenski, S.A.; Yaffe, K.; Aizenstein, H.J.; et al. Higher step length variability indicates lower gray matter integrity of selected regions in older adults. *Gait Posture* **2014**, *40*, 225–230. [CrossRef] [PubMed]
5. Studenski, S.; Perera, S.; Patel, K.; Rosano, C.; Faulkner, K.; Inzitari, M.; Brach, J.; Chandler, J.; Cawthon, P.; Connor, E.B.; et al. Gait speed and survival in older adults. *JAMA* **2011**, *305*, 50–58. [CrossRef] [PubMed]
6. Aubeck, F.; Isert, C.; Gusenbauer, D. Camera based step detection on mobile phones. In Proceedings of the International Conference on Indoor Positioning and Indoor Navigation (IPIN), Guimaraes, Portugal, 21–23 September 2011; pp. 1–7.
7. Cai, X.; Han, G.; Song, X.; Wang, J. Single-Camera-Based Method for Step Length Symmetry Measurement in Unconstrained Elderly Home Monitoring. *IEE Trans. Biomed. Eng.* **2017**, *64*, 2618–2627.
8. Xue, Z.; Ming, D.; Song, W.; Wan, B.; Jin, S. Infrared gait recognition based on wavelet transform and support vector machine. *Pattern Recognit.* **2010**, *43*, 2904–2910. [CrossRef]
9. Menz, H.B.; Latt, M.D.; Tiedemann, A.; San Kwan, M.M.; Lord, S.R. Reliability of the GAITRite® walkway system for the quantification of temporo-spatial parameters of gait in young and older people. *Gait Posture* **2004**, *20*, 20–25. [CrossRef]
10. Srinivasan, P.; Birchfield, D.; Qian, G.; Kidané, A. A pressure sensing floor for interactive media applications. In Proceedings of the ACM International Conference Proceeding Series, Valencia, Spain, 15–17 June 2005; pp. 278–281
11. Li, E.; Lin, X.; Seet, B.; Joseph, F.; Neville, J. Low Profile and Low Cost Textile Smart Mat for Step Pressure Sensing and Position Mapping. In Proceedings of the IEEE International Instrumentation and Measurement Technology Conference (I2MTC), Aukland, New Zealand, 20–23 May 2019; pp. 1–5
12. Nguyen, N.M.; Tran, L.C.; Safaei, F.; Phung, S.L.; Vial, P.; Huynh, N.; Cox, A.; Harada, T.; Barthelemy, J. Performance evaluation of non-GPS based localization techniques under shadowing effects. *Sensors* **2019**, *19*, 2633. [CrossRef]
13. Liu, J.; Wang, Z.; Yao, M.; Qiu, Z. VN-APIT: Virtual nodes-based range-free APIT localization scheme for WSN. *Wirel. Netw.* **2016**, *22*, 867–878. [CrossRef]
14. Zhu, X.; Feng, Y. RSSI-based Algorithm for Indoor Localization. *Commun. Netw.* **2013**, *5*, 37–42. [CrossRef]
15. Hamdoun, S.; Rachedi, A.; Benslimane, A. Comparative analysis of RSSI-based indoor localization when using multiple antennas in Wireless Sensor Networks. In Proceedings of the International Conference on Selected Topics in Mobile and Wireless Networking (MoWNeT), Montreal, QC, Canada, 19–21 August 2013; pp. 146–151.
16. Altoaimy, L.; Mahgoub, I.; Rathod, M. Weighted localization in Vehicular Ad Hoc Networks using vehicle-to-vehicle communication. In Proceedings of the Global Information Infrastructure and Networking Symposium (GIIS), Montreal, QC, Canada, 15–19 September 2014; pp. 1–5.
17. Poulose, A.; Kim, J.; Han, D.S. A sensor fusion framework for indoor localization using smartphone sensors and Wi-Fi RSSI measurements. *Appl. Sci.* **2019**, *9*, 4379. [CrossRef]

18. Yang, Z.; Tran, L.C.; Safaei, F. Step Length Measurements Using the Received Signal Strength Indicator. *Sensors* **2021**, *21*, 382. [CrossRef]
19. Wang, Q.; Ye, L.; Luo, H.; Men, A.; Zhao, F.; Huang, Y. Pedestrian stride-length estimation based on LSTM and denoising autoencoders. *Sensors* **2019**, *19*, 840. [CrossRef]
20. Wang, Q.; Luo, H.; Ye, L.; Men, A.; Zhao, F.; Huang, Y.; Ou, C. Personalized Stride-Length Estimation Based on Active Online Learning. *IEEE Internet Things J.* **2020**, *7*, 4885–4897. [CrossRef]
21. Vandermeeren, S.; Bruneel, H.; Steendam, H. Feature selection for machine learning based step length estimation algorithms. *Sensors* **2020**, *20*, 778. [CrossRef] [PubMed]
22. Renaudin, V.; Susi, M.; Lachapelle, G. Step length estimation using handheld inertial sensors. *Sensors* **2012**, *12*, 8507–8525. [CrossRef] [PubMed]
23. Köse, A.; Cereatti, A.; Della Croce, U. Bilateral step length estimation using a single inertial measurement unit attached to the pelvis. *J. Neuroeng. Rehabil.* **2012**, *9*, 1–10. [CrossRef]
24. Xing, H.; Li, J.; Hou, B.; Zhang, Y.; Guo, M. Pedestrian stride length estimation from IMU measurements and ANN based algorithm. *J. Sens.* **2017**, *2017*. [CrossRef]
25. Nouriani, A.; McGovern, R.A.; Rajamani, R. Step Length Estimation Using Inertial Measurements Units. In Proceedings of the American Control Conference (ACC), New Orleans, LA, USA, 25–28 May 2021; pp. 666–671.
26. Gu, F.; Khoshelham, K.; Yu, C.; Shang, J. Accurate step length estimation for pedestrian dead reckoning localization using stacked autoencoders. *IEEE Trans. Instrum. Meas.* **2018**, *68*, 2705–2713. [CrossRef]
27. Klein, I.; Asraf, O. StepNet—Deep learning approaches for step length estimation. *IEEE Access* **2020**, *8*, 85706–85713. [CrossRef]
28. Vezočnik, M.; Juric, M.B. Average step length estimation models' evaluation using inertial sensors: A review. *IEEE Sens. J.* **2018**, *19*, 396–403 [CrossRef]
29. Díaz, S.; Disdier, S.; Labrador, M. A. Step Length and Step Width Estimation using Wearable Sensors. In Proceedings of the 9th IEEE Annual Ubiquitous Computing, Electronics & Mobile Communication Conference (UEMCON), New York, NY, USA, 8–10 November 2018; pp. 997–1001.
30. Friis, H.T. A note on a simple transmission formula. *Proc. IRE* **1946**, *34*, 254–256. [CrossRef]
31. 802.15.4 IEEE Standard for Information Technology—Telecommunications and Information Exchange between Systems—Local and Metropolitan Area Networks—Specific Requirements Part 15.4: Wireless Medium Access Control (MAC) and Physical Layer (PHY) Specifications for Low-Rate Wireless Personal Area Networks (LR-WPANs). Available online: http://user.engineering.uiowa.edu/~mcover/lab4/802.15.4-2003.pdf (accessed on 27 January 2022)
32. Malyavej, V.; Udomthanatheera, P. RSSI/IMU sensor fusion-based localization using unscented Kalman filter. In Proceedings of the 20th Asia-Pacific Conference on Communication (APCC2014), Pattaya City, Thailand, 1–3 October 2014; pp. 227–232.

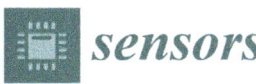

Article

Using a Portable Gait Rhythmogram to Examine the Effect of Music Therapy on Parkinson's Disease-Related Gait Disturbance

Emiri Gondo [1], Saiko Mikawa [2] and Akito Hayashi [1,2,*]

[1] Department of Rehabilitation, Juntendo University Graduate School of Medicine, 2-1-1 Hongo, Toyko 113-8421, Japan; emirigondo@gmail.com
[2] Department of Rehabilitation, Juntendo University Urayasu Hospital, 2-1-1 Tomioka, Urayasu 279-0021, Japan; sa-aiba@juntendo.ac.jp
* Correspondence: hayashi@juntendo.ac.jp

Abstract: External cues improve walking by evoking internal rhythm formation related to gait in the brain in patients with Parkinson's disease (PD). This study examined the usefulness of using a portable gait rhythmogram (PGR) in music therapy on PD-related gait disturbance. A total of 19 subjects with PD who exhibited gait disturbance were evaluated for gait speed and step length during a 10 m straight walking task. Moreover, acceleration, cadence, and trajectory of the center of the body were estimated using a PGR. Walking tasks were created while incorporating music intervention that gradually increased in tempo from 90 to 120 beats per minute (BPM). We then evaluated whether immediate improvement in gait could be recognized even without music after walking tasks by comparing pre- (pre-MT) and post-music therapy (post-MT) values. Post-MT gait showed significant improvement in acceleration, gait speed, cadence, and step length. During transitions throughout the walking tasks, acceleration, gait speed, cadence, and step length gradually increased in tasks with music. With regard to the trajectory of the center of the body, we recognized a reduction in post-MT medio-lateral amplitude. Music therapy immediately improved gait disturbance in patients with PD, and the effectiveness was objectively shown using PGR.

Keywords: portable gait rhythmogram; 3-D gait analysis; music therapy; Parkinson's disease; gait disturbance

1. Introduction

Parkinson's disease (PD) is a neurodegenerative condition among elderly populations [1] that develops through the degeneration of dopaminergic neurons in basal ganglia, causing a deficiency of such neurons [2]. The main symptoms of PD include resting tremors, rigidity, bradykinesia, postural instability [3], and gait disturbance—one of the most frequent and intractable motor disturbances [4]. Gait disturbance related to PD is an evolving condition with different patterns [5], such as reduced step length [6], slow speed, shuffling steps [7], and freezing of gait. Furthermore, gait disturbance not only decreases mobility and increases the risk of falling [8] but also restricts the functional independence and quality of life of people with PD (PwP) [9].

Although PD has been primarily treated through antiparkinsonian drugs and surgery with deep brain stimulation, evidence has shown that combining different rehabilitation approaches, such as physiotherapy, occupational therapy, and speech therapy, with antiparkinsonian drugs and surgical treatment can be more effective [10–12]. Apart from the mentioned therapies, music therapy, and a cue-based strategy that uses external sound rhythms to evoke walking rhythms in the brain [4,13], has also attracted attention in recent years. Among the various external cues (auditory, visual, and antennal cues), rhythmic auditory stimulation has been the most effective for gait disturbance treatment in PwP [3].

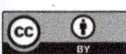

Moreover, reports have shown that gait training matched to metronomic rhythms can increase gait speed [14,15].

Over the years, there has been remarkable development in wearable devices and methods for investigating gait. The current study utilized a portable gait rhythmogram (PGR) that uses inertial sensors to evaluate three-dimensional (3-D) changes in the walking trajectory of the center of the body. The major advantages of inertial sensors include their small size, low cost, and long operating life, which allow for the unobtrusive monitoring of the walking pattern without interfering with the natural movement [16]. Moreover, a PGR allows us to easily monitor patient progress by drawing and visualizing the walking trajectory using gait data instead of simply comparing numerical values [16]. An objective and quantitative gait analysis system could, therefore, potentially improve the current practice (i.e., semi quantitative gait evaluation), which could aid in the diagnosis, symptom monitoring, therapeutic management, rehabilitation, fall risk assessment, and prevention of PD [17]. In addition to the medical field, a PGR can also be used in the field of music therapy, where it is difficult to quantify its overall effect on various diseases and there is still limited evidence-based research [18].

To investigate the effectiveness of music therapy as a rehabilitation approach for gait disturbance in PD, the current study utilized gait training with and without rhythmic auditory stimulation and examined whether immediate improvements occurred after training by evaluating the walking speed, acceleration, cadence, stride length, and walking trajectory of the center of the body.

Note that this is a small, open-label study with no long-term effects, therefore this is a pilot study describing the potential use of this method.

2. Materials and Methods

2.1. Subjects

A total of 19 PwP with mild gait disturbance (6 males and 13 females; mean age, 74.0 ± 6.7; H&Y, 2 or 3; duration, 6.0 ± 5.5 years; UPDRS-III, 17.3 ± 4.7) were included in this study. They had a gait score of 0 to 2 in the UPDRS-III and were able to walk without assistance. On examination, no one had freezing and no one had a high probability of falling. Regardless of the medication taken by the subjects, conventional treatments were provided without any changes.

2.2. Gait Analysis

Gait was analyzed using a PGR (MG-M 1110, LSI Medience Corporation, Tokyo, Japan), a small device ($8 \times 6 \times 2$ cm, weight; 80 g) that houses an accelerometer (Figure 1). As reported previously [19], gait-induced acceleration is extracted from limb and trunk movements using an automatic gait detection algorithm ("pattern matching method"), allowing for the 3-D measurement (a_x, a_y, a_z) of acceleration associated with voluntary limb and trunk movements, as well as acceleration induced by heel strike and toe-off when walking. As reported in detail previously [19], based on the "pattern matching method", the acceleration vectors associated with stepping can be distinguished from those associated with other limb and trunk movements or with unexpected artifacts. First, attention is focused on a relatively strong signal region (e.g., $a > 1$ m/s^2) in the acceleration time series, and a 3-D template wave (a_x, a_y, a_z) with a duration of about 0.5 s is arbitrarily chosen. Then, the cross-correlation $CC(t)$ between this wave and another wave with a time shift t chosen from the whole time series is computed using the following formula:

$$CC(t) = \frac{\frac{1}{p}\sum_{i=1}^{p}[a_x(i)a_x(i+t) + a_y(i)a_y(i+t) + a_z(i)a_z(i+t)]}{\left\{\frac{1}{p}\sum_{i=1}^{p}[a_x(i)^2 + a_y(i)^2 + a_z(i)^2]\right\}^{\frac{1}{2}} \left\{\frac{1}{p\sum_{i=1}^{p}[a_x(i+t)^2 + a_y(i+t)^2 + a_z(i+t)^2]}\right\}^{\frac{1}{2}}}$$

where t is the time index and p is the length of the template wave. If the acceleration change is caused by gait motion, the $CC(t)$ peaks exhibit alternate changes in magnitude with time due to left/right body sway during walking. Additionally, the cycle and amplitude are measured from the gait-induced acceleration signals. Since gait accelerations correlate with floor reaction forces, the amplitude of gait accelerations is selected as an index of floor reaction forces [20].

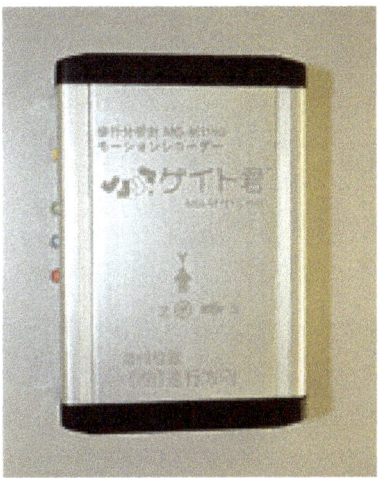

Figure 1. Portable gait rhythmogram (MG-M 1110, LSI Medience Corporation, Tokyo, Japan). Size = 8 × 6 × 2 cm. Weight = 80 g.

The device was secured at the center of subjects' waists using a Velcro band (Figure 2) and recorded the above signals at a sampling rate of 10 ms (100 Hz). The data were automatically stored on a microSD card. After transfer of the recorded data to a personal computer, the absolute values of acceleration vectors (a; $a^2 = a_x^2 + a_y^2 + a_z^2$) were calculated offline and graphically displayed on the monitor [16,21]. With the subject standing in the anatomical position, the three acceleration axes (X, Y, and Z) were oriented in the mediolateral (ML), vertical (VT), and anteroposterior (AP) directions, respectively. Accordingly, positive X, Y, and Z values indicated leftward, upward, and forward acceleration, respectively.

Gait analysis was conducted in a large indoor space. All subjects were requested to walk back and forth in a 5 m straight line [22] without assistance, in accordance with seven common walking tasks (details provided later). An extra 1 m distance was added before and after the walkway to minimize the influence of acceleration and deceleration. The time a subject took to walk along the 5 m and 10 m walkways was determined from the event marker recordings. The timing and number of stride events during this time interval were identified from the 3D acceleration signal using an automated peak detection algorithm [21]. In addition, the 5 m walking time and step count were measured for each task by an experimenter. While the subject was walking, an experimenter with a stopwatch followed slightly behind [16]. Videos of walking were also taken to observe the walking pattern, posture, and swinging of the arms. Based on these data, the basic gait characteristics (gait speed, cadence, step length) were calculated for each subject. Next, the 3-D acceleration signal was filtered by a high-pass filter $sT/(1 + sT)$ to remove slowly varying trends. The time constant was set at $T = 0.7$ s. Then, the acceleration magnitude $a_r(t)$ was calculated from the filtered components ($a_x(t)\ a_y(t)\ a_z(t)$) by $a_r(t) = (a_x(t)^2 + a_y(t)^2 + a_z(t)^2)_{0.5}$ [22].

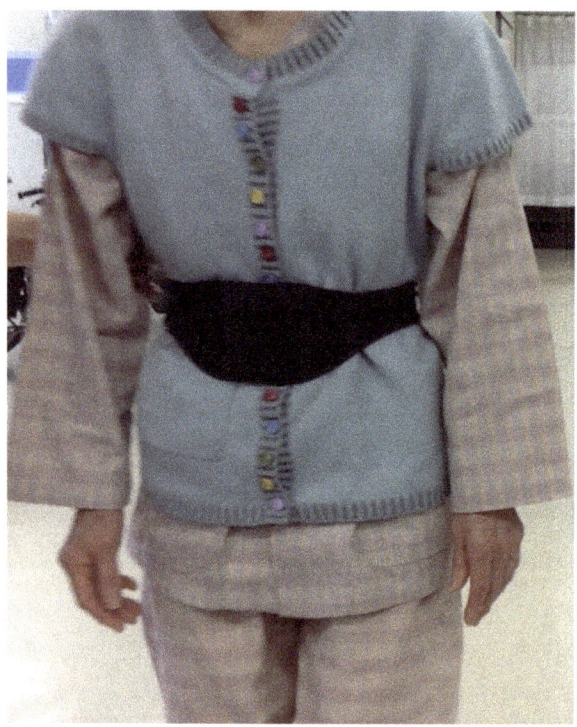

Figure 2. The device was secured at the center of subjects' waists using a Velcro band.

The common tasks were as follows: fast walking (walking as fast as possible without falling) (Task 1), self-paced walking with hand clapping (Task 2), walking in step with music at 90 beats per minute (BPM) (Task 3), 100 BPM (Task 4), 110 BPM (Task 5), and 120 BPM (Task 6), and fast walking again without music (Task 7). The instructions for each task were given as follows: "Please walk as fast as you can without falling". for Task 1, "Please walk at your own pace. I clap at your pace". for Task 2, "Next, music will be played. Please walk to the music". for Task 3, "Another track will be played. Please walk to the music again." for Tasks 4, 5, and 6, and "Next, there will be no music. Once again, please walk as fast as you can without falling". for Task 7. Thereafter, pre-MT (Task 1) values for acceleration (gait force), gait speed, cadence, step length, and gait trajectory of the center of the body were compared to post-MT (Task 7) values to evaluate whether improvement in gait occurred immediately after walking tasks with music (from Task 3 to Task 6), even without music. The hand clapping in Task 2 was performed in rhythm with the subjects' own pace and was observed by a separate experimenter. The music genres used in Tasks 3–6 included familiar classical music and Japanese traditional songs that matched metronomic rhythms (Japanese traditional song for BPM 90, classical music for BPM 100, Japanese traditional song for BPM 110, and classical music for BPM 120). The songs had no lyrics, and the melody was instrumentally edited by MIDI. The same tunes were used for all subjects. The music was played through the built-in speaker of a personal computer. Before starting the tasks, we played the music in fragments and checked if the subjects could hear it. All music was played at the same volume during the tasks. In each task, the four-beat metronome was played first and the participants were allowed to start walking at their own leisure after the music started.

2.3. Statistical Analysis

Significant differences between mean pre-MT and post-MT values of acceleration, gait speed, cadence, step length, and amplitude of the trajectory were evaluated using the paired *t*-test for normally distributed data. Statistical analysis was performed using StatPlus version 6.2.21 software for Macintosh (Apple Inc., Tokyo, Japan), with a *p* value of <0.05 indicating statistical significance.

Pre-MT and post-MT descriptive data were compared and analyzed using paired *t*-tests. An analysis of variance test was used to perform multiple comparisons among all seven tasks.

3. Results

After completing the tasks with music, subjects exhibited significant improvements in their acceleration (pre: 1.94 m/s^2; post: 2.44 m/s^2; $p < 0.001$; Table 1 and Figure 3A), gait speed (pre: 0.88 m/s; post: 0.97 m/s; $p < 0.04$; Table 1 and Figure 3B), cadence (pre: 117.3 steps/min; post: 122.9 steps/min; $p < 0.0001$; Table 1 and Figure 3C), and step length (pre: 41.55 cm; post: 46.70 cm; $p < 0.0001$; Table 1 and Figure 3D).

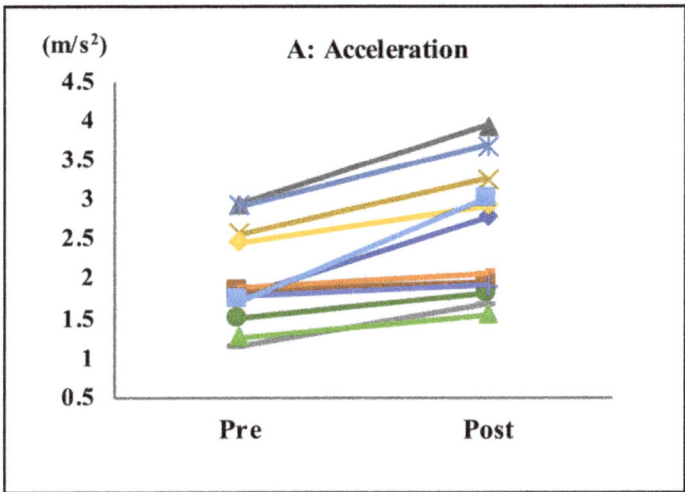

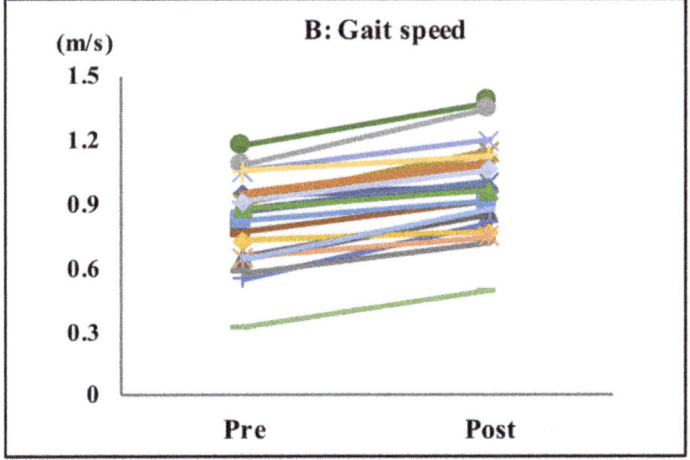

Figure 3. *Cont.*

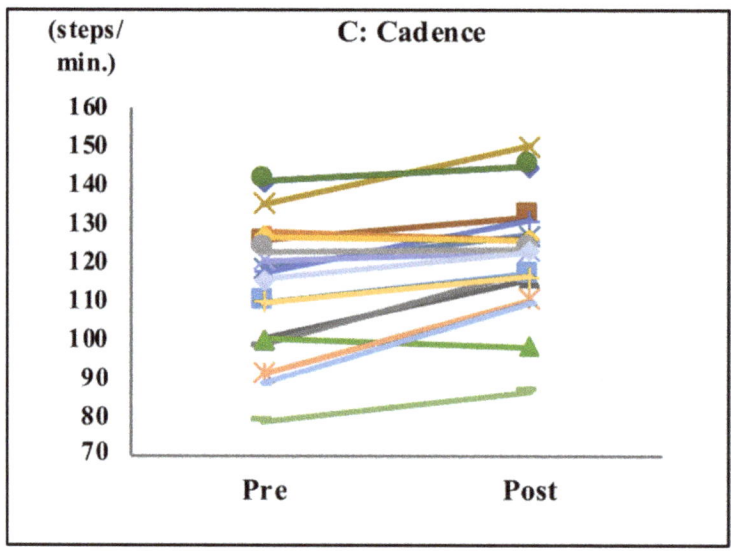
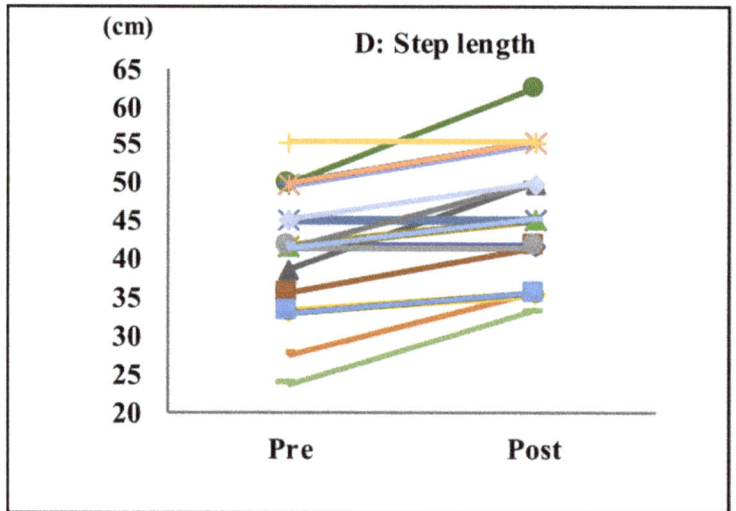

Figure 3. Gait parameters. Acceleration (**A**), gait speed (**B**), cadence (**C**), and step length (**D**). After the tasks with music, subjects showed significant improvements in their acceleration, gait speed, cadence, and step length.

Table 1. Comparison of gait characteristics before and after music therapy (MT).

	Pre-MT	Post-MT
Acceleration (m/s^2)	1.94 ± 0.56	2.44 ± 0.73 **
Speed (m/s)	0.88 ± 0.22	0.97 ± 0.22 **
Cadence (steps/min)	117.3 ± 17.74	122.9 ± 15.56 *
Step length (cm)	41.55 ± 8.38	46.70 ± 8.39 **

** $p < 0.001$, * $p < 0.05$.

Additionally, we compared the pre/post changes in acceleration, gait speed, cadence, and step length between the two groups of H&Y 2 (4 subjects) and 3 (15 subjects), but there was no significant difference between the different H&Y levels. Furthermore, the same comparison was made between the two groups with a gait score of one point (12 subjects) and two points (6 subjects) on the UPDRS-III, but there was no significant difference between these two groups (the remaining subject had zero point for Gait on the UPDRS-III).

During transitions in all walking tasks with music (from Tasks 3 to 6), the values of acceleration ($p < 0.05$), gait speed ($p < 0.08$), cadence ($p < 0.001$), and step length ($p < 0.6$) gradually increased. The best improvements were noted during Task 6 (music at 120 BPM), with the effects remaining in Task 7 even without music (Figure 4). Walking speed in Task 3 (music at 90 BPM) was slightly slower than that in Task 2 (with hand clapping), which was performed at the subjects' own pace. The rate of change in gait speed was $-8.66\% \pm 3.31\%$ for Task 3 (BPM 90), $3.82\% \pm 4.19\%$ for Task 4 (BPM 100), $7.13\% \pm 4.57\%$ for Task 5 (BPM 110), $16.04\% \pm 4.29\%$ for Task 6 (BPM 120), and $15.48\% \pm 4.8\%$ for Task 7 (post) ($p < 0.001$). The rate of change in acceleration was $-16.83\% \pm 2.49\%$ for Task 3 (BPM 90), $-0.8\% \pm 4.46\%$ for Task 4 (BPM 100), $4.04\% \pm 3.27\%$ for Task 5 (BPM 110), $15.52\% \pm 5.56\%$ for Task 6 (BPM 120), and $9.19\% \pm 4.44\%$ for Task 7 (post) ($p < 0.0001$).

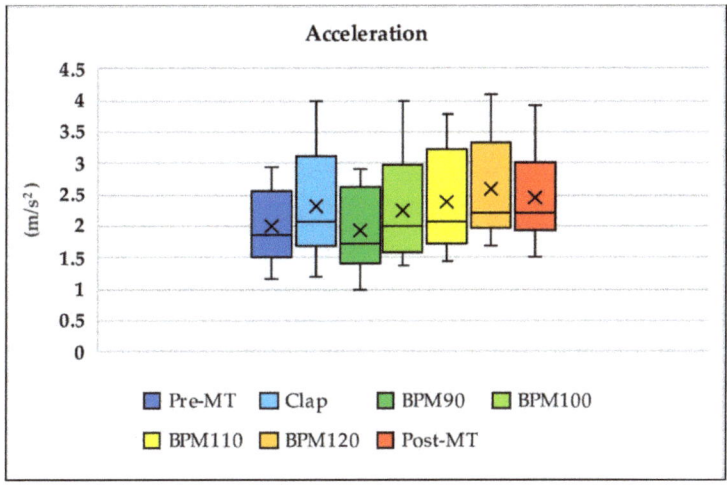

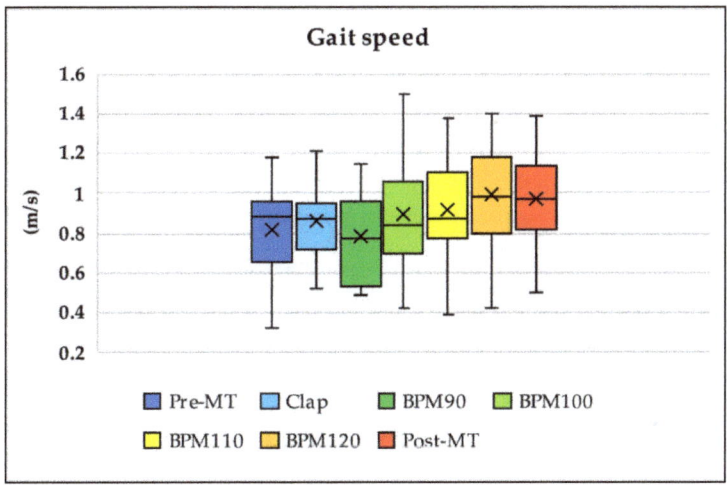

Figure 4. *Cont.*

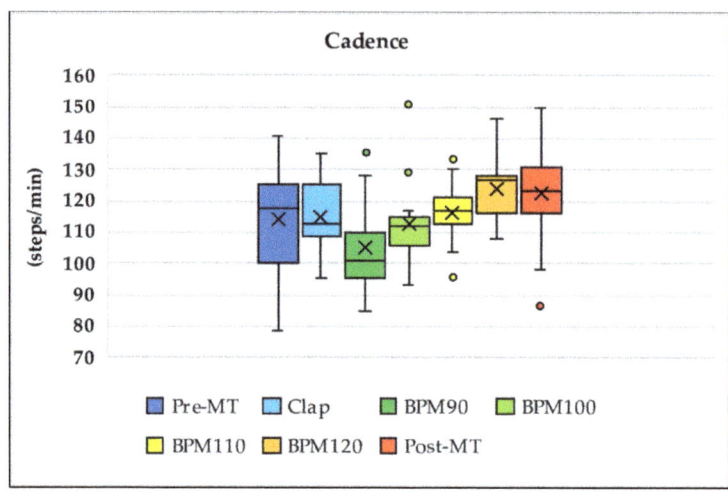
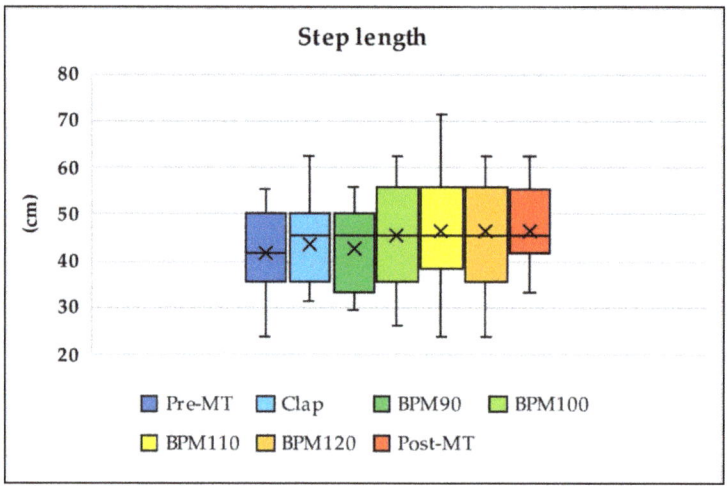

Figure 4. Transition throughout the entire walking task for acceleration, gait speed, cadence, and step length. During transitions in the walking tasks with music (from Tasks 3 to 6), values of acceleration, gait speed, cadence, and step length increased gradually. The best improvement was observed in Task 6 (music at 120 beats per minute (BPM)) and remained in Task 7 even without music. Walking speed in Task 3 (music at 90 BPM) was slightly slower than that in Task 2 (hand clapping while walking at the subjects' own pace).

With regard to the trajectory of the center of the body, the ML amplitude, which is typically large for PwP [23], was reduced significantly (pre: 1.88 ± 0.98 cm; post: 1.71 ± 0.84 cm; $p < 0.05$; Table 2, Figure 5).

Table 2. Changes in acceleration and amplitude over the three axes (mediolateral (ML), vertical (VT), and anteroposterior (AP)) before and after music therapy (MT).

	Acceleration (m/s^2)		Amplitude (cm)	
	Pre-MT	Post-MT	Pre-MT	Post-MT
Total	1.94 ± 0.56	2.44 ± 0.73	-	
ML	0.96 ± 0.22	1.13 ± 0.27	1.88 ± 0.98	1.71 ± 0.84
VT	1.96 ± 0.39	1.57 ± 0.47	1.07 ± 0.30	1.19 ± 0.36
AP	1.10 ± 0.31	1.15 ± 0.41	1.07 ± 0.99	1.23 ± 0.80

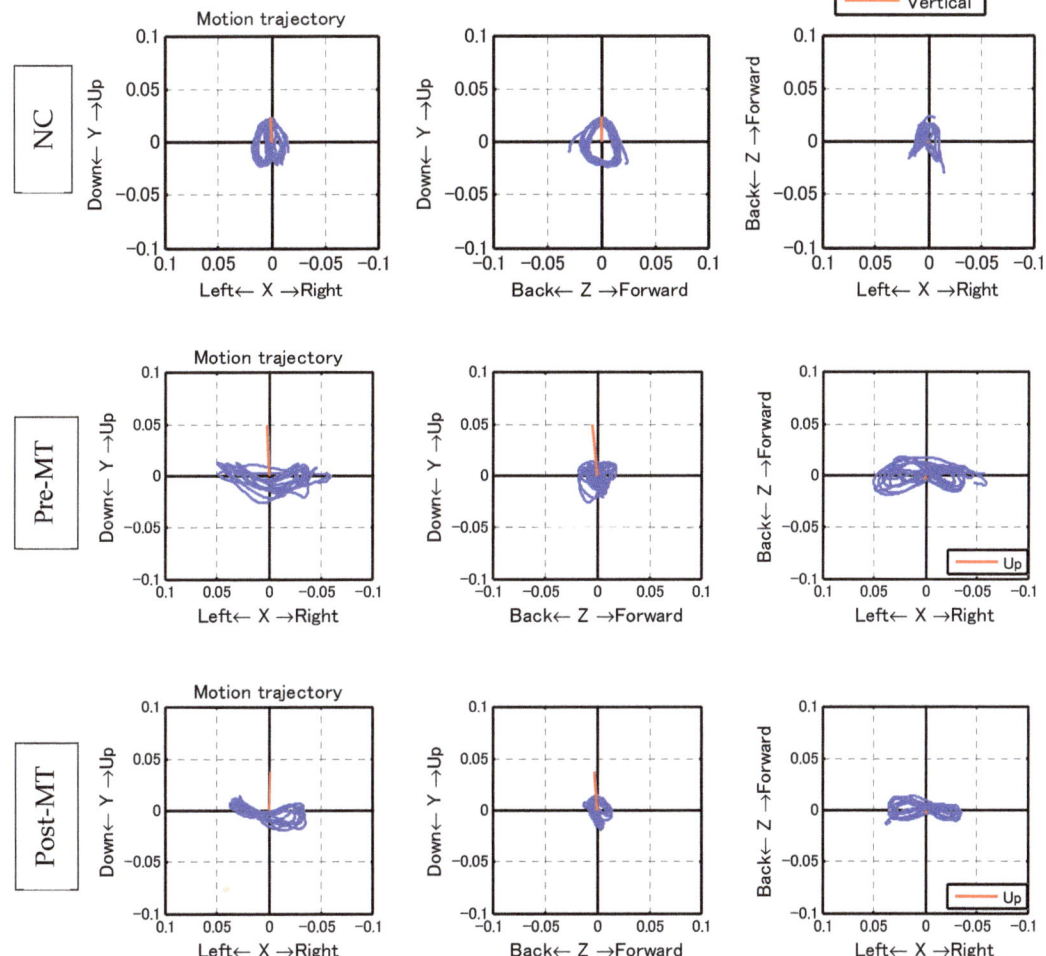

Figure 5. Walking trajectory. With regard to the trajectory of the center of the body, mediolateral (ML) amplitude, which is typically large for individuals with Parkinson's diseases, decreased significantly. Left row: coronal plane; middle row: sagittal plane; right row: horizontal plane. Upper row: the walking trajectory of a healthy 70-year-old woman. The trajectory was symmetrical and forms a butterfly pattern in the coronal and horizontal plane. On the sagittal plane, the trajectory forms a symmetrical circle. Middle row: Pre-MT walking trajectory of one subject. Lower row: Post-MT walking trajectory of the subject shown in the middle row.

4. Discussion

On comparing walking before and after rhythmic auditory stimulation with music, the current study found that music therapy had immediate effects for gait disturbance in PwP. Accordingly, significant improvements were observed in acceleration, gait speed, cadence, and step length, suggesting the efficacy of music therapy in reducing gait disturbance associated with PD. As such, music therapy can be expected to be utilized in the rehabilitation of PwP, particularly those with gait disturbance.

Comparing the gait of PwP with that of normal controls in another study (NC; normal gait at 70–79 years) [22] showed that the former had clearly lower values for acceleration, gait speed, cadence, and step length compared to the latter. Accordingly, PwP and NC had pre-MT values of 1.94 ± 0.56 and 3.38 ± 0.16 m/s^2 for acceleration, 0.88 ± 0.22 and 1.34 ± 0.01 m/s for gait speed, 109.99 ± 17.77 and 119.27 ± 2.05 steps/min for cadence, and 41.55 ± 8.38 and 67.43 ± 0.53 cm for step length, respectively. Music therapy was able to significantly improve gait disturbance in PD, which has been characterized as slow and small steps [5], a tendency observed herein.

PwP also exhibit a gait that has large amplitude in the ML direction, which can be observed from the trajectory of the PGR (Table 2, Figure 5). After music therapy, however, the gait force increased, whereas the ML/VT amplitude and ML/AP amplitude ratios decreased (Figure 6). The use of a PGR allows us to observe the data objectively in a manner that both the patient and therapist can easily understand, which can be useful from the perspective of personal communication. Apart from gait analysis in PD, studies have utilized the trajectory of the PGR to evaluate total hip arthroplasty [16,21] and cerebral infraction [24]. PGR analysis clearly showed that the ML amplitude of PwP was larger than the VT and AP amplitude ratio among NC. Nonetheless, music therapy was able to improve gait trajectory of PwP as well.

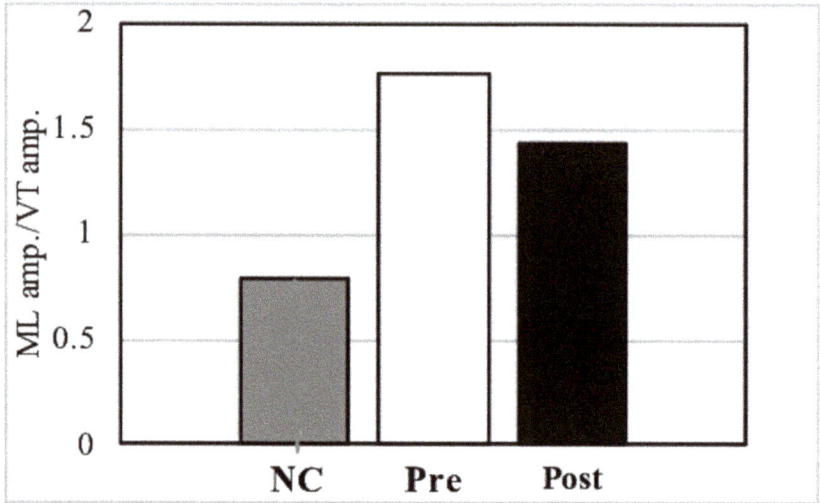

Figure 6. *Cont.*

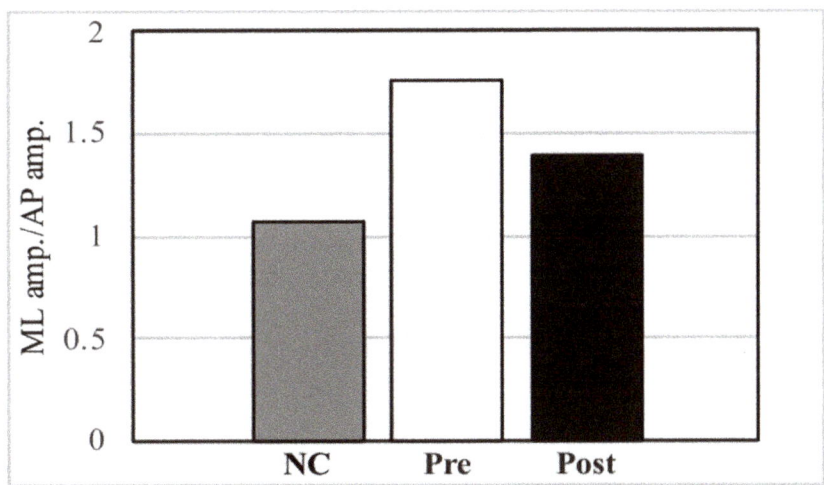

Figure 6. Comparison of the mediolateral (ML) amplitude/vertical (VT) amplitude ratio and ML amplitude/anteroposterior (AP) amplitude ratio between normal controls (NC) and pre- and post-music therapy individuals with Parkinson's disease.

Compared to NC, individuals with Parkinson's disease had a larger ML amplitude ratio among the three axes, although this decreased post-MT.

The current study considers the following two factors to have caused the immediate effect. First, music can act as external stimuli that normalized the destabilized processes of internal rhythmic formation [14]. External rhythmic cues can serve as surrogate cues for impaired internal timing [12]. Second, music can promote a pleasurable feeling by activating the limbic system, which facilitates dopamine release [25,26]. Salimpoor et al. reported that the intense pleasure experienced when listening to music was associated with dopamine activity in the mesolimbic reward system, which includes both the dorsal and ventral striatum [27]. Thus, it can be hypothesized that the mechanism by which music therapy promoted its effects included both aforementioned factors, indicating its utility for rehabilitation. Although the immediate effects were examined in the current study, in the future, based on this method, the long-term effects could also be evaluated using PGR. Furthermore, since a fully charged PGR can achieve 70 h of continuous recording [20], it is possible to observe not only gait in the short term but also the diurnal variation of Parkinson's disease patients and to detect freezing of gait.

Moreover, PD is commonly complicated by the existence of comorbid depression. In fact, Ito et al. [4] reported that simply listening to audio tapes at home without gait training for at least an hour daily over three to four weeks significantly decreased mean depression scale scores, suggesting that music could also be useful for improving depression as well as gait disturbance.

Rehabilitation plays a crucial role in maintaining quality of life associated with PD [4], the effects of which depend on the patients' own motivation. Therefore, rehabilitation techniques that patients can voluntarily perform by themselves are needed. Hence, music therapy together with other rehabilitation approaches can be beneficial.

The effectiveness of various nonpharmacological interventions, such as Tai Chi, robot-assisted gait training, Lee Silverman Voice Treatment, dance, video games, and virtual reality exercises, have also been reported [11,28]. In particular, music and dance have potential advantages in terms of noninvasive treatment and easy applicability [29].

Nowadays, telemedicine for PD has been receiving increasing attention [30]. In fact, reports have shown that rehabilitation can be provided through telemedicine [31] and that music therapy could also be used in that field.

5. Conclusions

The current study indicated in detail that gait training incorporating music via rhythmic auditory stimulation can be effective for treating gait disturbance associated with PD. Moreover, the objective and visualized data obtained using a PGR can aid in treating PD-associated gait disturbance. The rehabilitation process through music is simple, noninvasive, nonpharmacological, and inexpensive. Therefore, we believe that music therapy will become more utilized for the daily rehabilitation of PD-associated gait disturbance.

Author Contributions: Conceptualization: A.H.; Methodology: A.H.; Software: E.G.; Validation: E.G.; Formal analysis: E.G.; Investigation: S.M. and E.G.; Resources: S.M.; Data curation: S.M. and E.G.; Writing—original draft preparation: E.G.; Writing—review and editing: A.H. and E.G.; Visualization: E.G.; Supervision: A.H.; Project Administration: A.H. All authors have read and agreed to the published version of the manuscript.

Funding: This research received no external funding.

Institutional Review Board Statement: The study was conducted according to the guidelines of the Declaration of Helsinki and approved by the Research Ethics Committee, Faculty of Medicine, Juntendo University (protocol code 25-49).

Informed Consent Statement: Informed consent was obtained from all subjects involved in the study.

Data Availability Statement: The data presented in this study are available on request from the corresponding author. The data are not publicly available due to subjects' privacy.

Acknowledgments: The PGR was supplied by LSI Medience Corporation. This research did not receive any specific grant from any funding agency in the public, commercial, or not-for-profit sectors.

Conflicts of Interest: The authors declare no conflict of interest.

References

1. Mico-Amigo, M.E.; Kingma, I.; Faber, G.S.; Kunikoshi, A.; Van Uem, J.M.T.; Van Lummel, R.C.; Maetzler, W.; Van Dieën, J.H. Is the assessment of 5 meters of gait with a single body-fixed-sensor enough to recognize idiopathic Parkinson's disease-associated gait? *Ann. Biomed. Eng.* **2017**, *45*, 1266–1278. [CrossRef]
2. Ashoori, A.; Eagleman, D.M.; Jankovic, J. Effects of auditory rhythm and music on gait disturbances in Parkinson's disease. *Front. Neurol.* **2015**, *6*, 234. [CrossRef]
3. Lim, I.; Van Wegan, E.; De Goede, C.; Deutekom, M.; Nieuwboer, A.; Willems, A.; Jones, D.; Rochester, L.; Kwakkel, G. Effects of external rhythmical cueing on gait in patients with Parkinson's disease: A systematic review. *Clin. Rehabil.* **2005**, *19*, 695–713. [CrossRef] [PubMed]
4. Ito, N.; Hayashi, A.; Lin, W.; Ohkoshi, N.; Watanabe, M.; Shoji, S. Music therapy in Parkinson's disease: Improvement of parkinsonian gait and depression with rhythmic auditory stimulation. In *Integrated Human Brain Science: Theory, Method Application (Music)*; Nakada, T., Ed.; Elsevier: New York, NY, USA, 2000; pp. 435–443.
5. Mirelman, A.; Bonato, P.; Camicioli, R.; Ellis, T.D.; Giladi, N.; Hamilton, J.L.; Hass, C.J.; Hausdorff, J.M.; Pelosin, E.; Almeida, Q.J. Gait impairments in Parkinson's disease. *Lancet Neurol.* **2019**, *18*, 697–708. [CrossRef]
6. Pistacchi, M.; Gioulis, M.; Sanson, F.; De Giovannini, E.; Filippi, G.; Rossetto, F.; Marsala, S.Z. Gait analysis and clinical correlations in early Parkinson's disease. *Funct. Neurol.* **2017**, *32*, 28–34. [CrossRef] [PubMed]
7. Urquhart, D.M.; Morris, M.E.; Iansek, R. Gait consistency over a 7-day interval in people with Parkinson's disease. *Arch. Phys. Med. Rehabil.* **1999**, *80*, 696–701. [CrossRef]
8. Djaldetti, R.; Lorberboym, M.; Melamed, E. Primary postural instability: A cause of recurrent sudden falls in the elderly. *Neurol. Sci.* **2006**, *27*, 412–416. [CrossRef]
9. Agosti, V.; Vitale, C.; Avella, D.; Rucco, R.; Santangelo, G.; Sorrentino, P.; Varriale, P.; Sorrentino, G. Effects of global postural reeducation on gait kinematics in parkinsonian patients: A pilot randomized three-dimensional motion analysis study. *Neurol. Sci.* **2016**, *37*, 515–522. [CrossRef]
10. Mancini, M.; Fling, B.W.; Gendreau, A.; Lapidus, J.; Horak, F.B.; Chung, K.; Nutt, J.G. Effect of augmenting cholinergic function on gait and balance. *BMC Neurol.* **2015**, *15*, 264. [CrossRef]
11. Bloem, B.R.; De Vries, N.M.; Ebersbach, G. Nonpharmacological treatments for Parkinson's disease. *Mov. Disord.* **2015**, *30*, 1504–1520. [CrossRef]
12. Fox, S.H.; Katzenschlager, R.; Lim, S.Y.; Ravina, B.; Seppi, K.; Coelho, M.; Poewe, W.; Rascol, O.; Goetz, C.G.; Sampaio, C. The movement disorder society evidence-based medicine review update: Treatments for the motor symptoms of Parkinson's disease. *Mov. Disord.* **2011**, *26*, S2–S41. [CrossRef] [PubMed]

13. De Dreu, M.J.; Van der Wilk, A.S.D.; Poppe, E.; Kwakkel, G.; Wegen, E.E.H. Rehabilitation, exercise therapy and music in patients with Parkinson's disease: A meta-analysis of the effects of music-based movement therapy on walking ability, balance and quality of life. *Parkinsonism Relat. Disord.* **2012**, *18*, S114–S119. [CrossRef]
14. Freeman, J.S.; Cody, F.W.; Schady, W. The influence of external timing cues upon the rhythm of voluntary movements in Parkinson's disease. *J. Neurol. Neurosurg. Psychiatry* **1993**, *56*, 1078–1084. [CrossRef] [PubMed]
15. McIntosh, G.C.; Brown, S.H.; Rice, R.R.; Thaut, M.H. Rhythmic auditory-motor facilitation of gait patterns with Parkinson's disease. *J. Neurol. Neurosurg. Psychiatry* **1997**, *62*, 22–26. [CrossRef]
16. Gomi, M.; Maezawa, K.; Nozawa, M.; Yuasa, T.; Sugimoto, M.; Hayashi, A.; Mikawa, S.; Kaneko, K. Early clinical evaluation of total hip arthroplasty by three-dimensional gait analysis and muscle strength testing. *Gait Posture* **2018**, *66*, 214–220. [CrossRef] [PubMed]
17. Di Biase, L.; Di Santo, A.; Caminiti, M.L.; De Liso, A.; Shah, S.A.; Ricci, L.; Di Lazzaro, V. Gait analysis in Parkinson's disease: An overview of the most accurate markers for diagnosis and symptoms monitoring. *Sensors* **2020**, *20*, 3529. [CrossRef] [PubMed]
18. Mc Dermott, A. Science and Culture: At the nexus of music and medicine, some see treatments for disease. *Proc. Natl. Acad. Sci. USA* **2021**, *118*, e2025750118. [CrossRef]
19. Mitoma, H.; Yoneyama, M.; Orimo, S. 24-hour recording of Parkinsonian gait using a portable gait rhythmogram. *Intern. Med.* **2010**, *49*, 2401–2408. [CrossRef] [PubMed]
20. Mitoma, H.; Yoneyama, M. A newly developed wearable device for continuous measurement of gait-induced accelerations in daily activities. *Brain Disord. Ther.* **2014**, *3*, 4172. [CrossRef]
21. Sato, H.; Maezawa, K.; Gomi, M.; Kajihara, H.; Hayashi, A.; Maruyama, Y.; Nozawa, M.; Kaneko, K. Effect of femoral offset and limb length discrepancy on hip joint muscle strength and gait trajectory after total hip arthroplasty. *Gait Posture* **2020**, *77*, 276–282. [CrossRef] [PubMed]
22. Yoneyama, M.; Mitoma, H.; Hayashi, A. Effect of age, gender, and walkway length on accelerometry-based gait parameters for healthy adult subjects. *J. Mech. Med. Biol.* **2016**, *16*, 1650029. [CrossRef]
23. Hayashi, A.; Shimura, H.; Aiba, S.; Yoneyama, M.; Mitoma, H. Automatic detection of freezing index of Parkinson's disease using a portable gait rhythmogram. *J. Neurol. Sci.* **2013**, *333*, 97–98. [CrossRef]
24. De la Herran, A.M.; Zapirain, B.G.; Zorrilla, A.M. Gait analysis methods: An overview of wearable and non-wearable systems, highlighting clinical applications. *Sensors* **2014**, *14*, 3362–3394. [CrossRef]
25. Boso, M.; Politi, P.; Barale, F.; Emanuele, E. Neurophysiology and neurobiology of the musical experience. *Funct. Neurol.* **2006**, *21*, 187–191. [PubMed]
26. Menon, V.; Levitin, D.J. The rewards of music listening: Response and physiological connectivity of the mesolimbic system. *Neuroimage* **2005**, *28*, 175–184. [CrossRef] [PubMed]
27. Salimpoor, V.N.; Benovoy, M.; Larcher, K.; Dagher, A.; Zatorre, R.J. Anatomically distinct dopamine release during anticipation and experience of peak emotion to music. *Nat. Neurosci.* **2011**, *14*, 257–262. [CrossRef]
28. Aguiar, L.P.C.; Rocha, P.A.; Morris, M. Therapeutic dancing for Parkinson's disease. *Int. J. Gerontol.* **2016**, *10*, 64–70. [CrossRef]
29. Pereira, A.P.S.; Marinho, V.; Gupta, D.; Magalhaes, F.; Ayres, C.; Teixeira, S. Music therapy and dance as gait rehabilitation in patients with Parkinson disease: A review of evidence. *J. Geriatr. Psychiatry Neurol.* **2019**, *32*, 49–56. [CrossRef]
30. Achey, M.; Aldred, J.L.; Aljehani, N.; Bloem, B.R.; Biglan, K.M.; Chan, P.; Cubo, E.; Dorsey, E.R.; Goetz, C.G.; Guttman, M.; et al. The past, present, and future of telemedicine for Parkinson's disease. *Mov. Disord.* **2014**, *29*, 871–883. [CrossRef]
31. Howell, S.; Tripoliti, E.; Pring, T. Delivering the Lee Silverman Voice Treatment (LSVT) by web camera: A feasibility study. *Int. J. Lang. Commun. Disord.* **2009**, *44*, 287–300. [CrossRef]

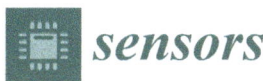

Article

Electromyography, Stiffness and Kinematics of Resisted Sprint Training in the Specialized SKILLRUN® Treadmill Using Different Load Conditions in Rugby Players

Antonio Martínez-Serrano [1,2], Elena Marín-Cascales [2], Konstantinos Spyrou [1,2,3], Tomás T. Freitas [1,2,3,4,*] and Pedro E. Alcaraz [1,2]

[1] UCAM Research Center for High Performance Sport, Catholic University of Murcia, 30107 Murcia, Spain; amartinez30@ucam.edu (A.M.-S.); kspyrou@ucam.edu (K.S.); palcaraz@ucam.edu (P.E.A.)
[2] Strength and Conditioning Society, 00118 Rome, Italy; elenamcascales@gmail.com
[3] Faculty of Sports Sciences, Catholic University of Murcia, 30107 Murcia, Spain
[4] NAR—Nucleus of High Performance in Sport, São Paulo 04753-060, Brazil
* Correspondence: tfreitas@ucam.edu; Tel.: +34-968-278-566

Abstract: This study's aim was to analyze muscle activation and kinematics of sled-pushing and resisted-parachute sprinting with three load conditions on an instrumentalized SKILLRUN® treadmill. Nine male amateur rugby union players (21.3 ± 4.3 years, 75.8 ± 10.2 kg, 176.6 ± 8.8 cm) performed a sled-push session consisting of three 15-m repetitions at 20%, 55% and 90% body mas and another resisted-parachute session using three different parachute sizes (XS, XL and 3XL). Sprinting kinematics and muscle activity of three lower-limb muscles (biceps femoris (BF), vastus lateralis (VL) and gastrocnemius medialis (GM)) were measured. A repeated-measures analysis of variance (RM-ANOVA) showed that higher loads during the sled-push increased (VL) ($p \leq 0.001$) and (GM) ($p \leq 0.001$) but not (BF) ($p = 0.278$) activity. Furthermore, it caused significant changes in sprinting kinematics, stiffness and joint angles. Resisted-parachute sprinting did not change kinematics or muscle activation, despite producing a significant overload (i.e., speed loss). In conclusion, increased sled-push loading caused disruptions in sprinting technique and altered lower-limb muscle activation patterns as opposed to the resisted-parachute. These findings might help practitioners determine the more adequate resisted sprint exercise and load according to the training objective (e.g., power production or speed performance).

Keywords: team-sports; performance; muscle activation; loaded sprint; sled-push

1. Introduction

Rugby union is a high contact team sport played worldwide which performance depends on the complex relationship between technique, tactics, cognition and physical capacities [1]. The game is based on collision and intermittent actions, where high-intensity activities (e.g., tackling, rucking, scrummaging, mauling) are interspersed with low-intensity activities (e.g., standing, walking, jogging) [2]. By analyzing the activity profile during a rugby union match, high-intensity actions, such as sprinting, are very frequent [3]. As such, linear sprint could be considered one of the most critical skills in this sport [4].

Sprint performance is determined by the athlete's capacity to generate and apply a great propulsive force during the acceleration phase and to maintain their maximum velocity for as long as possible during the maximum velocity phase [5]. In this regard, different non-specific strength-power exercises and methods have been used for the improvement of the acceleration phase of the sprint [6–8]. However, many coaches believe that training methods for improving sprint performance should also include specific strength exercises, so that the athlete can perform the desired movement with an added load [9]. This idea is supported by the training principle of specificity, which suggests that exercises should have

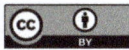

similar characteristics to the sport's requirements (i.e., type of action, movement patterns, velocity, muscle activation, etc.) [10]. Thus, resisted sprint training (RST) has been used as a specific training method for the enhancement of sprint performance in rugby and other team-sports, especially in the acceleration phase [11–14].

One of the most important variables considering RST is the selection of the training load. Most authors agree that RST is an effective training method for performance improvement, regardless of the load used [6,11,15,16]. Nevertheless, some argue that the use of tertiary methods does not replicate the sprint running movement [14,15] and the load must not be >20% body mass (BM) if the aim is to replicate sprint demands in terms of movement pattern, load, muscle activation and movement velocity [11]. These kinematics changes are mainly caused by a decrease in the lower limb stiffness, leading to a reduction of the force transmission ratio between the legs and the ground and therefore a lower acceleration and running speed [17].

When referring to RST, a wide variety of exercises and equipment can be used including sled and parachute towing, wearing a weighted vest and sprinting on sand or uphill [15]. From these, sled towing and pushing, along with resisted-parachute sprinting, are the most widely used in sports such as football, rugby and soccer. However, the scientific evidence regarding sled-pushing and resisted-parachute sprinting is limited in comparison to sled towing [18–22], particularly for variables such as muscle activation. In fact, only one study has analyzed muscle activation patterns in sled-pushing compared to squatting, finding a similar rectus and biceps femoris (BF) activation but higher gastrocnemius electromyographic (EMG) activity in the sled exercise [20].

A potential limitation of the RST is that it requires an exterior environment and facilities for its development, otherwise, a large interior space is needed. In addition, weather conditions can have a negative effect conducting the workout (e.g., wind conditions). Hence, alternative methods/equipment that can replicate the demands of RST indoor could be extremely valuable for coaches and athletes. In this context, a specialized treadmill SKILLRUN® (SR®) (Technogym, Cesena, Italy) capable of replicating RST has been recently developed with the aim of improving athlete's speed and power in a closed environment.

Given the lack of research, performing a muscle activity and kinematics analysis in sled-pushing and resisted-parachute sprinting on a treadmill with different loads would be interesting to determine which load in each of these exercises allows performing a sprinting effort without major disruptions of the muscle activity, movement pattern and leg stiffness. Hence, the aim of this study was to analyze the muscular activation and kinematics of sled-pushing and resisted-parachute sprinting with three load conditions on the instrumentalized treadmill. The secondary objective was to examine the effect of varying load on power production in these specific exercises. We hypothesized that: (1) the increased load would disrupt the kinematics of the exercises and cause increased gastrocnemius medialis (GM) and vastus lateralis (VL) muscle activation whereas BF would be reduced or maintained; and (2) moderate intensity loads would maximize power production.

2. Materials and Methods

Participants took part in a randomized crossover design pilot study consisting of: (1) one sled-push session in SR® treadmill using three different load conditions (i.e., 20%, 55% and 90% BM), and (2) one resisted-parachute session in SR® treadmill using three different parachute sizes (i.e., extra-small (XS), extra-large (XL) and triple extra-large (3XL)). Sled and parachute resistance were applied by the SR®; therefore, participants did not move across space but rather ran on the treadmill as depicted in Figure 1. Test distance and load selection were determined following a pilot study conducted at our facilities. An external researcher randomly determined the order of the sessions, the training intensity and parachute size. Each sled and parachute session were separated by 7-d due to team's training schedule during the season. Participants were asked to cease physical activity or training 24-h before the testing to ensure full recovery and all the tests were conducted in a similar time of the day (e.g., +/− 1-h) to minimize diurnal variations.

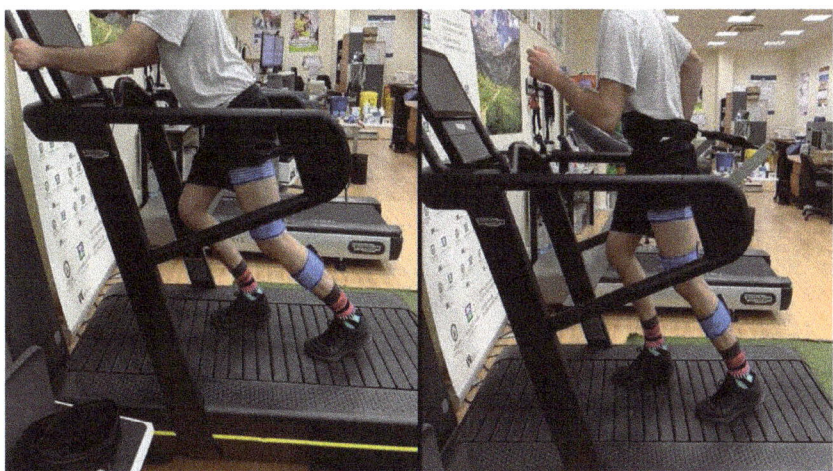

Figure 1. (left panel) Sled-push and, **(right panel)** resisted-parachute sprinting on the SR® treadmill.

2.1. Subjects

Nine male amateur rugby union players (age 21.3 ± 4.3 years, mass 75.8 ± 10.2 kg, height 176.6 ± 8.8 cm) participated in this study. Convenience sampling was used as the eligibility criteria. Over the course of the study, two participants suffered an injury and were unable to attend to the resisted-parachute session. Players were excluded if they: (1) were taking any medication or supplementation (e.g., caffeine 12-h prior to exercise) that could interfere with the results, (2) were suffering from any kind of disease and (3) had suffered from a lower limb injury six months prior to study enrollment. All subjects were familiar with performing the traditional sled-push and resisted-parachute sprinting exercises in their regular training. Participants read the information sheet and were informed of the benefits and risks of the investigation and signed the informed consent form before the study began. Parental or guardian informed consent form was obtained for those who were underage (n = 2). This study conforms with The Code of Ethics of the World Medical Association (Declaration of Helsinki) and it was approved by the local Ethics Committee (code: CE012009; date 31 January 2020).

2.2. Procedures

Anthropometric measurements (i.e., mass and height) were taken using a Tanita HD-313 scale (Tanita Corporation, Tokyo, Japan) and a stadiometer Seca 213 (Hamburg, Germany). Electrodes for the EMG analysis were placed on the VL, BF and GM muscles before volunteers performed a standardized warm-up which included: 8-min of cycling in a cycle ergometer, dynamic stretching of the lower limbs and one submaximal sled-push repetition with the participant's 20% BM over 15-m or a submaximal resisted-parachute sprint using XS parachute size over 15-m.

2.2.1. Sled-Push Test Protocol

In the SR® sled mode, the resistance is applied in such a way that it mimics the sensation of an over-ground sled-push. The treadmill resistance is higher during the initial phase of the run and decreases at a constant rate as velocity increases (accounting for inertia). Participants (n = 9) carried out three repetitions over 15-m and used three different training intensities: 20%, 55% and 90% BM. They had to run, "pushing" the treadmill belt, as fast as possible (speed was not kept constant by the treadmill but was rather determined by the athlete's running capabilities) with their hands fixed to the handles at the height they were most comfortable following manufacturer's recommendations. Starting position was established individually according to the subject's dominant leg and remained the same throughout all the sessions. Participants were encouraged to exert their maximum effort while performing the exercises. Resting time between repetitions was 3-min walking at 3 km/h.

2.2.2. Resisted-Parachute Test Protocol

In the SR® parachute mode, the sensation of sprinting outdoors with a parachute is also mimicked. The resistance is null at the start and increases progressively with running velocity. According to manufacturer specifications, the resistance deriving from the parachute is calculated analyzing different parameters (Equations (1)–(3)) that are used into a proprietary formula. The parameters are:

$$\text{Motor torque} = 0.01365 \times \left(v^2\right) \times \left(Pd^2\right) \times \left(10^{-6}\right) \tag{1}$$

$$\text{Force (N)} = F0 + 0.615752 \times \left(Pd^2\right) \times \left(v^2\right) \times \left(10^{-6}\right) \tag{2}$$

$$\text{Power (W)} = P0 + 0.615752 \times \left(Pd^2\right) \times \left(v^3\right) \times \left(10^{-6}\right) \tag{3}$$

In which F0 corresponds to the friction coefficient in N, v is the slat belt speed in m/s, P0 (W) is obtained by multiplying F0 by v, and Pd corresponds to the parachute diameter in mm. Resistance increases with the power of three relationship with speed (cubic relation).

Participants (n = 7) performed three repetitions over 15-m and used three different parachute sizes: XS, XL and 3XL. The parachute belt was buckled at waist level following manufacturer's recommendations. Participants were asked to run at maximum intensity and were encouraged over the course of the test. Resting time between repetitions was 3-min walking at 3 km/h.

2.2.3. Electromyography

The Surface ElectroMyoGraphy for the Non-Invasive Assessment of Muscles (SENIAM) protocol was used for skin preparation and sensor location [23]. Skin preparation included shaving areas where electrodes would be placed, removing dead epithelial cells using an abrasive paper and cleansing the area with alcohol, allowing it to vaporize. Two surface EMG electrodes (Ambu® BlueSensor N—Ambu A/S, Denmark) were placed 20 mm apart (electrode to electrode) on the participant's dominant leg over three muscles: (a) VL, (b) BF and (c) GM. The electrodes were placed superficially to each muscle belly and in the same orientation as the respective muscle fibers. This procedure was conducted before the beginning of the sled-push and resisted-parachute session. The placement of the electrodes was marked with a permanent marker to ensure that it was the same in both sessions. They were secured to the skin with adhesive tape and an elastic bandage in order to eliminate any movement artifact.

Muscle activation was measured via wireless surface EMG (Noraxon USA INC, Scottsdale, AZ, USA) at a sampling rate of 10,000 Hz with Noraxon MR 3.6.20 software (Noraxon, Scottsdale, AZ, USA). Raw EMG data was processed and filtered using the following settings: Filter: FIR, Window: 79 points, Type: Bandpass, Low frequency: 20 Hz, High frequency: 500 Hz, Window: Lancosh. Rectification and smoothing (Algorithm: RMS, Window: 100 ms) were also applied. Total muscle activation was analyzed with AcqKnowledge 3.9.1 software (BIOPAC Systems Inc., CA, USA) by calculating the average root-mean-square (RMS) of the whole gait cycle from the first 10 strides.

2.2.4. Performance Variables

Maximum velocity (V_{max}) and maximum power (P_{max}) were obtained from the specialized treadmill interface as performance variables. According to manufacturer specifications V_{max} (km/h) is directly measured from the rotational speed of the motor while P_{max} (W) is obtained by multiplying the rotational speed of the slat belt by the force applied by the athlete to the surface (deriving from the motor energetic absorption).

2.2.5. Kinematics

Running kinematics during the sled-push and parachute sessions were recorded using the camera of an iPhone XR running iOS 13.5 (Apple Inc., Cupertino, CA, USA) at a frequency of 240 Hz. The camera was placed sideways at a distance of 2-m from the treadmill on a 1-m height tripod recording the sagittal plane of the subject's dominant leg. Calibration frame was performed by measuring the length of one of the treadmill handles.

The following kinematic variables of the first ten strides of the participant's dominant leg were analyzed using Kinovea 0.9.1 (Kinovea.org, France): contact time (CT), flight time (FT), stride frequency (SF), stride length (SL), leg stiffness (K_{vert}) and ankle, knee and hip angles (A_{angle}, K_{angle}, H_{angle}, respectively) collected during the stance phase. Intraclass correlation coefficients (ICC) were determined for the different sled-push variables: CT (ICC ranging from 0.890 to 0.965), FT (from 0.744 to 0.940) and SL (from 0.883 to 0.945). Regarding resisted-parachute sprinting, ICCs ranging from 0.816 to 0.967, from 0.704 to 0.831 and from 0.765 to 0.911 were obtained for CT, FT and SL, respectively. K_{vert} was measured using the methods and calculations (Equations (4)–(6)) by Morin et al. [24]:

$$\hat{K}_{vert} = \hat{F}_{max} \cdot \Delta \hat{y}_c^{-1} \quad (4)$$

$$\hat{F}_{max} = mg \frac{\pi}{2} \left(\frac{t_f}{t_c} + 1 \right) \quad (5)$$

$$\Delta \hat{y}_c = \frac{\hat{F}_{max} t_c^2}{m \pi^2} + g \frac{t_c^2}{8} \quad (6)$$

In which $\Delta \hat{y}_c$ is the vertical center of mass displacement, m is the participant's body mass in kg, t_f is the flight time in s, and t_c is the contact time in s. Subsequently, the $\hat{K}_{vert}$ value obtained was multiplied by 1.0496 (i.e., a correction factor proposed by Coleman et al. [25]). Raw angle data from Kinovea was exported to Microsoft Excel 16.36 (Microsoft, USA) for further analysis.

2.3. Statistical Analysis

Data is shown as mean ± SD. The statistical analysis was performed using Jamovi® 1.1.9.0 for macOS. Shapiro–Wilk test and Levene's test were used for assessing the normality of the distribution of the variables and the homogeneity of variance. The EMG activity and kinematic variables during each load and exercises were determined using repeated-measures analysis of variance with Bonferroni post hoc comparisons. Partial eta squared was obtained from the repeated measures analysis and classified as: small (≤ 0.01), moderate (≤ 0.06) and large (≥ 0.14). Cohen's d effect sizes (ES) were calculated to provide qualitive descriptors of standardized effects using the following criteria: <0.2, 0.2–0.6, 0.6–1.2, 1.2–2, 2–4 and >4 for trivial, small, moderate, large, very large and near perfect, respectively [26]. Alpha-level was set at $p \leq 0.05$.

3. Results

3.1. Electromyography

Figure 2 displays the comparisons between EMG activation patterns of the different muscles in the sled-push and resisted-parachute sprinting in the different load conditions. Regarding sled-push, there was a statistically significant effect of increasing load on VL activation (F = 33.366; $p \leq 0.001$; η^2_P = 0.807). VL activation was significantly higher at 90% BM compared to 20 and 55% BM ($p \leq 0.001$, ES = 2.18; $p \leq 0.001$, ES = 2.39) respectively, and tended to increase from 20–55% BM (p = 0.054, ES = 0.90). In contrast, no significant differences were obtained on BF activation as load increased (F = 1.388; p = 0.278; η^2_P = 0.148). Increasing load had a statistically significant effect on GM activation (F = 14.439; $p \leq$ 0.001; η^2_P = 0.643). GM activation increased significantly from 20–55% BM (p = 0.012, ES = 1.07) and 20–90% BM ($p \leq$ 0.001, ES = 1.94) but not from 55–90% BM (p = 0.212, ES = 0.62) (Figure 2A). No significant differences were found in muscle activation of VL (F = 0.591; p = 0.569; η^2_P = 0.090), BF (F = 1.531; p = 0.256; η^2_P = 0.203) and GM (F = 0.879; p = 0.440; 0.128) using different parachute sizes (Figure 2B).

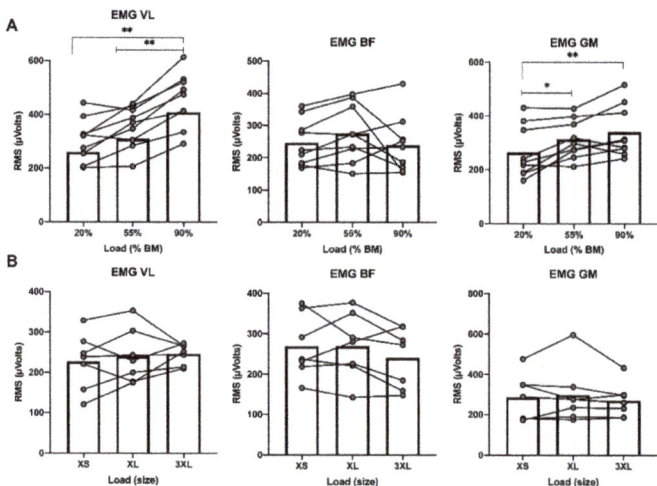

Figure 2. (**A**) Comparison of muscle activation of VL, BF and GM in sled-push under different load conditions. (**B**) Comparison of muscle activation of VL, BF and GM in resisted-parachute sprinting under different size conditions. * $p \leq$ 0.05; ** $p \leq$ 0.001; BF = biceps femoris; BM = body mass; EMG = electromyography; GM = gastrocnemius medialis; VL = vastus.

3.2. Kinematics

Table 1 depicts the descriptive analysis for the kinematic variables.

Table 1. Kinematics and performance variables of sled push and resisted-parachute sprinting with different load conditions, data is presented as mean ± SD.

	Sled Push			Parachute		
	20% BM	55% BM	90% BM	XS	XL	3XL
Kinematic Variables						
CT (s)	0.192 ± 0.012	0.241 ± 0.026	0.368 ± 0.115 **	0.186 ± 0.012	0.197 ± 0.009	0.196 ± 0.016
FT (s)	0.297 ± 0.019	0.291 ± 0.025	0.305 ± 0.042	0.283 ± 0.018	0.277 ± 0.016	0.279 ± 0.026
SF (Hz)	2.14 ± 0.18	1.89 ± 0.14	1.54 ± 0.29 **	2.13 ± 0.09	2.11 ± 0.08	2.11 ± 0.10
SL (cm)	62.63 ± 9.64	56.21 ± 9.05	46.39 ± 10.8 **	59.63 ± 7.41	58.43 ± 6.36	54.25 ± 5.49
K_{vert} (N/m)	16.14 ± 4.42	9.76 ± 2.08 **	4.72 ± 2.28 **	16.48 ± 4.33	14.37 ± 3.19	14.83 ± 4.02
Joint Angles						
A_{angle} (°)	106.73 ± 7.88	103.05 ± 11.04	99 ± 8.95 **	110.60 ± 2.99	108.76 ± 5.92	112.25 ± 6.58
K_{angle} (°)	142.27 ± 8.21	135.52 ± 9.64	127.63 ± 13.03 *	143.46 ± 11.07	141.30 ± 12.44	148.87 ± 7.03
H_{angle} (°)	142.52 ± 6.11	140.73 ± 10.69	135.03 ± 12.29 *	151.99 ± 6.50	149.37 ± 4.72	157.09 ± 3.78 *
Performance Variables						
P_{max} (W)	704.56 ± 107.37	900.89 ± 132.89 **	826.00 ± 121.04 *	440.71 ± 93.08	469.71 ± 85.19	533.14 ± 80.83 **
V_{max} (km/h)	17.36 ± 1.03	13.19 ± 1.02 **	8.81 ± 2.62 **	18.83 ± 1.62	16.80 ± 1.69*	15.96 ± 1.36 **

* $p \leq$ 0.05; ** $p \leq$ 0.001; η^2_P = significant difference between XL-3XL Aangle = ankle angle; BM = body mass; cm = centimeters; CT = contact time; FT = flight time; Hangle = hip angle; Hz = hertz; km/h = kilometers per hour; Kangle = knee angle; Kvert = stiffness vertical; s = seconds; SF = stride frequency; SL = stride length; Vmax = maximum velocity; W = watts; XS = extra-small; XL = extra-large; 3XL = triple extra-large.

Significant effects were found in CT (F = 16.367; $p \leq 0.001$; η^2_P = 0.672), SF (F = 16.543; $p \leq 0.001$; η^2_P = 0.674), SL (F = 12.505; $p \leq 0.001$; η^2_P = 0.610) and K_{vert} (F = 33.841; $p \leq 0.001$; η^2_P = 0.809) when pushing the sled. Higher CT were found from 20–90% BM ($p \leq 0.001$, ES = 1.42) and 55–90% BM (p = 0.003, ES = 1.20). Conversely, no changes were found in FT (F = 1.130; p = 0.347; η^2_P = 0.124). SF and SL increased significantly from 20–90 % BM ($p \leq 0.001$, ES = 1.52; $p \leq 0.001$, ES = 1.28) and 55–90% BM (p = 0.013, ES = 1.44; p = 0.025, ES = 0.92), respectively. K_{vert} decreased significantly in all load conditions 20–55% BM ($p \leq 0.001$, ES = 1.72), 20–90% BM ($p \leq 0.001$, ES = 1.98) and 55–90% BM (p = 0.007, ES = 2.21) (Figure 3).

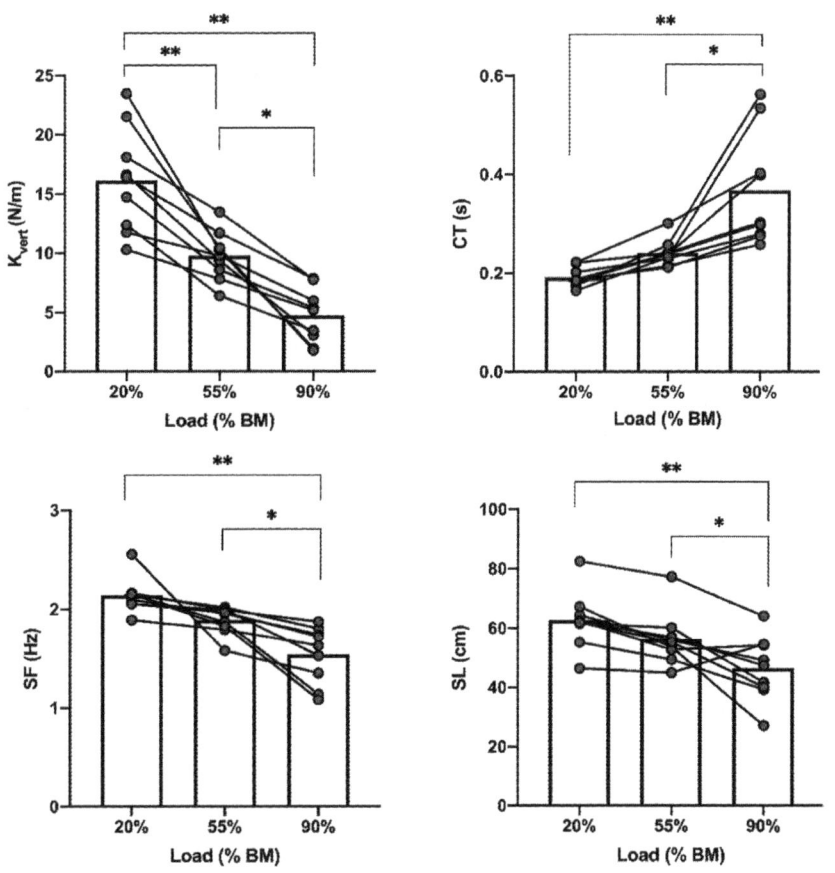

Figure 3. Comparison of sprinting K_{vert} and kinematics under different load conditions in sled-push. * $p \leq 0.05$; ** $p \leq 0.001$; BM = body mass; CT = contact time; FT = flight time; K_{vert} = vertical stiffness; SF = stride frequency; SL = stride length.

Increasing load had a significant effect on A_{angle} (F = 12.075; $p \leq 0.001$; η^2_P = 0.601), K_{angle} (F = 10.088; p = 0.001; η^2_P = 0.558) and H_{angle} (F = 4.611; p = 0.026; η^2_P = 0.366). A_{angle}, K_{angle} and H_{angle} decreased significantly from 20–90% BM ($p \leq 0.001$, ES = 1.46; p = 0.001, ES = 1.14; p = 0.031, ES = 0.79, respectively) and presented a non-significant decrease from 55–90% BM in A_{angle} (p = 0.062, ES = 0.99). No significant effects between kinematic variables and different parachute sizes in resisted-parachute sprinting were found in CT (F = 2.982; p = 0.089; η^2_P = 0.332), FT (F = 0.541; p = 0.595; η^2_P = 0.083), SF (F = 0.416; p = 0.669; 0.065), SL (F = 3.568; p = 0.061; 0.373) and K_{vert} (F = 3.109; p = 0.082;

$\eta^2_P = 0.341$). The only statistically significant difference was found from XL-3XL parachute size in H_{angle} ($p = 0.007$, ES = 1.64).

3.3. Performance

In sled-push, there were a statistically significant effect of increasing load on P_{max} (F = 27.101; $p \leq 0.001$; $\eta^2_P = 0.772$) and V_{max} (F = 86.972; $p \leq 0.001$; $\eta^2_P = 0.916$). P_{max} increased significantly from 20–55 % BM ($p \leq 0.001$, ES = 4.80), 20–90 % BM ($p = 0.001$, ES = 1.26) and decreased significantly from 55–90% BM ($p = 0.040$, ES = 0.81). On the other hand, V_{max} declined significantly between 20–55% BM ($p \leq 0.001$; ES = 3.35), 20–90% BM ($p \leq 0.001$; ES = 3.78) and 55–90% BM ($p \leq 0.001$; ES = 2.02). During resisted-parachute sprinting, we found a significant effect on P_{max} (F = 30.934; $p \leq 0.001$; $\eta^2_P = 0.838$) and V_{max} (F = 20.541; $p \leq 0.001$; $\eta^2_P = 0.774$). P_{max} increased significantly from XS to 3XL ($p \leq 0.001$, ES = 2.75) and XL to 3XL ($p \leq 0.001$, ES = 2.68), whereas V_{max} decreased significantly between XS-XL ($p = 0.003$, ES = 1.99) and XS-3XL ($p \leq 0.001$, ES = 1.91).

4. Discussion

The main findings of the study were that: (1) the muscle activation of the VL and GM (but not the BF) increased as a function of the load while pushing the sled but not when using parachutes of different sizes; (2) increasing the load in sled-push provoked several changes in running kinematics (i.e., increased CT and decreased SF, SL and K_{vert}, A_{angle}, K_{angle} and H_{angle}) whereas only an increase in the H_{angle} between XL-3XL sizes was detected in parachute running; and (3) the load conditions that produced the highest power output in sled-push and parachute were 55% BM and 3XL parachute size, respectively.

The reported EMG activity in VL while pushing the sled is supported by previous evidence suggesting there is an increase in knee torque due to increased horizontal concentric force during the acceleration phase of the sprint [27,28]. During this phase, the position of the trunk is leaning forward, bringing the body to a more horizontal position [29], similar to the one adopted to push the sled. In RST, athletes must adopt a more horizontal position [30] and lower their center of mass to increase the horizontal force application and ground CT and overcome the load [31]. This movement pattern defined as "Groucho running" [32] (i.e., increased trunk, knee and ankle flexion while running) could explain why VL and GM activation increased in all load condition whereas BF remained unchanged. Regarding GM, it is worth noting that this muscle plays an important role in the vertical and horizontal acceleration profiles during the stance phase in sprint acceleration [33]. The increased GM activity with heavier loads could be explained by its function as a dynamic muscle and by being the last segment of the kinetic chain trying to maintain linear momentum [20]. The present data is supported, at least in part, by Zabaloy et al. [34] that analyzed and compared the effects of unresisted and RST with 0%, 10%, 30% and 50% velocity loss (V_{loss}) in rugby players. The authors found that BF long head EMG decreased significantly as sled load increased whereas RF EMG increased. However, they did not notice any significant changes in GM and gluteus medius. Regarding resisted-parachute sprinting, it could be interesting to observe that EMG activity of the analyzed muscles remained unchanged during with different sizes. This might be related to the fact that no significant changes in running kinematics were found, despite the observed decrease in V_{max}. Still, these findings should be taken with caution as, to our knowledge, this is the first study investigating muscle activation in parachute-resisted sprinting.

Regarding kinematic analysis, the increased load caused a disruption in most variables during the sled-push. CT increased in all load conditions, as the athlete was "forced" to produce a greater muscular power and horizontal force at ground contact to overcome the higher resistance [30,34]. SL decreased even though no change in FT was found. This is not related to the idea that shorter SL is associated with decreased FT [30]. However, this exercise was performed on a treadmill; therefore, the relationship between the kinematic variables could be different than if it had been carried out overground [35]. Concerning the parachute condition, the findings herein are consistent with previous research [21], that reported that, despite parachute sprinting speed significantly decreasing by 4.4%, SF, SL, ground CT and joint angles (trunk, hip, knee and ankle) remained unchanged. In line with these results, Alcaraz et al. [15] established a 5% decreased running velocity in men and 6% on women with a medium size parachute compared to an unload sprint. Therefore, it appears that resisted-parachute sprinting caused an overload on the athlete without changing running kinematics and muscle activation patterns.

K_{leg} is a variable that plays an important role in sprint performance as it is associated with velocity, SF and energy cost [24]. In this regard, in the present study, K_{vert} decreased significantly with increasing loads. Nevertheless, caution is necessary when comparing sled-pushing and sled pulling since, despite both being effective RST exercises, they may offer different training stimuli [18]. Another aspect worth noting is that the significant reduction in A_{angle}, K_{angle} and H_{angle} herein could lead to an increased energy cost of the movement pattern as a result of a decline in the amount of stored and reused elastic energy [36]. This, together with an alteration of running kinematics and greater moments of force caused by the increased load, could raise the risk of sustaining an injury [37].

Of note, no previous research explored the use of different loads in sled-push and parachute running. Different authors have addressed this issue in other sled-resisted exercises (e.g., sled towing). For example, Cross et al. [38], using a sled towing protocol, found a range from 70–96% BM (recreational athletes: 70%; sprinters: 96%) to be optimal for power production. Opposite to these findings, Monte et al. [39] established maximal horizontal power production in male sprint athletes at 20% BM. In this study, although all kinematic parameters changed significantly with external load (CT, FT and SL), there was no variation in the angular parameters (i.e., in running technique). Importantly, caution is needed when discussing these values as optimal load is considered to be exercise-specific, therefore, the same relative intensity should not be applied to all sled-resisted exercises [40]. This could be explained by the fact that power production is affected by the biomechanical and neurophysiological characteristics of each exercise and the intrinsic characteristics of the athlete himself (training background, hypertrophy, distribution and type of fibers) [40,41]. Determining the load that maximized power production can be beneficial for programming the training; however, it is yet to be determined whether training with the optimal load in RST yields greater adaptations.

The main limitation of the present study is the small and heterogeneous sample size. A larger sample would have allowed us to get more statistical power. In addition, the non-normalization of muscle activation values could be considered a limitation. Nevertheless, the experimental context herein (i.e., comparison within a person and muscle, between different loads (within a session) without removing electrodes) allows the approach used (non-normalized data), as discussed elsewhere [42]. Future research should analyze the pattern of muscle activation during the different phases of the gait cycle while pushing the sled and sprinting with parachute so that it is possible to understand in which phases the lower limb muscles are more involved. Moreover, it would be interesting to study the long-term effects of RST on a variety of sport modalities (e.g., team-sports, athletics or endurance athletes).

5. Conclusions

In conclusion, the increased load in sled-push causes a disturbance in sprinting technique accompanied by changes in lower-limb muscle activation patterns. Conversely, sprinting with different parachute sizes does not change running kinematics and muscle activation, but it causes and overload on the athlete by increasing V_{loss}. As hypothesized, the load that maximized power production in sled-pushing was found at 55% BM. In resisted-parachute sprinting the biggest parachute size produced the highest power output.

From a practical perspective and based on our findings, increased load during the sled-push exercise in SR® treadmill modifies muscle activation, stiffness and kinematics. Therefore, depending on the training objective, we recommend strength and conditioning professionals to use: (1) very high loads (i.e., around 90% BM) to maximize the activation of the quadriceps and gastrocnemius muscles, (2) loads around 55% BM to maximize power production and (3) loads below or close to 20% BM if the objective is to improve velocity. Moreover, resisted-parachute sprinting in the SR® treadmill could be useful for improving sprint force production without compromising sprinting kinematics. The SR® treadmill was found to acutely modify muscle activation patterns and force production against the ground when performing RST. Therefore, this specialized treadmill seems to be a highly versatile device for training in different zones of the force-velocity curve.

Author Contributions: Conceptualization, A.M.-S. and P.E.A.; methodology, A.M.-S., E.M.-C. and K.S.; formal analysis, A.M.-S. and T.T.F.; investigation, A.M.-S., T.T.F. and E.M.-C.; resources, P.E.A. and E.M.-C.; data curation, A.M.-S. and K.S.; writing—original draft preparation, A.M.-S. and T.T.F.; writing—review and editing, E.M.-C., T.T.F. and P.E.A.; visualization, K.S.; supervision, P.E.A., T.T.F. and E.M.-C. All authors have read and agreed to the published version of the manuscript.

Funding: This research received no external funding.

Institutional Review Board Statement: The study was conducted according to the guidelines of the Declaration of Helsinki, and approved by the Ethics Committee of Universidad Católica San Antonio de Murcia (protocol code CE012009 and date of approval 31 January 2020).

Informed Consent Statement: Informed consent was obtained from all subjects involved in the study.

Data Availability Statement: The data presented in this study are available on request from the corresponding author.

Acknowledgments: Authors would like to thank the players and rugby club for their collaboration in the study and the company Technogym for the treadmill.

Conflicts of Interest: The authors declare no conflict of interest. The funders had no role in the design of the study; in the collection, analyses, or interpretation of data; in the writing of the manuscript, or in the decision to publish the results.

References

1. Cupples, B.; O'Connor, D. The Development of Position-Specific Performance Indicators in Elite Youth Rugby League: A Coach's Perspective. *Int. J. Sports Sci. Coach.* **2011**, *6*, 125–141. [CrossRef]
2. Duthie, G.M.; Pyne, D.B.; Marsh, D.J.; Hooper, S.L. Sprint patterns in rugby union players during competition. *J. Strength Cond. Res.* **2006**, *20*, 208–214. [CrossRef]
3. Gabbett, T.J.; Jenkins, D.G.; Abernethy, B. Physical demands of professional rugby league training and competition using microtechnology. *J. Sci. Med. Sport* **2012**, *15*, 80–86. [CrossRef]
4. Harries, S.K.; Lubans, D.R.; Buxton, A.; MacDougall, T.H.J.; Callister, R. Effects of 12-Week Resistance Training on Sprint and Jump Performances in Competitive Adolescent Rugby Union Players. *J. Strength Cond. Res.* **2018**, *32*, 2762–2769. [CrossRef]
5. von Lieres Und Wilkau, H.C.; Irwin, G.; Bezodis, N.E.; Simpson, S.; Bezodis, I.N. Phase analysis in maximal sprinting: An investigation of step-to-step technical changes between the initial acceleration, transition and maximal velocity phases. *Sports Biomech.* **2020**, *19*, 141–156. [CrossRef]
6. Lockie, R.G.; Murphy, A.J.; Callaghan, S.J.; Jeffriess, M.D. Effects of sprint and plyometrics training on field sport acceleration technique. *J. Strength Cond. Res.* **2014**, *28*, 1790–1801. [CrossRef]
7. Loturco, I.; Kobal, R.; Kitamura, K.; Cal Abad, C.C.; Faust, B.; Almeida, L.; Pereira, L.A. Mixed Training Methods: Effects of Combining Resisted Sprints or Plyometrics with Optimum Power Loads on Sprint and Agility Performance in Professional Soccer Players. *Front. Physiol.* **2017**, *8*, 1034. [CrossRef]
8. Delecluse, C. Influence of strength training on sprint running performance. Current findings and implications for training. *Sports Med.* **1997**, *24*, 147–156. [CrossRef]
9. Behm, D.G.; Sale, D.G. Intended rather than actual movement velocity determines velocity-specific training response. *J. Appl. Physiol.* **1993**, *74*, 359–368. [CrossRef]
10. Alcaraz, P.E.; Carlos-Vivas, J.; Oponjuru, B.O.; Martínez-Rodríguez, A. The Effectiveness of Resisted Sled Training (RST) for Sprint Performance: A Systematic Review and Meta-analysis. *Sports Med.* **2018**, *48*, 2143–2165. [CrossRef]
11. Lahti, J.; Jiménez-Reyes, P.; Cross, M.R.; Samozino, P.; Chassaing, P.; Simond-Cote, B.; Ahtiainen, J.P.; Morin, J.-B. Individual Sprint Force-Velocity Profile Adaptations to In-Season Assisted and Resisted Velocity-Based Training in Professional Rugby. *Sports* **2020**, *8*, 74. [CrossRef]
12. Spinks, C.D.; Murphy, A.J.; Spinks, W.L.; Lockie, R.G. The effects of resisted sprint training on acceleration performance and kinematics in soccer, rugby union, and Australian football players. *J. Strength Cond. Res.* **2007**, *21*, 77–85. [CrossRef]

13. Nicholson, B.; Dinsdale, A.; Jones, B.; Till, K. The Training of Short Distance Sprint Performance in Football Code Athletes: A Systematic Review and Meta-Analysis. *Sports Med.* **2021**, *51*, 1179–1207. [CrossRef]
14. Alcaraz, P.E.; Palao, J.M.; Elvira, J.L.; Linthorne, N.P. Effects of three types of resisted sprint training devices on the kinematics of sprinting at maximum velocity. *J. Strength Cond. Res.* **2008**, *22*, 890–897. [CrossRef]
15. Murray, A.; Aitchison, T.C.; Ross, G.; Sutherland, K.; Watt, I.; McLean, D.; Grant, S. The effect of towing a range of relative resistances on sprint performance. *J. Sports Sci.* **2005**, *23*, 927–935. [CrossRef]
16. Pareja-Blanco, F.; Pereira, L.A.; Freitas, T.T.; Alcaraz, P.E.; Reis, V.P.; Guerriero, A.; Arruda, A.F.S.; Zabaloy, S.; Sáez De Villarreal, E.; Loturco, I. Acute Effects of Progressive Sled Loading on Resisted Sprint Performance and Kinematics. *J. Strength Cond. Res.* **2020**. published ahead. [CrossRef]
17. Cahill, M.J.; Oliver, J.L.; Cronin, J.B.; Clark, K.P.; Cross, M.R.; Lloyd, R.S. Sled-Push Load-Velocity Profiling and Implications for Sprint Training Prescription in Young Athletes. *J. Strength Cond. Res.* **2020**, *35*, 3084–3089. [CrossRef]
18. Cahill, M.J.; Oliver, J.L.; Cronin, J.B.; Clark, K.P.; Cross, M.R.; Lloyd, R.S. Influence of resisted sled-push training on the sprint force-velocity profile of male high school athletes. *Scand. J. Med. Sci. Sports* **2020**, *30*, 442–449. [CrossRef]
19. Loturco, I.; Contreras, B.; Kobal, R.; Fernandes, V.; Moura, N.; Siqueira, F.; Winckler, C.; Suchomel, T.; Pereira, L.A. Vertically and horizontally directed muscle power exercises: Relationships with top-level sprint performance. *PLoS ONE* **2018**, *13*, e0201475. [CrossRef]
20. Maddigan, M.E.; Button, D.C.; Behm, D.G. Lower-limb and trunk muscle activation with back squats and weighted sled apparatus. *J. Strength Cond. Res.* **2014**, *28*, 3346–3353. [CrossRef]
21. Paulson, S.; Braun, W.A. The influence of parachute-resisted sprinting on running mechanics in collegiate track athletes. *J. Strength Cond. Res.* **2011**, *25*, 1680–1685. [CrossRef]
22. Seitz, L.B.; Mina, M.A.; Haff, G.G. A sled push stimulus potentiates subsequent 20-m sprint performance. *J. Sci. Med. Sport* **2017**, *20*, 781–785. [CrossRef]
23. Hermens, H.J.; Freriks, B.; Disselhorst-Klug, C.; Rau, G. Development of recommendations for SEMG sensors and sensor placement procedures. *J. Electromyogr. Kinesiol.* **2000**, *10*, 361–374. [CrossRef]
24. Morin, J.B.; Dalleau, G.; Kyröläinen, H.; Jeannin, T.; Belli, A. A simple method for measuring stiffness during running. *J. Appl. Biomech.* **2005**, *21*, 167–180. [CrossRef]
25. Coleman, D.R.; Cannavan, D.; Horne, S.; Blazevich, A.J. Leg stiffness in human running: Comparison of estimates derived from previously published models to direct kinematic-kinetic measures. *J. Biomech.* **2012**, *45*, 1987–1991. [CrossRef]
26. Hopkins, W.G.; Marshall, S.W.; Batterham, A.M.; Hanin, J. Progressive statistics for studies in sports medicine and exercise science. *Med. Sci. Sports Exerc.* **2009**, *41*, 3–13. [CrossRef]
27. Handsfield, G.G.; Knaus, K.R.; Fiorentino, N.M.; Meyer, C.H.; Hart, J.M.; Blemker, S.S. Adding muscle where you need it: Non-uniform hypertrophy patterns in elite sprinters. *Scand. J. Med. Sci. Sports* **2017**, *27*, 1050–1060. [CrossRef] [PubMed]
28. Tottori, N.; Suga, T.; Miyake, Y.; Tsuchikane, R.; Otsuka, M.; Nagano, A.; Fujita, S.; Isaka, T. Hip Flexor and Knee Extensor Muscularity Are Associated With Sprint Performance in Sprint-Trained Preadolescent Boys. *Pediatr. Exerc. Sci.* **2018**, *30*, 115–123. [CrossRef] [PubMed]
29. Nagahara, R.; Matsubayashi, T.; Matsuo, A.; Zushi, K. Kinematics of transition during human accelerated sprinting. *Biol. Open* **2014**, *3*, 689–699. [CrossRef] [PubMed]
30. Lockie, R.G.; Murphy, A.J.; Spinks, C.D. Effects of resisted sled towing on sprint kinematics in field-sport athletes. *J. Strength Cond. Res.* **2003**, *17*, 760–767. [CrossRef]
31. Bentley, I.; Sinclair, J.K.; Atkins, S.J.; Metcalfe, J.; Edmundson, C.J. Effect of Velocity-Based Loading on Acceleration Kinetics and Kinematics During Sled Towing. *J. Strength Cond. Res.* **2021**, *35*, 1030–1038. [CrossRef]
32. McMahon, T.A.; Valiant, G.; Frederick, E.C. Groucho running. *J. Appl. Physiol.* **1987**, *62*, 2326–2337. [CrossRef]
33. Hamner, S.R.; Delp, S.L. Muscle contributions to fore-aft and vertical body mass center accelerations over a range of running speeds. *J. Biomech.* **2013**, *46*, 780–787. [CrossRef]
34. Zabaloy, S.; Carlos-Vivas, J.; Freitas, T.T.; Pareja-Blanco, F.; Loturco, I.; Comyns, T.; Gálvez-González, J.; Alcaraz, P.E. Muscle Activity, Leg Stiffness, and Kinematics During Unresisted and Resisted Sprinting Conditions. *J. Strength Cond. Res.* **2020**. published ahead. [CrossRef] [PubMed]
35. Bailey, J.; Mata, T.; Mercer, J.A. Is the Relationship Between Stride Length, Frequency, and Velocity Influenced by Running on a Treadmill or Overground? *Int. J. Exerc. Sci.* **2017**, *10*, 1067–1075.
36. Turner, A.N.; Jeffreys, I. The Stretch-Shortening Cycle: Proposed Mechanisms and Methods for Enhancement. *Strength Cond. J.* **2010**, *32*, 87–99. [CrossRef]
37. Huygaerts, S.; Cos, F.; Cohen, D.D.; Calleja-González, J.; Guitart, M.; Blazevich, A.J.; Alcaraz, P.E. Mechanisms of Hamstring Strain Injury: Interactions between Fatigue, Muscle Activation and Function. *Sports* **2020**, *8*, 65. [CrossRef] [PubMed]
38. Cross, M.R.; Brughelli, M.; Samozino, P.; Brown, S.R.; Morin, J.B. Optimal Loading for Maximizing Power During Sled-Resisted Sprinting. *Int. J. Sports Physiol. Perform.* **2017**, *12*, 1069–1077. [CrossRef] [PubMed]
39. Monte, A.; Nardello, F.; Zamparo, P. Sled Towing: The Optimal Overload for Peak Power Production. *Int. J. Sports Physiol. Perform.* **2017**, *12*, 1052–1058. [CrossRef]

40. Izquierdo, M.; Häkkinen, K.; Gonzalez-Badillo, J.J.; Ibáñez, J.; Gorostiaga, E.M. Effects of long-term training specificity on maximal strength and power of the upper and lower extremities in athletes from different sports. *Eur. J. Appl. Physiol.* **2002**, *87*, 264–271. [CrossRef]
41. Soriano, M.A.; Jiménez-Reyes, P.; Rhea, M.R.; Marín, P.J. The Optimal Load for Maximal Power Production During Lower-Body Resistance Exercises: A Meta-Analysis. *Sports Med.* **2015**, *45*, 1191–1205. [CrossRef] [PubMed]
42. Besomi, M.; Hodges, P.W.; Clancy, E.A.; Van Dieën, J.; Hug, F.; Lowery, M.; Merletti, R.; Søgaard, K.; Wrigley, T.; Besier, T.; et al. Consensus for experimental design in electromyography (CEDE) project: Amplitude normalization matrix. *J. Electromyogr. Kinesiol.* **2020**, *53*, 102438. [CrossRef] [PubMed]

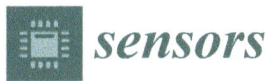

Article

Orientation-Invariant Spatio-Temporal Gait Analysis Using Foot-Worn Inertial Sensors

Vânia Guimarães [1,2,*], Inês Sousa [1] and Miguel Velhote Correia [2,3]

1 Fraunhofer Portugal AICOS, 4200-135 Porto, Portugal; ines.sousa@fraunhofer.pt
2 Faculty of Engineering, University of Porto, 4200-465 Porto, Portugal; mcorreia@fe.up.pt
3 Institute for Systems and Computer Engineering, Technology and Science (INESC TEC), 4200-465 Porto, Portugal
* Correspondence: vania.guimaraes@fraunhofer.pt

Abstract: Inertial sensors can potentially assist clinical decision making in gait-related disorders. Methods for objective spatio-temporal gait analysis usually assume the careful alignment of the sensors on the body, so that sensor data can be evaluated using the body coordinate system. Some studies infer sensor orientation by exploring the cyclic characteristics of walking. In addition to being unrealistic to assume that the sensor can be aligned perfectly with the body, the robustness of gait analysis with respect to differences in sensor orientation has not yet been investigated—potentially hindering use in clinical settings. To address this gap in the literature, we introduce an orientation-invariant gait analysis approach and propose a method to quantitatively assess robustness to changes in sensor orientation. We validate our results in a group of young adults, using an optical motion capture system as reference. Overall, good agreement between systems is achieved considering an extensive set of gait metrics. Gait speed is evaluated with a relative error of -3.1 ± 9.2 cm/s, but precision improves when turning strides are excluded from the analysis, resulting in a relative error of -3.4 ± 6.9 cm/s. We demonstrate the invariance of our approach by simulating rotations of the sensor on the foot.

Keywords: gait analysis; gait parameters; IMU; inertial sensors; orientation-invariant; sensor fusion

1. Introduction

Objective measurement of gait is fundamental for human motion analysis, with applications in clinical research, sports, rehabilitation, health diagnosis, and others [1]. The traditional approach for quantitative gait analysis, mostly based on the use of optical motion capture systems, was proven to be clinically relevant, however, these systems are often restricted to the laboratory setting [2]. In the clinical setting, visual observation, questionnaires or simple functional tests are commonly employed [2]. Although these evaluations require simple instruments and are easy to perform, subtle changes in spatio-temporal gait parameters (e.g., associated with geriatric syndromes like falls [3], cognitive impairment [4], or frailty [5]) can easily go undetected [2].

Inertial sensor-based gait analysis has become highly attractive in the past years, and constitutes a promising approach to assist clinical decision making for gait-related disorders in ageing [2]. Gait parameters such as gait speed, stride length, cadence, swing width, or foot clearance, can be obtained from the analysis of inertial sensor data [6–9], offering a cheaper and unrestricted alternative to gait analysis that may fit either assessment in clinical settings or continuous monitoring in daily life activities [2,10]. However, inertial sensors are susceptible to noise, and complex algorithms are needed to reliably measure gait parameters [11].

To handle errors, studies typically exploit the cyclic nature of gait and the hypothesis that the velocity of the sensor—when placed on the foot—is zero when the foot is in contact with the ground (i.e., at some point in stance) [12]. Zero velocity intervals (ZVIs) are then used to improve the methods for estimating sensor orientation [6,8,13] and reconstructing displacement [6–8,14–16]—required to evaluate spatio-temporal parameters of walking.

Even though the orientation of the sensor relative to the Earth frame can be obtained using appropriate sensor fusion methods [17,18], the orientation of the sensor relative to the movement direction or relative to the body part, is typically unknown. In some situations, for instance, when a smartphone is used to monitor users' motion, the sensor orientation and position relative to the body may be changing over time, which requires specific methods to identify the users' motion direction with respect to the sensor. Methods based on the ellipsoidal shape of horizontal components of acceleration [19], or based on sinusoidal approximations of the acceleration data [20] have been proposed in the literature, with direct applications on pedestrian dead reckoning. When the sensor is placed on the feet, other techniques can be used. Falbriard et al. [21] proposes an automatic calibration process, in which the Principal Component Analysis (PCA) is used to find the foot medio-lateral axis based on the angular rates acquired during gait. In [11], the foot orientation vector is estimated using a particle filter. Although [11,21] claim that the methods they propose enable the use of sensors in a robust and reproducible manner, reproducibility is not assessed by the authors.

Most studies assume that at least one sensor axis is aligned with the body—typically the medio-lateral axis when the sensor is placed on the feet. Based on this assumption, the medio-lateral angular rate and/or forward-anterior acceleration can be directly determined, and used to detect gait events [8,15]. Sagittal foot angle can also be obtained [14], from which heel and toe clearance metrics can be calculated [9,22]. The inertial coordinate system at the beginning of each gait cycle can be used as a base coordinate system (aligned with the medio-lateral and forward-anterior axis of the body), relative to which foot orientation and trajectories can be determined [15,16]. Besides assuming a known configuration, the extent to which algorithms depend on the precise alignment of the sensors has not yet been investigated.

Another approach for gait analysis relies on data-driven procedures. These methods require training in a relevant dataset, using features extracted from inertial sensor data [23] or, in case of using sufficiently deep architectures, regressing directly against raw sensor data [24]. In both cases, generalization is possible only if sufficient and representative data are given to the model, allowing it to learn from the data. Studies that employ data-driven approaches train their models without considering multiple sensor orientations [23,24], so their final models may not be robust to differences in orientation. However, assuming precise alignment of the sensors on the body seems unrealistic in practice.

In this paper, we approach the topic of orientation-invariance explicitly. We introduce an orientation-invariant gait analysis approach relying on inertial sensors placed on the shoes and validate results in a group of young adults, using an optical motion capture system as reference. We propose a method to quantitatively evaluate invariance to differences in orientation and demonstrate it by simulating rotations of the sensor on the foot. Experiments and results are presented in this work, together with a critical interpretation; findings are described considering the research problem being addressed and past work within the topic.

2. Materials and Methods
2.1. Wearable Sensors

Acceleration and angular rate were measured using two inertial measurement units (IMUs). The IMUs were developed in our lab, and incorporated a 32-bit Arm Cortex M4F processor (Nordic nRF52). The device was equipped with a tri-axial gyroscope and a tri-axial accelerometer (Bosch BMI160), and communicated with a computer via Bluetooth® Low Energy, enabling data collection at a sampling rate of 100 Hz. Sensors were placed on the shoes, near the foot instep, as shown in Figure 1.

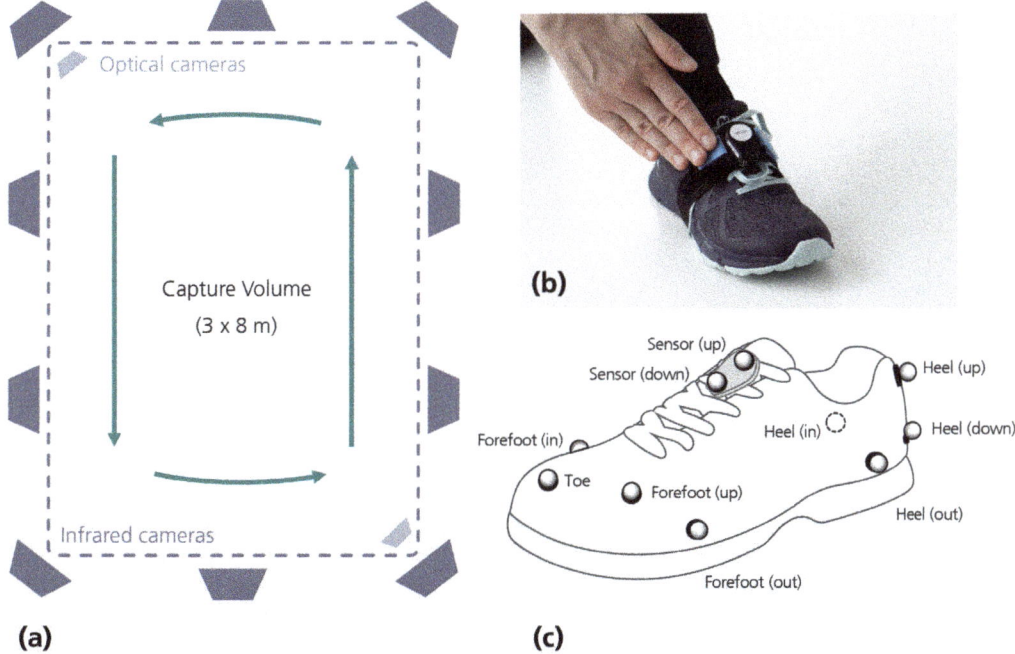

Figure 1. Wearable sensors and reference system: (**a**) Capture volume and camera installation. (**b**) Sensor placement. (**c**) Marker placement.

2.2. Reference System

As a reference system, we used an optical motion capture system (Vicon, Oxford Metrics). It consisted of 10 infrared cameras (Vicon Vero v2.2), plus 2 optical cameras (Vicon Vue), installed as illustrated in Figure 1, which resulted in a capture volume of around 3 per 8 m. Optical markers were placed on participants' shoes as illustrated in Figure 1.

The trajectories of the markers were captured at 100 Hz and post-processed using Vicon Nexus (Vicon Motion Systems Ltd., Version 2.10.1). Post-processing included automatic marker labelling, manual marker swapping correction and gap filling operations, using the methods of spline, rigid body and pattern fill available in Vicon Nexus.

After post-processing, gait parameters were automatically extracted from trajectories using a Python routine. The pipeline started with the identification of steady periods to segment signals into strides, which involved the application of thresholds to the velocity of the markers. It was followed by horizontal plane correction, where the normal (vertical) vector corresponded to the second principal axis obtained using Principal Component Analysis (PCA); PCA was applied to the position vectors–obtained from the heel (down) marker–formed between two successive steady states. Before determining gait events and calculating gait parameters, trajectories were low pass filtered using a zero-lag bidirectional first order Butterworth filter (cutoff of 20 Hz).

Initial foot contact (FC) and foot off (FO) were automatically detected, using as reference the trajectories from the markers on the heel (down) and toe. The FC instant was considered a minimum in heel vertical velocity [25], whereas the FO event was considered a maximum in vertical toe acceleration [26]. Temporal gait metrics—*stride, swing and stance duration*—were calculated as defined in [14]. *Cadence* was obtained as the inverse of stride duration, converted to the units of steps per minute.

The trajectories of the heel (down), toe and sensor centroid were used to evaluate spatial parameters, as illustrated in Figure 2: (i) *Stride length* (SL) was described as the linear distance obtained between two successive horizontal mid-stance sensor positions (as defined in [27]); (ii) *Turning angle* was defined as the angle (yaw) between two successive horizontal mid-stance foot vectors that were obtained from the positions of the heel and toe at mid-stance; (iii) *Swing width* (SW) was considered the maximum lateral excursion of the feet during swing, corresponding to the maximum-size vector perpendicular to the stride length direction; (iv) *Minimum toe clearance (MTC)* was obtained directly from toe trajectories, considered as the minimum peak vertical displacement during swing, to which the toe height at toe off was subtracted. *Gait speed* was obtained by dividing stride length by its corresponding stride duration.

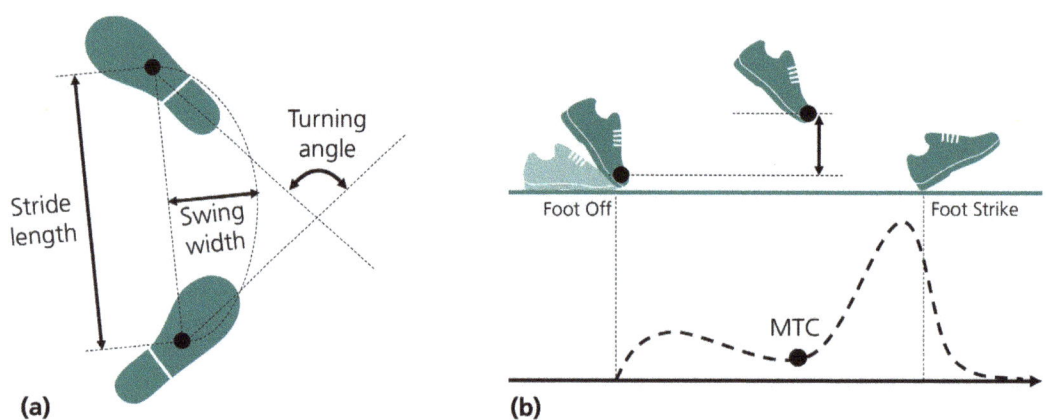

Figure 2. Illustration of spatial gait parameters: (**a**) Stride length, swing width and turning angle. (**b**) Minimum toe clearance (MTC).

All parameters were reported per stride, and calculated individually for each foot side.

2.3. Data Collection

A convenient sample of 26 healthy young adults (average age of 29.2 ± 5.3 years, 13 males and 13 females) participated in data collection activities. After calibrating Vicon cameras and preparing the system for data acquisition, we placed the sensors and markers on the shoes, as shown in Figure 1. This was followed by a short static subject calibration trial. Afterwards, we asked the participant to do three consecutive laps, during which Vicon and IMU data were collected simultaneously. In each lap, participants were requested to walk straight along the length of the capture volume (i.e., along the 8 m) and use the width of the capture volume to turn (as illustrated in Figure 1). Participants repeated the walking trials in both directions—clockwise and counterclockwise—walking at comfortable, slower and faster speeds (self-selected), which resulted in 6 acquisitions per participant. All conditions were then repeated once. The study received approval by the Ethical Committee of the University of Porto (81/CEUP/2019) and all participants provided written informed consent.

2.4. IMU Data Processing

The following sections describe the methods for IMU data processing, inspired by typical gait analysis routines—including the stages of zero velocity detection, orientation estimation, double integration, events detection, and gait parameters estimation. The processing pipeline included evaluation of different approaches for orientation estimation and double integration. Every stage was formulated using an orientation-invariant approach.

2.4.1. Zero Velocity Detection

Zero velocity intervals (ZVIs) were detected using the angular rate energy detector [28]. According to [28], angular rate provides rich information concerning the detection of ZVIs. Compared to other methods (e.g., the acceleration magnitude detector), the angular rate energy detector achieved the highest performance [28].

To calculate the energy of the angular rate magnitude, we used a sliding window with 0.15 s. The size of the window was experimentally set to ensure an appropriate energy result, i.e., not too smoothed, nor too noisy. The window size of 0.15 s resulted in a good compromise that could adapt to all walking speeds considered. To determine ZVIs, a threshold was applied to the energy of the angular rate magnitude. The threshold was calculated with basis on the average of the energy, to ensure that differences in walking speed (reflected as different signal amplitudes) would be considered. The threshold was experimentally set at 1/8 of the average, to ensure that all strides in all velocities would be captured by the method.

After roughly detecting ZVIs, we proceeded with a dynamic adjustment of the intervals. For each ZVI, we did a threshold refinement search: starting with a very low threshold, we have progressively increased it (in steps of 1/20 of the ZVI energy range), until a minimum interval size was obtained. The minimum interval size was set at 0.1 s, unless an interval lower than 0.1 s was registered in the trial. Using this process, we ensured a confident detection of all strides and, additionally, that all ZVIs were refined to potentially include only zero velocity instants. The remaining intervals, i.e., the moving intervals, were used to evaluate movement in the subsequent processing stages.

2.4.2. Orientation Estimation

Orientation, or attitude, of the sensor relative to the global frame of reference was expressed using quaternions. The global frame of reference was defined by two perpendicular horizontal axes (x and y)—arbitrarily set—and a vertical axis, z, pointing to the sky. To obtain quaternions, we tested three methods: gyroscope integration and two complementary filters (CFs)—Madgwick and Euston.

Gyroscope Integration

The gyroscope integration method takes advantage of the knowledge of the moving and not-moving intervals. When the sensor is not moving (i.e., during a ZVI)—when all measured accelerations are due to the Earth's gravity acceleration—the accelerometer signal is used to estimate sensor inclination. The vector $g_s = [\bar{a}_x, \bar{a}_y, \bar{a}_x]$, defined with the average acceleration values measured while the sensor is not moving, corresponds to the z-axis in the global frame of reference, i.e., the gravity axis. The horizontal axis—y-axis, perpendicular to gravity—is then defined arbitrarily. The initial quaternion is obtained from gravity and the horizontal vector, using the tri-axial attitude determination (TRIAD) algorithm [29].

The initial quaternion is updated each time the foot is in contact with the ground. During the intervals when the foot is moving, the quaternion $q(t)$ is updated resorting to the integration of angular rate $\omega(t)$ measured by the gyroscope, as described in [8,13]. This is performed as defined by Equations (1) and (2):

$$\dot{q}(t) = \frac{1}{2} q(t - \Delta t) \otimes p(\omega(t)) \tag{1}$$

$$q(t) = \frac{q(t - \Delta t) + \dot{q}(t)\Delta t}{||q(t - \Delta t) + \dot{q}(t)\Delta t||} \tag{2}$$

where $\dot{q}(t)$ is the quaternion derivative and Δt is the sampling interval. The function $p(.)$ denotes the quaternion representation of a vector and the $\otimes$ operator represents the quaternion product.

Madgwick CF

In Madgwick [30], the quaternion derivative $\dot{q}(t)$ used in Equation (2) is replaced by a corrected estimate $\dot{\hat{q}}(t)$ that incorporates orientation information provided by the accelerometer. The method is based on the calculation of the gradient descent, as shown in Equation (3).

$$\dot{\hat{q}}(t) = \dot{q}(t) - \beta \frac{\Delta \varepsilon(t)}{\|\Delta \varepsilon(t)\|} \quad \text{with} \quad \Delta \varepsilon(t) = J(\varepsilon(t))^T \varepsilon(t) \tag{3}$$

where J denotes the Jacobian, β is the filter gain and $\varepsilon(t)$ denotes the error term, obtained by subtracting the accelerometer measurement in the sensor frame $a_s(t)$ to the theoretical gravity vector in sensor coordinates $g_s(t)$ (obtained by transforming gravity in global coordinates to sensor coordinates). β can be defined as $\beta = \sqrt{3/4}\, \tilde{\omega}_{max} \pi / 180$, where $\tilde{\omega}_{max}$, expressed in degrees, represents the maximum gyroscope measurement error (mean zero gyroscope measurement error).

The Madgwick filter is applied at all instants of the signal (moving and not moving intervals) considering as basis the initial quaternion determined using TRIAD, as described previously.

Euston CF

The explicit complementary filter, also known as Euston filter, was implemented as described in [13,18]. In Euston, instead of replacing the value of the quaternion, the measured angular rate $\omega(t)$ is replaced by a corrected angular rate signal, resulting in the following filter dynamics:

$$\dot{\hat{q}}(t) = \frac{1}{2}\hat{q}(t - \Delta t) \otimes p(\omega(t) + \delta(t)) \tag{4}$$

in which the error term δ is obtained following Equations (5) and (6), where the term $e(t)$ describes the angular mismatch between theoretical ($g_s(t)$) and measured ($a_s(t)$) direction of gravity [18].

$$e(t) = \frac{g_s(t)}{\|g_s(t)\|} \times \frac{a_s(t)}{\|a_s(t)\|} \tag{5}$$

$$\delta(t) = k_P e(t) + k_I \int e(t) dt \tag{6}$$

The Euston filter has two adjustable parameters, the proportional gain k_P—to separate low- and high-frequency estimates of orientation—and the integrator gain k_I—to compensate for gyroscope bias [13,18]. Similarly to the Madgwick filter, we apply Euston to all instants of the signal, considering as basis the initial quaternion determined using TRIAD [29].

2.4.3. Double Integration

After obtaining orientation quaternions, $q(t)$, we calculate linear acceleration in global coordinates, hereinafter represented as $a(t)$ for simplicity. To that purpose, we first estimate the value of the gravity vector in global coordinates, $g_w = [0, 0, \bar{a}_{zv}]$, where $\bar{a}_{zv}$ is the average acceleration magnitude measured during ZVIs. Linear acceleration is then obtained as shown in Equation (7).

$$a(t) = q(t) \otimes p(a_s(t)) \otimes q^{-1}(t) - g_w \tag{7}$$

where $a_s(t)$ represents raw acceleration, as measured by the sensor.

To obtain displacements, we integrate linear acceleration two times. On the first integration, an estimate of velocity, $\hat{v}(t)$, is obtained. Integrals are computed using the Trapezoidal Rule, as shown in Equation (8).

$$\hat{v}(t) \approx \sum_i \frac{a_i + a_{i-1}}{2} \Delta t \qquad (8)$$

To bound the errors, two different methods—linear dedrifting and direct and reverse integration—are employed, as we explain next. After obtaining trajectories, a novel approach to correct the final vertical position (assuming walking on a flat surface) is tested. The method rotates the trajectories so that the final height of each stride is zero. To that purpose, a rotation quaternion is calculated, using as basis the angle with the horizontal plane at the end of the stride and the rotation vector calculated as the cross product between the vertical axis and the stride displacement vector. The rotation quaternion is used to rotate trajectories within each moving interval.

Linear Dedrifting

Double integration is performed between ZVIs, on a stride-by-stride basis. To fulfil the zero-velocity assumption—on which moving intervals are bounded by zero velocity instants—a linear drift function ($d_v(t)$) is estimated and subtracted from the estimated velocity, as described in [14] and shown in Equation (9).

$$v(t) = \hat{v}(t) - d_v(t) \qquad (9)$$

Trajectory $s(t)$ is obtained by integrating again velocity $v(t)$.

Direct and Reverse Integration

The direct and reverse integration method fuses the regular integral with a time-reversed integral so that the boundary conditions, in this case, the zero-velocity conditions, are satisfied in the initial and final values of the integral [15,16]. The result of direct ($v_\rightarrow(t)$) and reverse ($v_\leftarrow(t)$) integration is combined using a sigmoid weighting function ($w(t)$), as shown in Equation (10).

$$v(t) = (1 - w(t))v_\rightarrow(t) + w(t)v_\leftarrow(t) \qquad (10)$$

The sigmoid $w(t)$, specified in Equation (11), is shaped using the steepness parameter, η, and the inflection point, t_i, defined between the temporal bounds t_n and t_{n+1} of each moving interval. To define t_i, a proportion α_i, between 0 and 1, of the moving interval is used.

$$w(t) = \frac{h(t) - h(t_n)}{h(t_{n+1}) - h(t_n)} \quad \text{with} \quad h(t) = \left(1 + \exp\left(-\frac{t - t_i}{\eta}\right)\right)^{-1} \qquad (11)$$

Position is estimated by integrating velocity.

2.4.4. Events Detection

To detect gait events avoiding the need of determining angular rate or acceleration in body coordinates (where the alignment of the sensor on the body would need to be known [8,15,16]), we used acceleration magnitude and the vertical component of acceleration (in global coordinates).

We observed that FO events can generally be found in an acceleration magnitude perturbation before swing. To approximate this instant, we filtered acceleration magnitude using a zero-lag bidirectional 2nd order Butterworth low-pass filter with a cutoff of 7 Hz. The cutoff frequency was experimentally chosen to ensure that (i) the perturbations were smoothed resulting in a single peak value, and (ii) the resultant peak approximates the acceleration magnitude perturbation where annotated FO events are observed. The FO event was considered the first maximum peak above the average of the moving interval appearing between two ZVIs (i.e., the first value above the average surrounded by two values with lower magnitude), as illustrated in Figure 3.

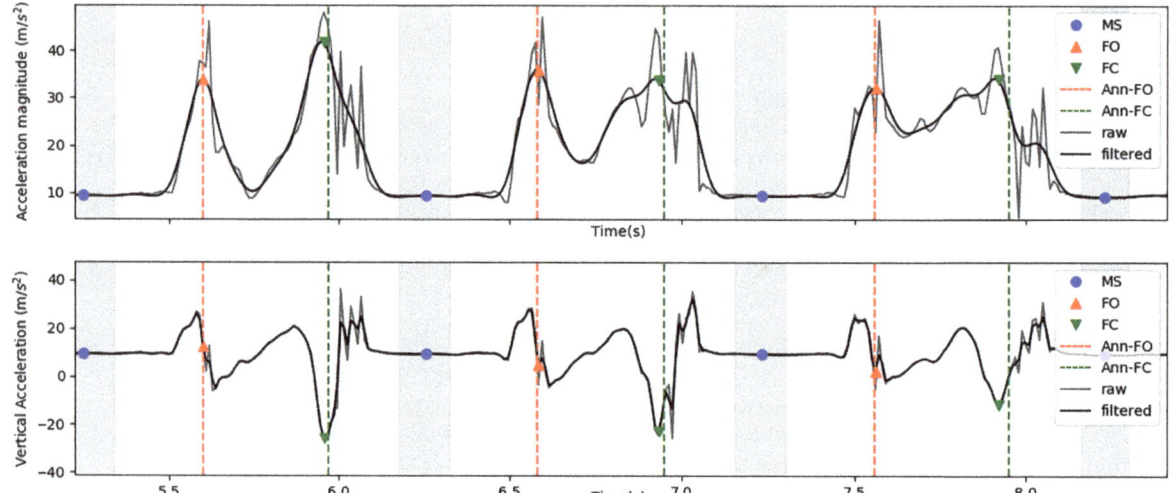

Figure 3. Events detection from low pass filtered acceleration magnitude and low pass filtered vertical acceleration (*FO*—Foot off; *FC*—Initial foot contact; *MS*—Mid-stance; *Ann-FO*—Annotated FO; *Ann-FC*—Annotated FC).

FCs are detected between FOs and the beginnings of the next ZVIs. FCs were considered the absolute minimum of vertical acceleration measured between these two instants (Figure 3). Before detecting FC events, vertical acceleration was low-pass filtered using a zero-lag bidirectional 1st order Butterworth filter with a cutoff of 30 Hz. The cutoff frequency was experimentally chosen to ensure the attenuation of high frequency noise that could hinder the detection of FC events.

2.4.5. Gait Parameters Estimation

After calculating orientation, position and determining FO and FC events, temporal and spatial parameters were estimated for each gait cycle n. Temporal parameters—stride, swing and stance duration—were determined as defined in [14]. Cadence was obtained as the inverse of stride duration, expressed in steps per minute. Spatial parameters (illustrated in Figure 2) were calculated using information of moving intervals, defined by the temporal bounds of t_n and t_{n+1}. To estimate SL and SW, we used trajectories on the horizontal plane, s_{xy}, as determined by Equations (12) and (13), where $\vec{s}_n(t)$ represents a displacement vector relative to the final stride position at t_{n+1}, obtained as $s_{xy}(t_{n+1}) - s_{xy}(t)$). In Equation (13), the symbol $\angle$ denotes the angle between two vectors.

$$SL_n = \|\vec{s}_n(t_n)\| \tag{12}$$

$$SW_n = \max_{t \in \{FO_n : FC_{n+1}\}} \|\vec{s}_n(t)\| \sin(\angle(\vec{s}_n(t_n), \vec{s}_n(t)) \tag{13}$$

Gait speed was obtained by dividing SL by its corresponding stride duration.

To calculate MTC, we used a method inspired on the work by Kanzler, C. [9]. To estimate toe trajectory, we have first estimated the distance between the sensor and the toe, r, using as a basis the angle produced by the foot at FO, $\alpha(FO_n)$, in each gait cycle n, as illustrated in Figure 4.

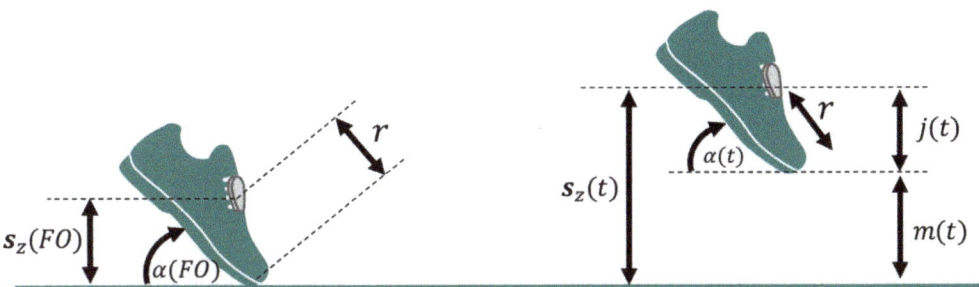

Figure 4. Variables involved in the calculation of toe trajectory.

To obtain the angle $\alpha(t)$, we did a series of vector transformations. First, we have converted the vertical vector $[0, 0, 1]$ to sensor coordinates, using the quaternion at the beginning of the moving interval, i.e., at the foot flat at t_n. Then, we transformed the resultant vector back to global coordinates using the quaternion at FO. This vector, $\vec{v}_w$, was used to estimate the medio-lateral vector, $\vec{l}_w$, using the cross product between $\vec{v}_w$ and $[0, 0, 1]$. The forward vector, $\vec{f}_w$, was calculated using the cross product between $[0, 0, 1]$ and $\vec{l}_w$, which was then converted back to sensor coordinates using the quaternion at t_n. This vector, $\vec{f}_s$, parallel to the ground at foot flat and pointing forward towards the toes, was used to estimate the angle $\alpha(t)$, as depicted in Equation (14).

$$\alpha(t) = \angle([0,0,1], \vec{v}) - \alpha(t_n) \quad \text{with} \quad \vec{v} = q(t) \otimes p(\vec{f}_s) \otimes q(t)^{-1} \quad \text{and} \quad t \in [t_n : t_{n+1}] \quad (14)$$

The distance between the sensor and the toe (r) was obtained by the average of the values determined in each stride n, as shown in Equation (15).

$$r = \frac{1}{N} \sum_{n=1}^{N} \frac{s_z(FO_n)}{\sin(\alpha(FO_n))} \quad (15)$$

where N is the total number of strides and $s_z(t)$ represents the z component of the trajectory of the sensor (i.e., its vertical displacement). MTC was considered the minimum peak vertical toe displacement measured during the swing phase of walking. This vertical displacement, $m(t)$, was estimated as shown in Equation (16), where $r \times \sin(\alpha(t))$ represents the vertical distance between the sensor and the toe (shown as $j(t)$ in Figure 4).

$$MTC_n = \min_{t \in \{FO_n : FC_{n+1}\}} m(t) \quad \text{with} \quad m(t) = \begin{cases} s_z(t) - r \times \sin(\alpha(t)) & \text{if } \alpha(t) > 0 \\ s_z(t) + r \times \sin(\alpha(t)) & \text{otherwise} \end{cases} \quad (16)$$

To calculate turning angles, we converted an arbitrary horizontal vector (e.g., the vector $[0, 1, 0]$) to sensor coordinates, using as basis the quaternions estimated at t_n and at t_{n+1}. The resultant vectors represented the orientation of the sensor in the horizontal plane, so that the angle between these two vectors corresponded to the turning angle.

2.5. Experiments

One hundred and sixty of the collected samples were post-processed using Vicon Nexus, and used as reference for IMU-based gait analysis evaluation. To avoid overfitting, we split data into development and validation sets. Approximately 30% of the samples, from uniquely randomly selected users, were included in the development set, and used for algorithm design, debug and optimization. The remaining 70% were used for validation and orientation-invariance proof. The resulting dataset split is shown in Table 1.

Table 1. Dataset characteristics after splitting.

Metric	Development Set (7 Subjects/45 Samples)	Validation Set (19 Subjects/115 Samples)
Height (cm)	168.9 ± 7.7	172.5 ± 9.2
Gender (female/male)	4/3	9/10
Weight (kg)	67.3 ± 15.4	71.1 ± 14.7
Foot size (cm)	27.4 ± 1.6	27.8 ± 2.0

To compare gait parameters extracted from the IMU with those extracted from Vicon, systems were first synchronized. To this purpose, we used the cross-correlation between acceleration magnitude—obtained from the IMU—and the centroid of the sensor markers—obtained after deriving the centroid trajectory two times; the maximum cross-correlation was used to compensate for the time-shift between data sources, as in [6].

A tolerance of 0.1s was employed to classify FC events (and its corresponding stride gait parameters) as true positive cases. Only the strides whose FC time was consistent with those obtained with Vicon were considered for comparison. Reference strides without any corresponding IMU-derived candidate were classified as not detected.

2.5.1. Parameter Tuning and Algorithm Selection

The development set was used to tune parameters, and select the most reliable methods for orientation estimation and double integration. As shown in Section 2.4.2, the possible orientation estimation methods were the Madgwick CF, the Euston CF and the gyroscope integration, which could be used in combination with two possible double integration methods: the direct and reverse integration, and the linear dedrifting—both presented in Section 2.4.3. Additionally, the horizontal correction method presented in Section 2.4.3 could or not be employed. Each method—with the exception of gyroscope integration and linear dedrifting—included a set of parameters (also detailed in Sections 2.4.2 and 2.4.3) that needed to be optimized in view to improve the performance of the gait analysis method. Using a grid-search approach, all possible combination of methods (i.e., orientation estimation and double integration methods) and a set of candidate parameters could be tested, where the number of resultant combinations depended on the number for parameters tested. For this reason, parameter tuning was first performed using a coarse grid of parameters—i.e., a small amount of candidate parameters covering a wider range of values. The most promising combinations of parameters and methods were used to define a finer grid that considered candidate parameters defined in the neighbourhood of the best parameter configurations. Parameters tested within coarse (resulting in 140 combinations) and fine grid-search (resulting in 105 combinations) are shown in Table 2.

Table 2. Methods and parameters used in coarse and fine grid-search.

Type	Methods	Coarse Grid-Search	Fine Grid-Search
Orientation estimation	Madgwick CF	$\bar{\omega}_{max} = \{2, 4, 6\}$	$\bar{\omega}_{max} = \{1.0, 1.5, 2.0, 2.5, 3.0\}$
	Euston CF	$k_P = \{0.2, 0.4, 0.6\}$ $k_I = \{0, 0.05\}$	$k_P = \{0.15, 0.2, 0.25\}$ $k_I = \{0, 0.01\}$
Double integration	Gyroscope integration	Not applicable	Not applicable
	Direct and reverse integration	$\eta = \{0.1, 0.2\}$ $\alpha_i = \{0.4, 0.5, 0.6\}$	$\eta = \{0.15, 0.2, 0.25\}$ $\alpha_i = 0.55, 0.6, 0.65$
	Linear dedrifting	Not applicable	Not applicable
	Horizontal correction	{True, False}	{True}

To select the best combination of parameters and methods, we calculated the root mean square error (RMSE) between IMU-derived and reference gait parameters. The RMSE of each parameter was normalized by the average of the reference, and then averaged to obtain a single score per configuration. The minimum normalized RMSE defined the most appropriate set of parameters and methods.

2.5.2. Instrument Comparison and Validation

We compared gait parameters extracted from the IMU with those extracted from Vicon using the validation set. For each cycle, we estimated the difference between IMU-derived and reference gait parameters. Accuracy (mean of relative and absolute error) and precision (standard deviation of relative and absolute error) were reported for each parameter. Agreement between the two instruments was assessed using 95% limits of agreement, as introduced by Bland Altman [31]. Data were assessed for normal distribution using Shapiro–Wilk tests, to decide for the use of parametric or non-parametric tests. Correlation between instruments was calculated using the correlation coefficients of Pearson (r_p)—in case of normal distribution—or Spearman (r_s)—when data could not be assumed to be normally distributed. We have also reported RMSE and equivalence tests using an equivalence zone of ±5% of the average of the metric. Equivalence tests were based on Paired T-test (T)—for parametric—or Wilcoxon signed-rank test (W)—for non-parametric.

To validate results in a scenario where only straight walking is considered for gait assessment (as required to assess several gait disorders [32]), we repeated validation tests without including turns. For this purpose, a turning stride was considered a stride where the turning angle (as measured by the reference system) was above 20 degrees (as in [7]).

A significance level (p-value) of 5% was used to evaluate results.

2.5.3. Orientation Invariance

To test for orientation invariance, we simulated multiple rotations of the IMU on the shoes. For that purpose, we sampled uniform random rotations (quaternions), as suggested by Shoemake, K. [33], and used those quaternions to synthetically rotate raw inertial sensor data. To evaluate the performance of the system when IMUs were placed at random rotations, we compare gait parameters extracted from the original sensor orientation with those extracted from a rotated version of the sensor. To quantify differences, we calculated the Root Mean Square Deviation (RMSD), correlation (using Pearson-parametric- or Spearman-non-parametric) and equivalence tests using a stricter equivalence zone of ±1% of the average of the metric. Equivalence tests were based on Paired T-test (T)—for parametric—or Wilcoxon signed-rank test (W)—for non-parametric. To choose an appropriate test, samples were first tested for normal distribution using Shapiro–Wilk; non-parametric tests were chosen in case of non-normal distribution. A significance level (p-value) of 5% was used to evaluate results.

3. Results

3.1. Algorithm Selection and Parameter Tuning

The most promising combinations of parameters and methods were defined by the results of the coarse grid-search. We selected the best performing combinations considering the minimum normalized RMSE achieved by each candidate method. The best combinations in coarse grid-search were: (i) the Madgwick CF ($\tilde{\omega}_{max} = 2.0$) combined with direct and reverse integration ($\eta = 0.2$, $\alpha_i = 0.6$) or with linear dedrifting methods; (ii) the Euston CF ($k_P = 0.2$, $k_I = 0$) combined with direct and reverse integration ($\eta = 0.2$, $\alpha_i = 0.6$); and (iii) the gyroscope integration combined with linear dedrifting, all with active horizontal correction. The second optimization was performed using a finer grid of parameters (shown in Table 2), defined on the vicinity of the best performing combinations. The resulting best combination of methods and parameters was the Euston CF ($k_P^{opt} = 0.15$, $k_I^{opt} = 0$) with direct and reverse integration ($\eta^{opt} = 0.25$, $\alpha_i^{opt} = 0.55$) and active horizontal correction. The RMSE values obtained in the development set using this parameter configuration are shown in Table 3.

Table 3. Performance on the development set, using the best combination of methods and parameters (n = 2788 strides). Shown are mean values (standard deviation) and RMSE.

Metric	IMU	VICON	Rel. Error	Abs. Error	RMSE
Stride dur. (s)	1.23 (0.27)	1.23 (0.27)	0.00 (0.03)	0.02 (0.03)	0.03
Swing dur. (s)	0.41 (0.08)	0.40 (0.07)	0.01 (0.04)	0.03 (0.03)	0.04
Stance dur. (s)	0.82 (0.21)	0.83 (0.21)	−0.01 (0.03)	0.02 (0.02)	0.03
Cad. (st/min)	101.8 (21.0)	101.7 (20.9)	0.1 (2.6)	1.7 (1.9)	2.6
SL (cm)	112.4 (25.2)	114.9 (26.0)	−2.5 (7.3)	5.3 (5.6)	7.7
Speed (cm/s)	97.8 (35.9)	100.2 (37.9)	−2.3 (6.9)	4.8 (5.4)	7.3
SW (cm)	8.9 (8.1)	9.2 (8.5)	−0.3 (1.3)	0.9 (1.0)	1.3
MTC (cm)	1.7 (0.8)	1.7 (0.6)	0.1 (0.8)	0.6 (0.5)	0.8
Turn angle (°)	36.0 (40.3)	35.3 (40.3)	0.7 (1.4)	1.0 (1.2)	1.6

3.2. Validation

The best combination of methods and parameters was used to generate results for validation. In the analysis, 7015 strides out of 7142 (i.e., approximately 98.2%) were included, meaning that only 127 strides (i.e., 1.8%) were classified as not detected. FC events were detected with an average relative error of -0.01 ± 0.02 s and limits of agreement of -0.06 and 0.04 s. FO events were detected with an average relative error of -0.01 ± 0.05 s and limits of agreement of -0.11 and 0.08 s. FC and FO events were detected with the same average relative error, but the dispersion of the errors in FO detection was higher, as evidenced by the standard deviation and limits of agreement.

The comparison of IMU-derived and reference gait parameters, obtained in the validation set, is shown in Table 4.

Table 4. Performance on the validation set, including turns (n = 7015 strides). Shown are mean values (standard deviation), limits of agreement, RMSE, correlation and equivalence interval (p-value). [†] All correlations were based on Spearman and have $p < 0.01$. [‡] Equivalence tests were based on Wilcoxon signed-rank test.

Metric	IMU	VICON	Rel. Error	Abs. Error	Lim. Agr.	RMSE	Corr.[†]	Equival.[‡]
Stride dur. (s)	1.22 (0.23)	1.23 (0.24)	0.00 (0.05)	0.02 (0.05)	[−0.11, 0.11]	0.05	0.99	±0.06 (0.0)
Swing dur. (s)	0.41 (0.08)	0.41 (0.06)	0.01 (0.05)	0.03 (0.04)	[−0.08, 0.09]	0.05	0.87	±0.02 (0.0)
Stance dur. (s)	0.81 (0.18)	0.82 (0.19)	−0.01 (0.05)	0.03 (0.05)	[−0.11, 0.10]	0.05	0.98	±0.04 (0.0)
Cad. (st/min)	101.2 (17.5)	101.1 (17.4)	0.1 (3.1)	1.8 (2.5)	[−6.0, 6.1]	3.1	0.99	±5.05 (0.0)
SL (cm)	120.8 (25.1)	124.2 (26.5)	−3.5 (9.7)	6.4 (8.0)	[−22.5, 15.6]	10.3	0.94	±6.21 (0.0)
Speed (cm/s)	103.6 (33.9)	106.7 (36.3)	−3.1 (9.2)	5.8 (7.8)	[−21.1, 15.0]	9.7	0.98	±5.33 (0.0)
SW (cm)	9.9 (9.2)	10.2 (10.1)	−0.4 (4.4)	1.5 (4.2)	[−9.0, 8.3]	4.4	0.93	±0.51 (0.0)
MTC (cm)	1.7 (1.0)	1.9 (0.7)	−0.2 (0.8)	0.6 (0.6)	[−1.9, 1.4]	0.9	0.55	±0.10 (1.0)
Turn angle (°)	37.3 (41.0)	36.4 (41.0)	0.9 (8.6)	2.3 (8.4)	[−16.0, 17.8]	8.7	0.97	±1.82 (0.0)

According to the classification proposed in [34], high (i.e., between 70 and 90) to very high (i.e., above 90) correlation was obtained in all variables, except MTC that had a moderate correlation ($r_s = 0.55$). Equivalence tests revealed all metrics to be practically equivalent (with $p < 0.01$), except MTC, considering equivalence intervals corresponding to 5% of the average of the metric. Average absolute errors in stride duration of 0.02 ± 0.05 s were obtained, which represents an average error of two samples considering the sampling rate of 100 Hz. SL had an average relative error of -3.5 ± 9.7 cm (Table 4).

Results excluding turns are shown in Table 5, where about 2% of the reference strides (i.e., 78 strides) are considered as not detected, resulting in the analysis of 3785 strides. Correlations between variables are high (i.e., between 70 and 90) or very high (i.e., above 90), except for MTC and turning angles where Spearman correlations are of 0.55 and 0.68, respectively, and classified as moderate. Accordingly, equivalence tests reveal all metrics to be practically equivalent (with $p < 0.01$), except for MTC and turning angles. Average relative errors of 0.00 ± 0.04 s and -3.9 ± 6.2 cm were obtained for stride duration and SL, respectively (Table 5).

Table 5. Performance on the validation set, excluding turning strides (n = 3785 strides). Shown are mean values (standard deviation), limits of agreement, RMSE, correlation and equivalence interval (p-value). [†] All correlations were based on Spearman and have $p < 0.01$. [‡] Equivalence tests were based on Wilcoxon signed-rank test.

Metric	IMU	VICON	Rel. Error	Abs. Error	Lim. Agr.	RMSE	Corr.[†]	Equival.[‡]
Stride dur. (s)	1.22 (0.24)	1.22 (0.24)	0.00 (0.04)	0.02 (0.04)	[−0.08, 0.08]	0.04	0.99	±0.06 (0.0)
Swing dur. (s)	0.41 (0.07)	0.40 (0.06)	0.00 (0.04)	0.02 (0.04)	[−0.08, 0.09]	0.04	0.89	±0.02 (0.0)
Stance dur. (s)	0.81 (0.19)	0.82 (0.19)	0.00 (0.04)	0.02 (0.03)	[−0.09, 0.08]	0.04	0.98	±0.04 (0.0)
Cad. (st/min)	101.8 (17.6)	101.5 (17.4)	0.3 (2.5)	1.5 (2.1)	[−4.7, 5.2]	2.5	0.99	±5.08 (0.0)
SL (cm)	129.8 (18.3)	133.7 (20.7)	−3.9 (6.2)	4.6 (5.8)	[−16.1, 8.2]	7.4	0.98	±6.69 (0.0)
Speed (cm/s)	112.0 (31.9)	115.3 (35.1)	−3.4 (6.9)	4.4 (6.3)	[−17.0, 10.2]	7.7	0.99	±5.77 (0.0)
SW (cm)	4.9 (3.2)	4.7 (2.2)	0.1 (2.8)	0.9 (2.7)	[−5.4, 5.6]	2.8	0.84	±0.24 (0.0)
MTC (cm)	1.4 (0.7)	1.8 (0.6)	−0.4 (0.7)	0.6 (0.5)	[−1.7, 0.9]	0.8	0.55	±0.09 (1.0)
Turn angle (°)	6.4 (7.0)	5.1 (4.8)	1.2 (5.1)	1.5 (5.1)	[−8.8, 11.3]	5.3	0.68	±0.26 (1.0)

3.3. Orientation Invariance

The comparison of gait parameters extracted using the original sensor orientation and using simulated rotations is shown in Table 6. As can be observed, all parameters, except turning angle, present the same values when the sensor is rotated, i.e., all parameters have a RMSD of 0.0, except turning angle that has a RMSD of 1.5°. The correlation between turning angles extracted using the original orientation and random rotations of the sensor is very high ($r_s = 0.99$). The performance of the system when data are synthetically rotated remains practically equivalent (equivalence tests have $p < 0.01$ for all gait metrics, considering an equivalence interval of 1% of the average of the metric).

Table 6. Orientation invariance results (n = 7138 strides). Shown are mean values (standard deviation), RMSD, Correlation—with Spearman or Pearson—and equivalence interval (p-value). [†] All correlations have $p < 0.01$. [‡] All equivalence tests are based on Paired T-test, except for turning angle, which is based on Wilcoxon signed-rank test.

Metric	Original Orientation	Random Rotations	RMSD	Correlation[†]	Equivalence[‡]
Stride dur. (s)	1.23 (0.26)	1.23 (0.26)	0.0	$r_p = 1.0$	±0.01 (0.0)
Swing dur. (s)	0.41 (0.08)	0.41 (0.08)	0.0	$r_p = 1.0$	±0.00 (0.0)
Stance dur. (s)	0.82 (0.20)	0.82 (0.20)	0.0	$r_p = 1.0$	±0.01 (0.0)
Cad. (st/min)	100.7 (17.9)	100.7 (17.9)	0.0	$r_p = 1.0$	±1.01 (0.0)
SL (cm)	120.4 (25.5)	120.4 (25.5)	0.0	$r_p = 1.0$	±1.20 (0.0)
Speed (cm/s)	102.9 (34.3)	102.9 (34.3)	0.0	$r_p = 1.0$	±1.03 (0.0)
SW (cm)	9.8 (9.2)	9.8 (9.2)	0.0	$r_p = 1.0$	±0.10 (0.0)
MTC (cm)	1.7 (1.0)	1.7 (1.0)	0.0	$r_p = 1.0$	±0.02 (0.0)
Turn angle (°)	37.4 (41.0)	37.4 (41.0)	1.5	$r_s = 0.99$	±0.37 (0.0)

Figure 5 allows further (visual) inspection of the generated rotations and their relationship with the differences in measured turning angles (the only metric that presented some differences when the sensor was synthetically rotated). As can be observed, rotations are uniformly distributed across all 3D space. The differences in turning angles are randomly distributed through the space, showing no particular tendency towards a specific region.

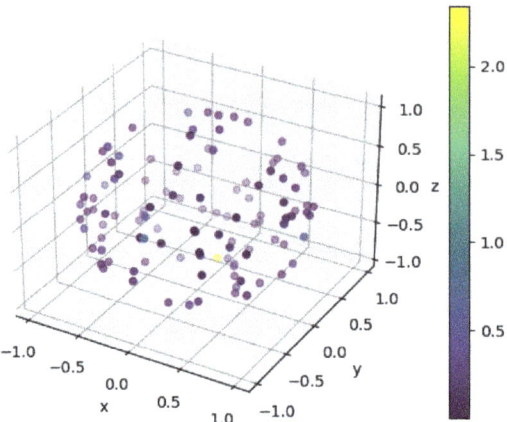

Figure 5. Synthetically generated rotations and their relationship with differences in measured turning angles. Colours represent the absolute difference in turning angles, presented in degrees.

4. Discussion

In this work, we proposed an orientation-invariant gait analysis approach: sensor alignment on the foot is unknown and can be anything. We based our approach in previously studied methods, where some adaptations were introduced in view to maintaining all methods independent to differences in sensor orientation.

To this purpose, orientation-invariant signals were used. To detect ZVIs, we relied on the energy of angular rate, as in [28]. To detect gait events (FC and FO), instead of using medio-lateral angular rate and/or forward acceleration (as proposed by [8,15] or [16]), we used features from acceleration magnitude and from the vertical component of acceleration, obtained in global coordinates.

Instead of representing trajectories using the body coordinate system (as proposed by [15,16]), we evaluated trajectories in global coordinates, from which SL and SW could be estimated. However, to calculate MTC, we estimated a medio-lateral and a forward axis, that were defined with basis on the medio-lateral rotation produced by the foot when moving from foot-flat to FO. These axes were required to estimate the angle $\alpha(t)$—as shown in Equation (14)—and could be used to obtain sensor data in body coordinates—similar to the use of PCA, as proposed by Falbriard et al. [21].

The proposed approach was tested in a group of young adults, without any visible gait disorder, using an optical motion capture system as reference. We tested multiple orientation estimations and double integration approaches. Based on the results achieved on the development set, we selected the Euston CF ($k_P^{opt} = 0.15$, $k_I^{opt} = 0$), combined with direct and reverse integration ($\eta^{opt} = 0.25$, $\alpha_i^{opt} = 0.55$) with active horizontal correction. With an η^{opt} of 0.25, the sigmoid used in direct and reverse integration (Equation (11)) approximates the linear shape. Yet, the results achieved with the linear and reverse integration were better than the results achieved with the linear dedrifting method. According to [13,18], the $k_I^{opt} = 0$ used in Euston CF is an appropriate choice due to the short integration times (below 5–10 min) and the slow dynamics of the movements involved. The horizontal correction mechanism allowed for a compensation of the final vertical position achieved in each stride, assuming walking on a flat surface. Although it improved the results in our study, the method can only be applied when walking on a flat surface, and cannot be generalized to walking in inclined surfaces or stairs.

In [13], the same orientation estimation and double integration methods were benchmarked, using a dataset comprising 20 healthy subjects (between 16 and 80 years old), all using the same shoe model and walking straight at multiple speeds in a path with 10 m.

According to the authors, the best performing orientation estimation method (evaluated by the angles obtained in each axis) was Madgwick CF ($\bar{\omega}_{max} = 3.04$), followed by gyroscope integration and Euston CF ($k_P = 0.0046$, $k_I = 0$); but the performance of the three methods did not differ much. For double integration, the direct and reverse integration ($\eta = 0.08$, $\alpha_i = 0.6$) was the best performing method, which is also according to our results. The optimal set of parameters differed from ours, which may be explained by differences in datasets, namely due to different sensor characteristics, subjects, and protocol. While we apply orientation estimation methods at all instants of the signal, in [13] acceleration data are only used when the magnitude of the acceleration approximates the value of the gravity (i.e., the sensor is roughly static). Moreover, the criteria for evaluating methods performance differed from ours. In [13], orientation estimation methods were optimized first based on the measured angles; double integration methods were optimized after selecting the best orientation estimation method, using as criteria the error distribution of estimated velocities and clearance parameters [13]. In our study, we considered that orientation estimation methods have an impact on the performance of double integration methods, which, altogether, have an impact on all gait metrics considered. Therefore, optimizing for a single metric could penalize the performance of the other metrics. For this reason, we opted for the jointly selection of methods and the tuning of parameters based on the overall results achieved in all metrics considered.

The results achieved on the development set with the optimized set of methods and parameters is shown in Table 3. Even though optimization was performed in this set, some of the metrics differ by some units from the reference system. Table 4 shows the results on the validation set. As expected, the central tendency and the dispersion of the errors are lower on the development set where algorithm selection and parameter tuning occurred. The generalization of the method can only be effectively evaluated using the validation set, which included data from unique users never seen during the optimization process.

Using the sensor on foot instep, Mariani et al. [35] tested gait event detection using multiple candidate features (i.e., minimum, maximum or zero-crossing) and multiple signals—including signals that are independent of IMU orientation, namely acceleration magnitude and the derivative of angular rate magnitude. According to their results, the best candidate features are observed in the acceleration magnitude signal [35], close to the instants we propose to detect FC and FO in this work. On average, FO and FC events were detected 0.01 s (i.e., one sample) before the annotations, but the dispersion of the errors was higher for FO detection. While FCs can generally be well perceived on acceleration signals (they represent an impact of the foot on the ground), TO events may be less evident, which may justify the results. Nevertheless, event detection errors are, in general, low, causing a small impact on estimated temporal parameters.

Our event detection method resulted in absolute errors between 0.02 s and 0.03 s in temporal parameters, with precision between 0.03 s and 0.05 s (as shown in Tables 4 and 5). These errors represent average differences of just two or three samples at 100 Hz, not differing much whether we include turns or not, which demonstrates the robustness of the method. In [8], relative errors of 0.00 ± 0.07 s, -0.01 ± 0.04 s, and 0.01 ± 0.07 s are obtained for stride, swing and stance duration in a group of geriatric inpatients, where events are determined based on the analysis of medio-lateral angular rate and forward acceleration, assuming a fixed alignment of the sensor on the shoes. In [16], sensors are placed on the shanks, obtaining relative errors of 0.00 ± 0.02 s in stride duration in a group of young adults. Although the performance on temporal parameters is more or less consistent between studies, it is worth mentioning that while studies differ in subjects and protocols applied, the procedures to estimate reference gait events are also different, which hinders comparison of results. Moreover, these studies are conducted in a laboratory setting, ensuring the precise alignment of the sensors on the body. For this reason, they may not represent the results that would be achieved in a more realistic clinical setting.

In our study, relative errors of -3.5 ± 9.7 cm and -3.1 ± 9.2 cm/s were obtained for SL and gait speed, respectively. When we exclude turns from the analysis, the precision is improved, resulting in relative errors of -3.9 ± 6.2 cm for SL and of -3.4 ± 6.9 cm/s for gait speed. Additionally, RMSE values are lowered and correlations increase (see Tables 4 and 5). These results show that increased errors in SL (reflected also as increased errors in gait speed) may be related with differences imposed by gait patterns while turning, so that evaluation of these metrics in straight walking seems more reliable. Results would possibly improve if parameter optimization was performed using straight walking exclusively, however, at the cost of making the method less robust.

In [7], relative errors of 1.3 ± 3.0 cm and of 2.8 ± 2.4 cm/s were obtained for SL and speed, respectively, in a group of patients with Parkinson's Disease and age-matched elderly subjects, after discarding turning, initiation and termination cycles. In [8], relative errors of -0.3 ± 8.4 cm were obtained for SL in a group of geriatric inpatients walking straight. Using the same dataset, Hannink et al. [24] achieved relative errors of 0.0 ± 5.4 cm, using a deep convolutional neural network. In [16], SL and gait speed had a performance of 5.4 ± 3.1 cm and 3.4 ± 3.9 cm/s, considering only data from young adults obtained while walking straight. In a group of young and elderly volunteers, Mariani et al. [6] achieved performance of 1.5 ± 6.8 cm for SL and 1.4 ± 5.6 cm/s for speed, using a protocol that included assessment with U-turn and 8-turn. As we can see from the literature, results are highly heterogeneous and comparison of performance in a fair and robust way is not possible due to the different protocols, subjects, and reference systems employed. Yet, considering that these metrics had very high correlations with the reference system in our study, we can consider our approach appropriate to assess movement performance. This is especially true when we consider straight walking tests, where precision is improved.

Although the precision of SW is improved when turns are excluded (relative error of -0.4 ± 4.4 cm versus 0.1 ± 2.8 cm when turns are excluded) and RMSE is lowered (4.4 cm versus 2.8 cm), the correlation between IMU-based and reference-based SW is worse when turns are excluded. We also observe that, when we exclude turns, the average and standard deviation of the metric decreases, meaning that curves may be associated with increased SW necessary to describe the trajectory of the turn. When we exclude turns, the values of SW are more consistent (closer to the mean) and, as such, harder to correlate, which may justify the results. The same observation is also valid for turning angles where we can see that even though precision is improved (relative error of $0.9 \pm 8.6°$ versus $1.2 \pm 5.1°$), the correlation decreases when we exclude turns (see Tables 4 and 5). In [7], relative errors of 0.15 ± 2.13 cm and $0.12 \pm 3.59°$ are obtained for SW and turning angle, considering only straight and steady walking.

MTC is one of the metrics with highest errors, considering their relation to the average of the metric. Relative errors of -0.2 ± 0.8 cm and -0.4 ± 0.7 cm are obtained for MTC when turns are included and excluded, respectively; we observe a small improvement in precision and RMSE when turns are excluded, which again, highlights the challenging conditions possibly imposed by the turns.

In [22], a method is proposed to determine toe trajectories that requires the size of the shoe as an input; using this method, authors achieved relative errors of 1.3 ± 0.9 cm in MTC, in a group of healthy adults walking straight, where only steady walking was included in the analysis. In [9], prior information about shoe dimensions was not required, and relative errors of 1.7 ± 0.7 cm were obtained in a group of young, mid-age and old subjects, where conditions for straight or turning walking are not specified. Although the reported relative errors are similar to our results, higher correlations (0.91) are documented by the authors [9]. However, to achieve these results, Kanzler et al. [9] employ a correction that adjusts the amplitude of toe clearance trajectories—possibly penalizing generalization of the method. Moreover, authors discuss that the assumption of the rigid shoe model may not be realistic due to the bending of the shoe at FO, which may also constitute a source of errors in our approach. These errors, combined with a poor estimation of sensor-to-toe distance and errors imposed by the reference—due to a toe marker that is not placed precisely at the tiptoe—can possibly justify the results.

All gait metrics extracted using the IMU present moderate, high or very high correlation with the reference system. Metrics are also practically equivalent, except for MTC and for turning angle when turns are excluded (Tables 4 and 5). Based on these results, we can state that, overall, there is a good agreement between both systems, which denotes the potential of the solution. Sensor wireless capabilities, combined with a flexible alignment on the foot—fostered by the orientation-invariant approach—makes the proposed solution promising for use at clinics and ambulatory settings.

Although the reference system used in this study is currently considered the gold standard for gait analysis [6,7,9,15,16], possible errors can be introduced by the reference. For instance, due to errors in markers labelling or gap filling operations, trajectories of the markers may not always reliably replicate the actual trajectories performed. Additionally, detection of events from trajectories may also display errors that can impact temporal parameters used as reference [26].

Despite our efforts to make the process completely invariant to differences in sensor orientation, we can observe some differences in turning angles when we synthetically rotate sensor data (see Table 6). These differences have no apparent correlation with the generated rotations, as can be visually confirmed in Figure 5. Moreover, rotations were uniformly sampled to ensure a uniform distribution along all possible 3D transformations (Figure 5), which avoided bias on observations—i.e., ensuring that the method is truly invariant to changes in sensor orientation, no matter how it is oriented relative to the feet. The differences in turning angle, not observed in any other metric extracted, may be explained by the sensor fusion process employed to estimate sensor orientation relative to the global frame. While the estimation of the vertical axis employs corrections based on measured acceleration values, in the horizontal plane no correction mechanisms can be employed, and only integration of angular rates are used to estimate changes in orientation (or heading) over time. This may lead to cumulative error propagation due to the integration process, which may differ depending on sensor orientation: different sensor orientations may lead to distinct error propagation profiles. Given the random nature of the noise properties of gyroscope measurements [36], no particular tendency for an increased error towards a specific rotation can be observed. All gait parameters extracted using synthetically rotated data remained practically equivalent (see Table 6), which demonstrates the invariance of the method to differences in orientation. Based on these results, we can state that our method does not require careful alignment of the sensor on the foot, which may increase trust and potentially simplify the data acquisition process in the context of clinics.

Future work should address spatio-temporal gait analysis in specific groups (e.g., older adults or groups with a specific pathology), so that validity and robustness of the method to different walking pattern characteristics may be assessed, demonstrating its possible application in real scenarios.

5. Conclusions

Foot-worn inertial sensors were used to evaluate a comprehensive set of spatio-temporal gait metrics in a group of young adults. To avoid restrictions on sensor alignment, we proposed an orientation-invariant gait analysis approach, and assessed its performance using an optical motion capture system as reference. Overall, good agreement between both systems was achieved in our study, demonstrating the robustness and reliability of the proposed approach. Additionally, we demonstrated the invariance of the method by simulating rotations of the sensor on the foot. Taking advantage of this feature, and considering the wireless capabilities of the sensor, we postulate that the proposed solution is highly attractive for use at clinics and ambulatory settings. Its flexibility, combined with low errors achieved in the evaluation of gait parameters, may leverage trust and potentially simplify the data acquisition process. The solution should be evaluated with people with gait-related disorders, so that it may support clinical decision making in real scenarios.

Author Contributions: Conceptualization, V.G.; methodology, V.G.; software, V.G.; data curation, V.G.; validation, V.G.; formal analysis, V.G.; supervision, I.S. and M.V.C.; writing—original draft preparation, V.G.; writing—review and editing, V.G., I.S. and M.V.C. All authors have read and agreed to the published version of the manuscript.

Funding: This work was performed in the context of the project VITAAL (AAL-2017-066), funded under the AAL Programme and co-funded by the European Commission and the National Funding Authorities of Portugal, Switzerland and Belgium.

Institutional Review Board Statement: The study was conducted according to the guidelines of the Declaration of Helsinki, and approved by the Ethics Committee of the University of Porto (81/CEUP/2019, approved on 9 December 2019).

Informed Consent Statement: Informed consent was obtained from all subjects involved in the study.

Data Availability Statement: Not applicable.

Acknowledgments: The authors would like to thank the collaboration of all volunteers who participated in data collection.

Conflicts of Interest: The authors declare no conflict of interest.

Abbreviations

The following abbreviations are used in this manuscript:

CF	Complementary filter
FC	Initial foot contact
FO	Foot off
IMU	Inertial measurement unit
MTC	Minimum toe clearance
PCA	Principal component analysis
RMSD	Root mean square deviation
RMSE	Root mean square error
SL	Stride length
SW	Swing width
TRIAD	Tri-axial attitude determination
ZVI	Zero velocity interval

References

1. Akhtaruzzaman, M.; Shafie, A.A.; Khan, M.R. Gait analysis: Systems, technologies, and importance. *J. Mech. Med. Biol.* **2016**, *16*, 1630003. [CrossRef]
2. Chen, S.; Lach, J.; Lo, B.; Yang, G.Z. Toward Pervasive Gait Analysis with Wearable Sensors: A Systematic Review. *IEEE J. Biomed. Health Inform.* **2016**, *20*, 1521–1537. [CrossRef]
3. Marques, N.R.; Spinoso, D.H.; Cardoso, B.C.; Moreno, V.C.; Kuroda, M.H.; Navega, M.T. Is it possible to predict falls in older adults using gait kinematics? *Clin. Biomech.* **2018**, *59*, 15–18. [CrossRef]
4. Chhetri, J.K.; Chan, P.; Vellas, B.; Cesari, M. Motoric Cognitive Risk Syndrome: Predictor of Dementia and Age-Related Negative Outcomes. *Front. Med.* **2017**, *4*. [CrossRef] [PubMed]
5. Schoon, Y.; Bongers, K.; Van Kempen, J.; Melis, R.; Olde Rikkert, M. Gait speed as a test for monitoring frailty in community-dwelling older people has the highest diagnostic value compared to step length and chair rise time. *Eur. J. Phys. Rehabil. Med.* **2014**, *50*, 693–701. [PubMed]
6. Mariani, B.; Hoskovec, C.; Rochat, S.; Büla, C.; Penders, J.; Aminian, K. 3D gait assessment in young and elderly subjects using foot-worn inertial sensors. *J. Biomech.* **2010**, *43*, 2999–3006. [CrossRef] [PubMed]
7. Mariani, B.; Jiménez, M.C.; Vingerhoets, F.J.G.; Aminian, K. On-Shoe Wearable Sensors for Gait and Turning Assessment of Patients With Parkinson's Disease. *IEEE Trans. Biomed. Eng.* **2013**, *60*, 155–158. [CrossRef]
8. Rampp, A.; Barth, J.; Schülein, S.; Gaßmann, K.G.; Klucken, J.; Eskofier, B.M. Inertial sensor-based stride parameter calculation from gait sequences in geriatric patients. *IEEE Trans. Biomed. Eng.* **2015**, *62*, 1089–1097. [CrossRef]
9. Kanzler, C.M.; Barth, J.; Rampp, A.; Schlarb, H.; Rott, F.; Klucken, J.; Eskofier, B.M. Inertial sensor based and shoe size independent gait analysis including heel and toe clearance estimation. In Proceedings of the 2015 37th Annual International Conference of the IEEE Engineering in Medicine and Biology Society (EMBC), Milan, Italy, 25–29 August 2015; pp. 5424–5427. [CrossRef]

10. Petraglia, F.; Scarcella, L.; Pedrazzi, G.; Brancato, L.; Puers, R.; Costantino, C. Inertial sensors versus standard systems in gait analysis: A systematic review and meta-analysis. *Eur. J. Phys. Rehabil. Med.* **2019**, *55*, 265–280. [CrossRef]
11. Tunca, C.; Pehlivan, N.; Ak, N.; Arnrich, B.; Salur, G.; Ersoy, C. Inertial Sensor-Based Robust Gait Analysis in Non-Hospital Settings for Neurological Disorders. *Sensors* **2017**, *17*, 825. [CrossRef]
12. Peruzzi, A.; Della Croce, U.; Cereatti, A. Estimation of stride length in level walking using an inertial measurement unit attached to the foot: A validation of the zero velocity assumption during stance. *J. Biomech.* **2011**, *44*, 1991–1994. [CrossRef]
13. Hannink, J.; Ollenschläger, M.; Kluge, F.; Roth, N.; Klucken, J.; Eskofier, B.M. Benchmarking Foot Trajectory Estimation Methods for Mobile Gait Analysis. *Sensors* **2017**, *17*, 1940. [CrossRef]
14. Sabatini, A.M.; Martelloni, C.; Scapellato, S.; Cavallo, F. Assessment of walking features from foot inertial sensing. *IEEE Trans. Biomed. Eng.* **2005**, *52*, 486–494. [CrossRef] [PubMed]
15. Kluge, F.; Gaßner, H.; Hannink, J.; Pasluosta, C.; Klucken, J.; Eskofier, B.M. Towards Mobile Gait Analysis: Concurrent Validity and Test-Retest Reliability of an Inertial Measurement System for the Assessment of Spatio-Temporal Gait Parameters. *Sensors* **2017**, *17*, 1522. [CrossRef] [PubMed]
16. Hori, K.; Mao, Y.; Ono, Y.; Ora, H.; Hirobe, Y.; Sawada, H.; Inaba, A.; Orimo, S.; Miyake, Y. Inertial Measurement Unit-Based Estimation of Foot Trajectory for Clinical Gait Analysis. *Front. Physiol.* **2019**, *10*, 1530. [CrossRef] [PubMed]
17. Madgwick, S.O.H.; Harrison, A.J.L.; Vaidyanathan, R. Estimation of IMU and MARG orientation using a gradient descent algorithm. In Proceedings of the 2011 IEEE International Conference on Rehabilitation Robotics, Zurich, Switzerland, 29 June–1 July 2011; pp. 1–7. [CrossRef]
18. Euston, M.; Coote, P.; Mahony, R.; Jonghyuk Kim.; Hamel, T. A complementary filter for attitude estimation of a fixed-wing UAV. In Proceedings of the 2008 IEEE/RSJ International Conference on Intelligent Robots and Systems, Nice, France, 22–26 September 2008; pp. 340–345. [CrossRef]
19. Basso, M.; Martinelli, A.; Morosi, S.; Sera, F. A Real-Time GNSS/PDR Navigation System for Mobile Devices. *Remote Sens.* **2021**, *13*, 1567. [CrossRef]
20. Leonardo, R.; Rodrigues, G.; Barandas, M.; Alves, P.; Santos, R.; Gamboa, H. Determination of the Walking Direction of a Pedestrian from Acceleration Data. In Proceedings of the 2019 International Conference on Indoor Positioning and Indoor Navigation (IPIN), Pisa, Italy, 30 September–3 October 2019; pp. 1–6. [CrossRef]
21. Falbriard, M.; Meyer, F.; Mariani, B.; Millet, G.P.; Aminian, K. Accurate Estimation of Running Temporal Parameters Using Foot-Worn Inertial Sensors. *Front. Physiol.* **2018**, *9*. [CrossRef] [PubMed]
22. Mariani, B.; Rochat, S.; Büla, C.J.; Aminian, K. Heel and toe clearance estimation for gait analysis using wireless inertial sensors. *IEEE Trans. Biomed. Eng.* **2012**, *59*, 3162–3168. [CrossRef] [PubMed]
23. Byun, S.; Lee, H.J.; Han, J.W.; Kim, J.S.; Choi, E.; Kim, K.W. Walking-speed estimation using a single inertial measurement unit for the older adults. *PLoS ONE* **2019**, *14*, e0227075. [CrossRef] [PubMed]
24. Hannink, J.; Kautz, T.; Pasluosta, C.F.; Barth, J.; Schülein, S.; Gaßmann, K.; Klucken, J.; Eskofier, B.M. Mobile Stride Length Estimation With Deep Convolutional Neural Networks. *IEEE J. Biomed. Health Inform.* **2018**, *22*, 354–362. [CrossRef]
25. Lambrecht, S.; Harutyunyan, A.; Tanghe, K.; Afschrift, M.; De Schutter, J.; Jonkers, I. Real-Time Gait Event Detection Based on Kinematic Data Coupled to a Biomechanical Model. *Sensors* **2017**, *17*, 671. [CrossRef] [PubMed]
26. Hreljac, A.; Marshall, R.N. Algorithms to determine event timing during normal walking using kinematic data. *J. Biomech.* **2000**, *33*, 783–786. [CrossRef]
27. Huxham, F.; Gong, J.; Baker, R.; Morris, M.; Iansek, R. Defining spatial parameters for non-linear walking. *Gait Posture* **2006**, *23*, 159–163. [CrossRef] [PubMed]
28. Skog, I.; Nilsson, J.; Händel, P. Evaluation of zero-velocity detectors for foot-mounted inertial navigation systems. In Proceedings of the 2010 International Conference on Indoor Positioning and Indoor Navigation, Zurich, Switzerland, 15–17 September 2010; pp. 1–6. [CrossRef]
29. Shuster, M.D.; Oh, S.D. Three-axis attitude determination from vector observations. *J. Guid. Control* **1981**, *4*, 70–77. [CrossRef]
30. Madgwick, S.O.H. *An Efficient Orientation Filter for Inertial and Inertial/Magnetic Sensor Arrays*; Technical Report, Report x-io; University of Bristol (UK): Bristol, UK, 2010.
31. Altman, D.G.; Bland, J.M. Measurement in Medicine: The Analysis of Method Comparison Studies. *Statistician* **1983**, *32*, 307. [CrossRef]
32. Ravi, D.K.; Gwerder, M.; König Ignasiak, N.; Baumann, C.R.; Uhl, M.; van Dieën, J.H.; Taylor, W.R.; Singh, N.B. Revealing the optimal thresholds for movement performance: A systematic review and meta-analysis to benchmark pathological walking behaviour. *Neurosci. Biobehav. Rev.* **2020**, *108*, 24–33. [CrossRef]
33. Shoemake, K. Uniform Random Rotations. In *Graphics Gems III (IBM Version)*; Elsevier: Amsterdam, The Netherlands, 1992; pp. 124–132. [CrossRef]
34. Mukaka, M. A guide to appropriate use of Correlation coefficient in medical research. *Malawi Med. J.* **2012**, *24*, 69–71.
35. Mariani, B.; Rouhani, H.; Crevoisier, X.; Aminian, K. Quantitative estimation of foot-flat and stance phase of gait using foot-worn inertial sensors. *Gait Posture* **2013**, *37*, 229–234. [CrossRef] [PubMed]
36. Han, S.; Meng, Z.; Omisore, O.; Akinyemi, T.; Yan, Y. Random Error Reduction Algorithms for MEMS Inertial Sensor Accuracy Improvement—A Review. *Micromachines* **2020**, *11*, 1021. [CrossRef]

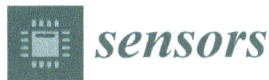

Communication

Are the Assioma Favero Power Meter Pedals a Reliable Tool for Monitoring Cycling Power Output?

Víctor Rodríguez-Rielves [1,2], José Ramón Lillo-Beviá [1], Ángel Buendía-Romero [1], Alejandro Martínez-Cava [1], Alejandro Hernández-Belmonte [1], Javier Courel-Ibáñez [1] and Jesús G. Pallarés [1,*]

[1] Human Performance and Sports Science Laboratory, University of Murcia, 30100 Murcia, Spain; Victor.RRielves@uclm.es (V.R.-R.); jr.lillo@ua.es (J.R.L.-B.); Angel.buendiar@um.es (Á.B.-R.); Alejandro.martinez12@um.es (A.M.-C.); alejandro.hernandez7@um.es (A.H.-B.); courel@um.es (J.C.-I.)
[2] Exercise Physiology Laboratory, University of Castilla-La Mancha, 13001 Toledo, Spain
* Correspondence: jgpallares@um.es

Abstract: This study aimed to examine the validity and reliability of the recently developed Assioma Favero pedals under laboratory cycling conditions. In total, 12 well-trained male cyclists and triathletes (VO$_{2max}$ = 65.7 ± 8.7 mL·kg^{-1}·min^{-1}) completed five cycling tests including graded exercises tests (GXT) at different cadences (70–100 revolutions per minute, rpm), workloads (100–650 Watts, W), pedaling positions (seated and standing), vibration stress (20–40 Hz), and an 8-s maximal sprint. Tests were completed using a calibrated direct drive indoor trainer for the standing, seated, and vibration GXTs, and a friction belt cycle ergometer for the high-workload step protocol. Power output (PO) and cadence were collected from three different brand, new pedal units against the gold-standard SRM crankset. The three units of the Assioma Favero exhibited very high within-test reliability and an extremely high agreement between 100 and 250 W, compared to the gold standard (Standard Error of Measurement, SEM from 2.3–6.4 W). Greater PO produced a significant underestimating trend ($p < 0.05$, Effect size, ES ≥ 0.22), with pedals showing systematically lower PO than SRM (1–3%) but producing low bias for all GXT tests and conditions (1.5–7.4 W). Furthermore, vibrations ≥ 30 Hz significantly increased the differences up to 4% ($p < 0.05$, ES ≥ 0.24), whereas peak and mean PO differed importantly between devices during the sprints ($p < 0.03$, ES ≥ 0.39). These results demonstrate that the Assioma Favero power meter pedals provide trustworthy PO readings from 100 to 650 W, in either seated or standing positions, with vibrations between 20 and 40 Hz at cadences of 70, 85, and 100 rpm, or even at a free chosen cadence.

Keywords: cycling; mobile power meter; testing; load monitoring

Citation: Rodríguez-Rielves, V.; Lillo-Beviá, J.R.; Buendía-Romero, Á.; Martínez-Cava, A.; Hernández-Belmonte, A.; Courel-Ibáñez, J.; Pallarés, J.G. Are the Assioma Favero Power Meter Pedals a Reliable Tool for Monitoring Cycling Power Output? *Sensors* **2021**, *21*, 2789. https://doi.org/10.3390/s21082789

Academic Editor: Felipe García-Pinillos

Received: 12 March 2021
Accepted: 13 April 2021
Published: 15 April 2021

Publisher's Note: MDPI stays neutral with regard to jurisdictional claims in published maps and institutional affiliations.

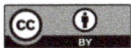

Copyright: © 2021 by the authors. Licensee MDPI, Basel, Switzerland. This article is an open access article distributed under the terms and conditions of the Creative Commons Attribution (CC BY) license (https://creativecommons.org/licenses/by/4.0/).

1. Introduction

The use of power meters in cycling has been on the rise in recent years, making accessible, valuable information for training, that was only available with impractical and expensive ergometers [1,2]. Portable power meter devices overcome important drawbacks of laboratory testing, allowing the use of cyclists' own bicycles, so that decisive metrics such as the crank width (Q–factor), crank length, and geometry-related variables are replicated in the test [3]. Commercial indoor stationary cycle training, cycling treadmills, or rollers are a valid and reliable alternative to recreate outdoor cycling conditions, both for testing [4–6] and training [7]. While these tools simulate outdoor cycling, they do not allow recording during real outdoor environments (e.g., missing air drag and downhill sections or increasing dehydration), which may alter the metrics [8,9] and limit to apply the results to real-life situations.

The development of wearable power meters with micro-sensors attached to the bicycle crank, pedals or wheel, constitutes a milestone for cycling, giving rise to the creation of new devices, which can track cyclists' performance in real settings. The first approach was the SRM (professional model; Schoberer Rad Messtechnik, Julich, Germany) crankset (strain gauges), which remains as the Gold-Standard to measure the bicycle power output (PO) outside the laboratory [10–12]. Since then, emerging alternatives have been demonstrated to be valid and reliable, such as the wheels Powertap Hub [13–15] or the pedals Garmin Vector [1,15–18] and Powertap P1 [19–21]. In particular, due to their quick installation and use [1,15–21], the pedal power meters would represent a high practical technology to be used interchangeably in different bicycles (e.g., track, road, and time trials). Additionally, pedals are likely to reduce the loss of PO due to mechanical connections [12]. Recently, a new brand of pedal power meters called Assioma Favero (Favero Electronics SRL, Arcade TV, Italy) has been launched on the market. In addition to reduced weight and size, the lower of this device compared to the traditional SRM makes the PO measurement more affordable for practitioners. Nevertheless, there is scarce information about the measurement errors of this commercially available technology.

In practice, the main goal of tracking PO is to quantify the real effort incurred during training or competition, and also to determine changes in performance throughout the season [22]. For this purpose, it is essential to determine the measurement error of the device in use to guarantee that these errors are narrow enough to determine the true PO achieved by the cyclists [23,24]. Accordingly, if the error exceeds the expected changes, the device renders it completely useless for its intended purpose [25]. Hence, to be sure of the certainty of the outcomes, emerging power meter devices should be repeatedly tested across a variety of cycling conditions to determine how well they respond to changes in the cadence, the pedaling position (seated or stand), the PO, or the vibration [15].

Therefore, considering the practical advantages that the pedals power meter would provide to the PO prescription and monitoring, as well as the need to comprehensively analyze the suitability of this type of technologies to be used on the daily basis, this study aimed to examine the validity and reliability of the recently developed Assioma Favero pedals under laboratory cycling conditions.

2. Materials and Methods

2.1. Experimental Design

This study followed a repeated measures design to determine the validity and test–retest reliability of three units of the new power meter pedals Assioma Favero against the gold-standard SRM crankset. After a familiarization session, each participant completed the following cycling tests: three counterbalanced, graded exercises tests (GXT) at different cadences (70, 85, 100 revolutions per minute, rpm) and sub-maximal workloads (100, 150, 200, 250, 300, 350 Watts, W) in a seated position, three GXT at four sub-maximal workloads (free cadence; 250, 350, 450, 550 W) in a standing position, and a ramp vibration protocol (from 20 to 40 Hz) at constant workload (200 W; 85 rpm). Finally, all cyclists performed a high-workload step protocol (450, 550, 650 W, in seated position, 85 rpm), as well as an 8-s maximal sprint test.

2.2. Subjects

A total of 12 well-trained male cyclists and triathletes volunteered to take part in this study. (M ± SD: age 27.9 ± 9.5 years; height 180.0 ± 7.8 cm; body mass 78.0 ± 16.4 kg; VO_{2max} = 65.7 ± 8.7 mL·kg^{-1}·min^{-1} [26]). All subjects had more than 5 years of cycling training experience and followed a training routine of 6 h per week during the 12 months preceding the study. Athletes were all older than 18 years, were informed of the experimental procedures, and signed a written informed consent agreeing to participate in the study. Participants were asked to avoid strenuous exercise, caffeine, or alcohol for at least 24 h before each testing session. The study was conducted according to the Declaration of Helsinki, and was approved by the Bioethics Commission of Local University.

2.3. Testing Procedures

All tests were performed in the same facilities under standardized conditions (23.8 ± 2.4 °C; 39 ± 5% humidity). For the seated and standing GXTs, as well as the vibration tests, the SRM 172.5 mm crank power meter was fixed on a medium-size road bicycle (2010 Giant Giant-Bicycles, Taiwan; Aluminum alloy frame with carbon fiber fork). The rear wheel of the bicycle was removed and attached to a calibrated Cycleops Hammer [6] device with 10 speed (11–25 tooth) rear gear ratio and 39 to 53 tooth front gear ratio. For all tests, the gear ratio 53 × 15 was selected, and cyclists were not allowed to change it to prevent a potential effect of this variable on pedaling technique. The zero–offset of the Assioma Favero power meter pedals was set before each testing session. For the vibration tests, the whole system (Bike trainer and bicycle) was installed over a vibrating plate (Merit Fitness V2000) with the front fork of the bicycle attached to a Kickr Climb Indoor Grade Simulator (Wahoo Fitness, Atlanta, GA, USA) for stability and to compensate the height of the vibration platform (0% slope). The bicycle seat height position was matched to the cyclist's training geometry. For the high-workload step protocol (GXT $\geq$ 450 W) and the 8-s maximal sprint, the SRM crankset unit was installed in a friction belt cycle ergometer (Monark 847E Varberg, Sweden) to achieve the required mechanical resistance. The saddle and handlebar positions of the cycle ergometer were also matched to the cyclist's training geometry. Data were transmitted to display units (Garmin 520, Garmin International Inc., Olathe, KS, USA) fixed on the handlebars. Calibration and set-up were conducted according to the manufacturer's recommendations. Cyclists used their cycling shoes fitted with Look cleats.

2.4. Cyclings Tests

Subjects visited the laboratory on four separate occasions to test the three Assioma Favero power meter pedals. All tests began with a standardized warm-up of 5 min at 75 W with a free chosen cadence and the Hammer set in the hyperbolic mode. Thereafter, subjects performed three randomized and counterbalanced 1-min GXT in seated position, one for each selected fixed cadence (70, 85, and 100 rpm), at six sub-maximal workloads (i.e., 100, 150, 200, 250, 300, and 350 W), separated by 4 min of recovery at 75 W with free chosen cadence [6] (Figure 1). The order of the three cadence levels was randomized to ensure that results were not altered due to increments on the ergometer break temperature or by the cyclists' fatigue. After recovery, cyclists performed three 1-min GXT in standing pedaling position at 250, 350, 450 W, and 550 W with free chosen cadence. After 2 min of recovery at 75 W, subjects performed a vibration test, simulating common vibrations in road cycling [27]. The test consisted of a 1 min ramp exercise, bouts on a vibrating plate by steps of 10 Hz, increasing from 20 to 40 Hz, at 200 W with a pedaling cadence of 85 rpm. This complete protocol was repeated on three different occasions in a randomized and counterbalanced way, one for each Assioma Favero pedal units (Figure 1). In the fourth visit to the laboratory, subjects performed a 30-s, seated position, high-load GXT at 85 rpm in a friction belt cycle ergometer, with the resistances required to produce 450 W (5.3 kp), 550 W (6.4 kp), and 650 W (7.6 kp). Each step was followed by 3 min of recovery with 1 kp (85 W). Following a further 5-min recovery period, subjects were required to complete an 8-s maximal sprint test (verbally encouraged, all-out effort) starting from a complete stop with the pedal of the dominant leg placed at 90° from the vertical and against the resistance of 7.5% of the subject's body mass (body mass × 0.075 kg) [28]. The four sessions were conducted at the same time of the day (10:00–13:30 h), and under similar environmental conditions (21–22 °C and 53–62% humidity) [29].

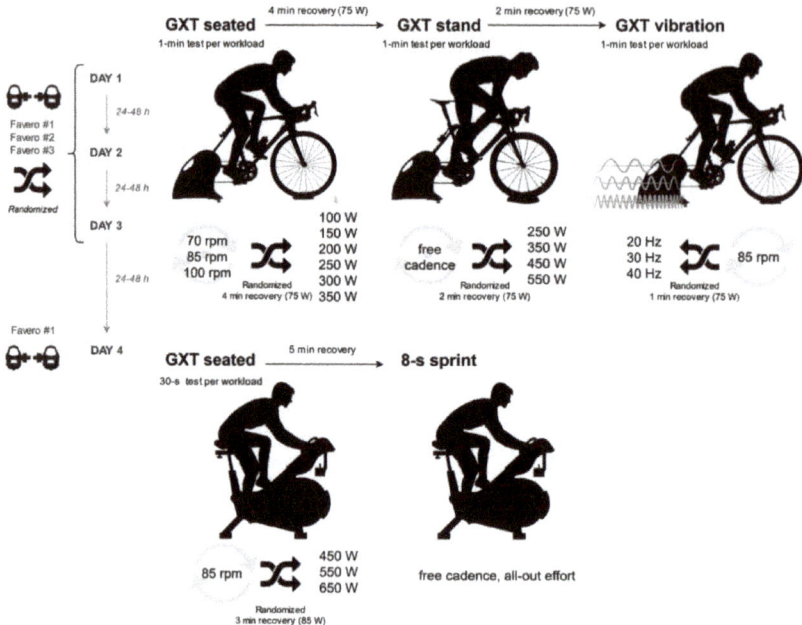

Figure 1. Experimental design including the five cycling tests.

2.5. Data Collection

Records for PO (W) and cadence (rpm) were collected at 1 Hz using a Garmin 520 cycling computer for the Assioma Favero pedals and the Power Control VIII (professional model, Schoberer Rad Messtechnik, Julich, Germany) for the SRM crankset. Data for GXT and vibration tests included the 15th to the 55th s of each 60 s steps, to allow the ergometer enough time to stabilize the assigned breaking load [12]. Similarly, data from the 8th and the 28th s of each 30 s steps were considered for the high-load GXT tests, while peak PO and the mean PO for the first 6 s of the sprints were included. Data were exported and analyzed using the publicly available software (Golden Cheetah, version 3.5) and Microsoft Excel 2016.

2.6. Statistical Analysis

Standard statistical methods were used for the calculation of means, standard deviations (SD), coefficient of variation (CV), and standard error of measurement (SEM) [30]. Intraclass correlation coefficients (ICC) were used to determine the relationship between the power outcomes of the SRM and the Assioma Favero pedals. Bland–Altman plots were used to examine heteroscedasticity and assess the systematic errors and their 95% limits of agreement (LoA = bias ± 1.96 SD) [31]. Levels of acceptable disagreement were proposed at ≤2% to identify true changes in performance after a training intervention [24]. Homoscedasticity was confirmed by Levene's test. Repeated-measures ANOVA was conducted to determine the statistical effects of the different devices in the PO metrics across the different GXT tests. Partial eta squared was calculated to estimate the effect size (ES), interpreted as small (0.02), medium (0.13), and large (0.26) [32]. Statistical significance was set as $p \leq 0.05$. Analyses were performed using GraphPad Prism 6.0 (GraphPad Software, Inc., San Diego, CA, USA), SPSS software version 19.0 (SPSS, Chicago, IL, USA), and Microsoft Excel 2016 (Microsoft Corp, Redmond, WA, USA).

3. Results

The three Favero Assioma pedals exhibited very high reliability during the tests (CV from 1.5 to 13.8%) comparable to the SRM (CV differences < 2%), and high ICC (from 0.741 to 0.999). SRM crankset and the three Favero Assioma showed similar PO in most conditions (Table 1), with extremely high agreement when pedaling between 100 and 250 W (SEM from 2.3 to 6.4 W). Greater PO produced a significant underestimating trend, especially in GXT seated at 300 W/70 rpm, GXT seated at 350 W/80 rpm, and GXT standing > 450 W ($p < 0.05$, ES > 0.22), with Favero showing from 1 to 3% lower PO than SRM consistently. In turn, all devices showed similar PO during [30], the GXT seated ≥ 450 W in the Monark. Vibrations ≥ 20 Hz significantly increased the differences up to 4% ($p < 0.05$, ES > 0.24). Peak and mean PO differed importantly between devices during the sprints ($p < 0.03$, ES > 0.39). Bland–Altman plots (Figure 2) confirmed that Favero Assioma pedals showed systematically lower PO than SRM, but produced low bias (1.5 and 7.4 W) and SD (4.7 and 10.0 W) for all testing conditions.

Table 1. Power outcomes for SRM crack set and the three Favero Assioma pedals.

	Mean (SD)		SEM	Mean (SD)		SEM	Mean (SD)		SEM	Within-Device Effect	
	SRM	Favero #1		SRM	Favero #2		SRM	Favero #3		p-Value	ES
GXT seated [70 rpm]											
100 W	100 (6)	97 (6)	2.3	100 (8)	97 (8)	2.8	98 (3)	96 (4)	2.7	0.399	0.078
150 W	250 (6)	143 (5)	2.5	250 (6)	145 (8)	2.6	250 (4)	142 (5)	3.2	0.132	0.165
200 W	200 (7)	197 (7)	2.9	200 (5)	197 (6)	3.1	199 (4)	194 (5)	3.8	0.165	0.155
250 W	249 (6)	246 (5)	3.1	250 (6)	246 (6)	3.6	249 (4)	244 (4)	3.9	0.1	0.186
300 W	300 (5)	296 (5)	3.3	300 (3)	296 (4)	3.3	299 (3)	294 (5)	4.0	0.046 *	0.269
350 W	350 (6)	348 (5)	3.1	350 (5)	346 (7)	3.8	349 (4)	344 (5)	4.0	0.071	0.209
GXT seated [85 rpm]											
100 W	100 (9)	98 (8)	2.8	100 (7)	97 (8)	3.1	99 (3)	96 (4)	3.5	0.454	0.066
150 W	149 (7)	146 (7)	3.3	149 (5)	147 (7)	2.6	148 (5)	145 (6)	3.9	0.377	0.085
200 W	201 (7)	197 (6)	3.2	200 (3)	196 (4)	3.4	200 (4)	195 (6)	4.6	0.099	0.2
250 W	250 (9)	246 (9)	3.9	250 (6)	246 (8)	4.0	250 (5)	244 (5)	5.1	0.152	0.162
300 W	300 (8)	296 (7)	4.1	299 (7)	294 (7)	4.1	300 (4)	294 (6)	5.5	0.109	0.186
350 W	350 (7)	345 (7)	4.3	350 (4)	345 (6)	4.4	350 (6)	343 (6)	6.1	0.035 *	0.275
GXT seated [100 rpm]											
100 W	100 (14)	98 (14)	2.1	100 (11)	97 (12)	4.2	100 (6)	96 (7)	3.8	0.647	0.034
150 W	150 (8)	147 (6)	3.3	149 (6)	145 (8)	5.1	151 (6)	146 (7)	4.0	0.153	0.153
200 W	199 (10)	195 (8)	3.7	200 (6)	195 (7)	5.2	199 (4)	193 (4)	5.3	0.08	0.202
250 W	249 (11)	245 (8)	4.7	250 (8)	245 (7)	4.6	250 (6)	242 (6)	6.4	0.08	0.202
300 W	300 (11)	293 (9)	5.5	300 (12)	294 (11)	5.6	300 (7)	292 (7)	6.7	0.102	0.18
350 W	349 (14)	343 (12)	5.3	350 (11)	342 (11)	6.5	350 (5)	340 (6)	7.4	0.124	0.178
GXT stand [free cadence]											
250 W	250 (9)	251 (7)	2.1	250 (9)	250 (9)	1.4	249 (8)	244 (7)	4.3	0.352	0.091
350 W	350 (7)	350 (6)	1.9	350 (8)	350 (9)	1.7	350 (8)	343 (9)	5.7	0.15	0.156
450 W	451 (10)	452 (12)	4.2	450 (7)	452 (9)	2.8	449 (10)	442 (10)	6.3	0.050 *	0.221
550 W	551 (14)	554 (16)	4.1	550 (10)	554 (13)	5.0	542 (28)	537 (24)	9.2	0.045 *	0.235
GXT vibration [85 rpm]											
20 Hz	200 (6)	196 (5)	4.4	200 (6)	195 (9)	4.4	201 (7)	193 (8)	5.7	0.106	0.186
30 Hz	200 (7)	196 (8)	3.8	200 (7)	193 (7)	5.8	201 (7)	193 (9)	5.9	0.043 *	0.244
40 Hz	200 (8)	194 (7)	5.0	200 (5)	194 (8)	5.3	201 (6)	192 (8)	6.3	0.024 *	0.272
GXT seated [85 rpm]											
450 W	449 (6)	449 (8)	3.5	—	—		—	—		0.708	0.013
550 W	544 (7)	545 (6)	3.0	—	—		—	—		0.671	0.017
650 W	645 (11)	647 (11)	3.4	—	—		—	—		0.306	0.095
6-s sprints											
Peak PO	1268 (278)	1156 (171)	127.5	—	—		—	—		0.023 *	0.386
Mean PO	1082 (181)	921 (119)	130.5	—	—		—	—		<0.001 *	0.758

SEM: Standard error of measurement. GXT: graded exercises tests, rpm: revolutions per minute. ES: Effect size. * Significant differences compared to the SRM device ($p < 0.05$).

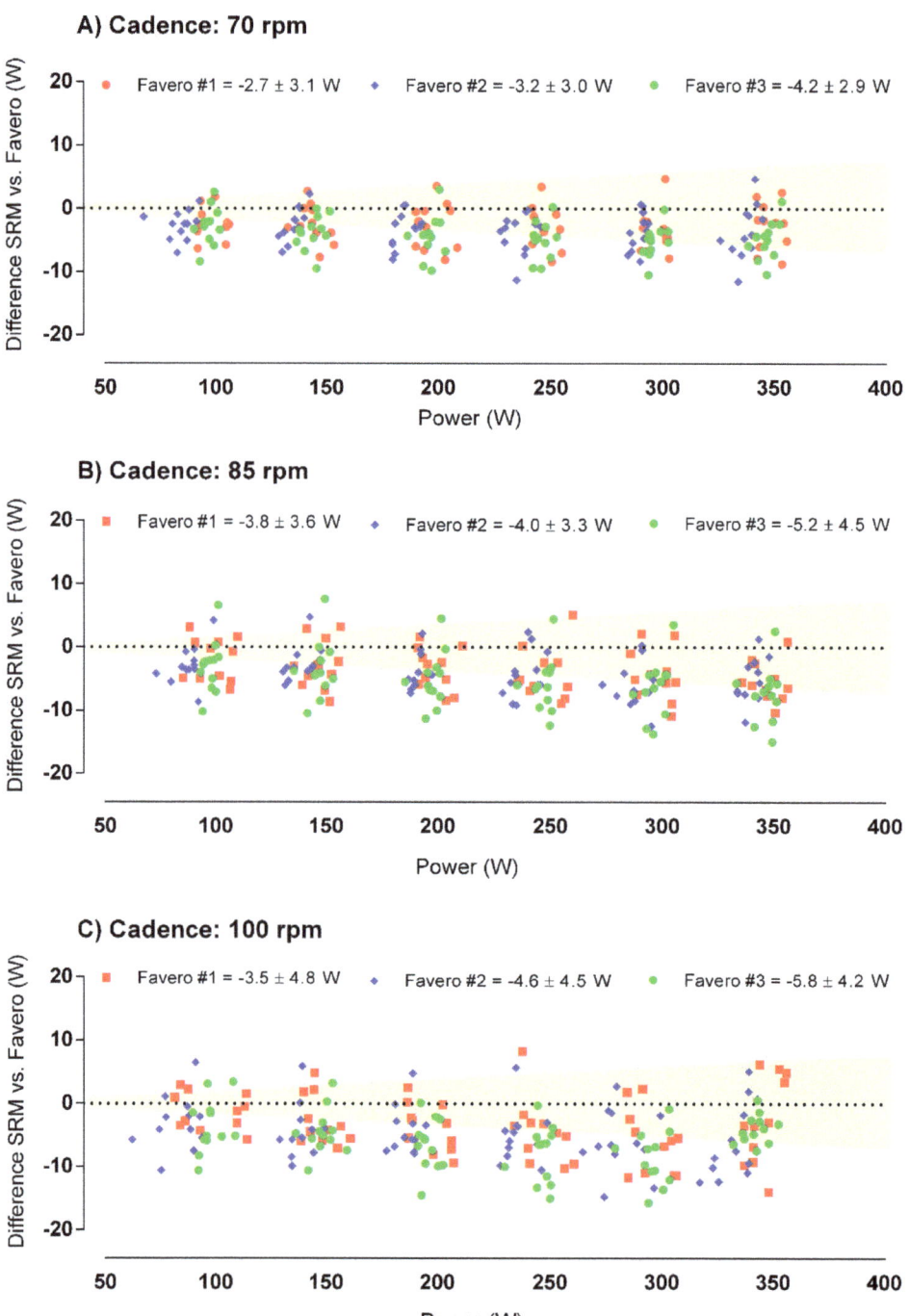

Figure 2. Bland–Altman plots showing the level of agreement between the three Favero Assioma pedals (markers) and the gold standard SRM crankset, during the seated graded exercises tests (GXT). Area shaded in yellow indicates an acceptable level of agreement ≤ 2% [24].

4. Discussion

The results of this study indicate that the Assioma Favero Pedals are a highly suitable tool for monitoring cycling performance in a wide range of workloads (100 to 650 W) and cadences (70, 85, and 100 rpm), different pedaling positions (seated and standing), and under vibration stress (20, 30, and 40 Hz). Importantly, the pedals slightly underestimated the PO compared with SRM readings, but errors are low enough to be handled in practice. To the best of our knowledge, this is the first study examining the validity and reliability of the recently commercialized Assioma Favero pedals. Stemming from this comprehensive research, coaches and researchers may be confident in using these portable power meters for cycling training and testing and benefit from their practical advantages.

The SRM crankset constitutes the best alternative available to laboratory cycle ergometers, with extremely low variability (<1.0% for a 20-strain-gauge model, and <2.0% for the 4-strain-gauge model) [12]. According to our findings, the Assioma Favero readings were very similar to the SRM across the variety of conditions examined, considering a systematic underestimation of PO readings (from -2.7 ± 5.8 W to -6.0 ± 9.9 W), probably due to the strain gauges' sensitivity or the signal processing [15]. These disparities are comparable to previously validated devices such as the Powertap P1 pedals (from -2.4 ± 4.8 W to -9.0 ± 5.3 W) [19], Garmin Vector Pedals (0.6 $\pm$ 6.2 W, 11.6 to 12.7 W; -11.6 to 12.7 W, -3.7 to 9.5 W) [1,15], Powertap Hub (2.9 $\pm$ 3.3 W; -3.7 to 9.5 W) [13], and Look Keo Power Pedal (4.6 $\pm$ 0.4 W; -15.9 to 13.9 W) [33]. Our results suggest that Assioma Favero pedals are therefore not only useful but also reliable for cycling load monitoring. In addition to the lower price in comparison with the SRM technology (>1.500 US), these pedal power meters have key advantages such as maintaining the usual riding position, the wheelset, and the crankset, as well as the reduced extra weight (microsensors attached to the pedals). Moreover, from a practical view, the ease installation of the Assioma Favero pedals allows athletes to use them interchangeably in different bicycles (e.g., track, road, and time trial). On the other hand, in comparison with other brands of pedal power meters, the features of the Assioma Favero pedals (cost ~800 US; weight ~151.5 g) make them a more affordable technology than the Garmin Vector (cost ~1400 US; weight ~156 g), as well as a lighter option than the Powertap P1 (cost ~750 US; weight ~194.5 g).

An important contribution of the present study is that we examined a large variety of testing conditions, allowing us to conclude the effects of three big cycling concerns: pedaling positions, vibration, and extremely high loads. Whereas previous studies have included some of these conditions [1,15–17,21,34], this is the first time they have all been examined in the same experiment. Of interest, there was no substantial difference in the readings between standing and seated pedaling positions, even though it is known that standing pedaling causes lateral sways and affects the biomechanics of pedaling [35]. Furthermore, testing the device performance under vibration stress is quite important considering that 88% of the excitation power during a ride on the granular rough road falls within a 10–50 Hz frequency bandwidth [27]. Our results showed that Assioma Favero pedals had similar CV, bias, and SD of bias than SRM under vibration conditions, including high ICC values. However, readings could be altered ~4% by vibrations > 20 Hz.

The fact that the Assioma Favero pedals produce errors of ~2% compared to the SRM suggests that they are sufficiently accurate to track performance changes over time [24]. This result is similar to those observed in the Powertap Hub (1.7 to 2.7%) [13] and better than the ones found in the Garmin 3.1% [1] and Vector pedals (8.5 $\pm$ 4.0%) [17]. Despite the practical advantages they offer, the Assioma Favero Pedals are limited concerning their calibration. Static calibration is not possible because the pedals need a reading of the cadence [36]. Thus, the slope of the power curve cannot be adjusted, meaning that they will always be limited by the factory calibration. Accordingly, the pedal measurement should be checked regularly against a calibrated scientific SRM crankset. Given that the current experiment was conducted under laboratory settings, future research should address the reliability of the Assioma Favero Pedals in field conditions [15].

5. Conclusions

This study confirms that the new Assioma Favero pedals are valid and reliable mobile power meters to measure PO in cyclists. This portable power meter provides an alternative to more expensive laboratory ergometers while allowing cyclists to use their bicycles for testing, training, or competition purposes. The results demonstrate that the Assioma Favero power meter pedals provide trustworthy PO readings from 100 to 650 W, in either seated or standing positions, with vibrations between 20 and 40 Hz at cadences of 70, 85, and 100 rpm, or even at a free chosen cadence. Of note, pedals consistently underestimated the SRM readings by up to 4%, with differences depending on the cycling condition.

Author Contributions: Conceptualization, V.R.-R., J.R.L.-B., and J.G.P.; methodology, V.R.-R., J.R.L.-B., Á.B.-R., A.M.-C., A.H.-B., J.C.-I., and J.G.P.; formal analysis, Á.B.-R., A.M.-C., A.H.-B., and J.C.-I.; investigation, J.R.L.-B., Á.B.-R., A.M.-C., A.H.-B.; resources, V.R.-R., J.R.L.-B., and J.G.P.; data curation, Á.B.-R. and A.M.-C.; writing—original draft preparation, J.R.L.-B., J.C.-I., and J.G.P.; writing—review and editing, V.R.-R., J.R.L.-B., and J.G.P.; visualization, J.C.-I.; supervision, J.G.P.; All authors have read and agreed to the published version of the manuscript.

Funding: This research received no external funding.

Institutional Review Board Statement: The study was conducted according to the guidelines of the Declaration of Helsinki, and approved by the Institutional Ethics Committee of the University of Murcia (ID: 2504/2019).

Informed Consent Statement: Informed consent was obtained from all subjects involved in the study.

Data Availability Statement: The data presented in this study are available on request from the corresponding author. The data are not publicly available due to privacy.

Acknowledgments: We thank the participants for their involvement in the study.

Conflicts of Interest: The authors declare no conflict of interest.

References

1. Nimmerichter, A.; Schnitzer, L.; Prinz, B.; Simon, D.; Wirth, K. Validity and Reliability of the Garmin Vector Power Meter in Laboratory and Field Cycling. *Int. J. Sports Med.* **2017**, *38*, 439–446. [CrossRef] [PubMed]
2. Peiffer, J.J.; Losco, B. Reliability/Validity of the Fortius Trainer. *Int. J. Sports Med.* **2011**, *32*, 353–356. [CrossRef] [PubMed]
3. Disley, B.X.; Li, F.X. The effect of Q Factor on gross mechanical efficiency and muscular activation in cycling. *Scand. J. Med. Sci. Sports* **2014**, *24*, 117–121. [CrossRef] [PubMed]
4. Zadow, E.K.; Kitic, C.M.; Wu, S.S.X.; Smith, S.T.; Fell, J.W. Validity of Power Settings of the Wahoo KICKR Power Trainer. *Int. J. Sports Physiol. Perform.* **2016**, *11*, 1115–1117. [CrossRef]
5. Zadow, E.K.; Kitic, C.M.; Wu, S.S.X.; Fell, J.W. Reliability of Power Settings of the Wahoo KICKR Power Trainer After 60 Hours of Use. *Int. J. Sports Physiol. Perform.* **2017**, 1–13. [CrossRef]
6. Lillo-Bevia, J.R.; Pallarés, J.G. Validity, and reliability of the Cycleops hammer cycle ergometer. *Int. J. Sports Physiol. Perform.* **2018**, *13*, 853–859. [CrossRef] [PubMed]
7. Muriel, X.; Courel-Ibáñez, J.; Cerezuela-Espejo, V.; Pallarés, J.G. Training Load and Performance Impairments in Professional Cyclists During COVID-19 Lockdown. *Int. J. Sports Physiol. Perform.* **2020**, 1–4. [CrossRef] [PubMed]
8. Jeffries, O.; Waldron, M.; Patterson, S.D.; Galna, B. An Analysis of Variability in Power Output during Indoor and Outdoor Cycling Time Trials. *Int. J. Sports Physiol. Perform.* **2019**, *14*, 1273–1279. [CrossRef]
9. González-Alonso, J.; Mora-Rodríguez, R.; Coyle, E.F. Stroke volume during exercise: Interaction of environment and hydration. *Am. J. Physiol. Hearth Circ. Physiol.* **2000**, *278*, H321–H330. [CrossRef] [PubMed]
10. Passfield, L.; Doust, J.H. Changes in cycling efficiency and performance after endurance exercise. *Med. Sci. Sports Exerc.* **2000**, *32*, 1935–1941. [CrossRef] [PubMed]
11. Martin, J.C.; Milliken, D.L.; Cobb, J.E.; McFadden, K.L.; Coggan, A.R. Validation of a mathematical model for road cycling power. *J. Appl. Biomech.* **1998**, *14*, 276–291. [CrossRef]
12. Jones, S.M.; Passfield, L. Dynamic calibration of bicycle power measuring cranks. *Eng. Sport* **1998**, 265–274.
13. Bertucci, W.; Duc, S.; Villerius, V.; Pernin, J.N.; Grappe, F. Validity and reliability of the PowerTap mobile cycling powermeter when compared with the SRM device. *Int. J. Sports Med.* **2005**, *26*, 868–873. [CrossRef] [PubMed]
14. Gardner, A.S.; Stephens, S.; Martin, D.T.; Lawton, E.; Lee, H.; Jenkins, D. Accuracy of SRM and power tap power monitoring systems for bicycling. *Med. Sci. Sports Exerc.* **2004**, *36*, 1252–1258. [CrossRef] [PubMed]

15. Bouillod, A.; Pinot, J.; Soto-Romero, G.; Bertucci, W.; Grappe, F. Validity, Sensitivity, Reproducibility, and Robustness of the PowerTap, Stages, and Garmin Vector Power Meters in Comparison with the SRM Device. *Int. J. Sports Physiol. Perform.* **2017**, *12*, 1023–1030. [CrossRef] [PubMed]
16. Dickinson, T.; Wright, J. The reliability and accuracy of the Garmin Vector 3 power pedals. *Proc. Inst. Mech. Eng. Part P J. Sport. Eng. Technol.* **2020**. [CrossRef]
17. Hutchison, R.; Klapthor, G.; Edwards, K.; Bruneau, K.; Mocko, G.; Vahidi, A. Validity and Reproducibility of the Garmin Vector Power Meter When Compared to the SRM Device. *J. Sport. Sci.* **2017**, *5*, 235–241.
18. Novak, A.R.; Dascombe, B.J. Agreement of Power Measures between Garmin Vector and SRM Cycle Power Meters. *Meas. Phys. Educ. Exerc. Sci.* **2016**, *20*, 167–172. [CrossRef]
19. Pallarés, J.G.; Lillo-Bevia, J.R. Validity and Reliability of the PowerTap P1 Pedals Power Meter. *J. Sports Sci. Med.* **2018**, *17*, 305–311.
20. Whittle, C.; Smith, N.; Jobson, S.A. Validity of PowerTap P1 Pedals during Laboratory-Based Cycling Time Trial Performance. *Sport* **2018**, *6*, 92. [CrossRef]
21. Wright, J.; Walker, T.; Burnet, S.; Jobson, S.A. The reliability and validity of the Powertap P1 power pedals before and after 100 hours of use. *Int. J. Sports Physiol. Perform.* **2019**, *14*, 855–858. [CrossRef] [PubMed]
22. Bertucci, W.; Duc, S.; Villerius, V.; Grappe, F. Validity and reliability of the axiom powertrain cycle ergometer when compared with an SRM powermeter. *Int. J. Sports Med.* **2005**, *26*, 59–65. [CrossRef] [PubMed]
23. Vanpraagh, E.; Bedu, M.; Roddier, P.; Coudert, J. A simple calibration method for mecanically braked cycle ergometers. *Int. J. Sports Med.* **1992**, *13*, 27–30. [CrossRef] [PubMed]
24. Paton, C.D.; Hopkins, W.G. Tests of cycling performance. *Sport Med.* **2001**, *31*, 489–496. [CrossRef]
25. Jeukendrup, A.E.; Craig, N.P.; Hawley, J.A. The bioenergetics of World Class Cycling. *J. Sci. Med. Sport* **2000**, *3*, 414–433. [CrossRef]
26. Storer, T.W.; Davis, J.A.; Caiozzo, V.J. Accurate prediction of VO2(max) in cycle ergometry. *Med. Sci. Sports Exerc.* **1990**, *22*, 704–712. [CrossRef] [PubMed]
27. Lepine, J.; Champoux, Y.; Drouet, J.M. A Laboratory Excitation Technique to Test Road Bike Vibration Transmission. *Exp. Tech.* **2016**, *40*, 227–234. [CrossRef]
28. Hernández-Belmonte, A.; Buendía-Romero, Á.; Martínez-Cava, A.; Courel-Ibáñez, J.; Mora-Rodríguez, R.; Pallarés, J.G. Wingate test, when time and overdue fatigue matter: Validity and sensitivity of two time-shortened versions. *Appl. Sci.* **2020**, *10*, 8002. [CrossRef]
29. Pallarés, J.G.; López-Samanes, A.; Fernández-Elías, V.E.; Aguado-Jiménez, R.; Ortega, J.F.; Gómez, C.; Ventura, R.; Segura, J.; Mora-Rodríguez, R. Pseudoephedrine and circadian rhythm interaction on neuromuscular performance. *Scand. J. Med. Sci. Sport.* **2015**, *25*, e603–e612. [CrossRef] [PubMed]
30. Atkinson, G.; Nevill, A. Statistical methods for asssing measurement Error (reliability) in variables relevant to sports medicine. *Sport Med.* **1998**, *26*, 217–238. [CrossRef] [PubMed]
31. Bland, J.M.; Altman, D.G. Measuring agreement in method comparison studies. *Stat. Methods Med. Res.* **1999**, *8*, 135–160. [CrossRef] [PubMed]
32. Cohen, J. *Statistical Power Anaylsis for the Behavioral Sciences*, 2nd ed.; Lawrence Erlbaum: Hillsdale, MI, USA, 1988; ISBN 0805802835.
33. Sparks, S.A.; Dove, B.; Bridge, C.A.; Midgley, A.W.; McNaughton, L.R. Validity and Reliability of the Look Keo Power Pedal System for Measuring Power Output During Incremental and Repeated Sprint Cycling. *Int. J. Sports Physiol. Perform.* **2015**, *10*, 39–45. [CrossRef] [PubMed]
34. Granier, C.; Hausswirth, C.; Dorel, S.; Yann, L.M. Validity and Reliability of The Stages Cycling Power Meter. *J. Strength Cond. Res.* **2017**. [CrossRef] [PubMed]
35. Stone, C.; Hull, M.L. Rider bicycle interaction loads durinig standing treadmill cycling. *J. Appl. Biomech.* **1993**, *9*, 202–218. [CrossRef]
36. Bini, R.R.; Hume, P.A. Assessment of bilateral asymmetry in cycling using a commercial instrumented crank system and instrumented pedals. *Int. J. Sports Physiol. Perform.* **2014**, *9*, 876–881. [CrossRef] [PubMed]

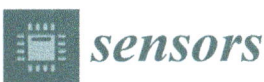

Article

The Relationship between VO$_2$max, Power Management, and Increased Running Speed: Towards Gait Pattern Recognition through Clustering Analysis

Juan Pardo Albiach [1,*], Melanie Mir-Jimenez [1,2], Vanessa Hueso Moreno [3], Iván Nácher Moltó [2] and Javier Martínez-Gramage [2]

1. Embedded Systems and Artificial Intelligence Group, Universidad Cardenal Herrera-CEU, CEU Universities, 46115 Valencia, Spain; melanie.mir@alumnos.uchceu.es
2. Department of Physiotherapy, Universidad Cardenal Herrera-CEU, CEU Universities, 46115 Valencia, Spain; ivan.nacher.molto@gmail.com (I.N.M.); jmg@uchceu.es (J.M.-G.)
3. Triathlon Technification Program, Valencian Community Triathlon Federation, 46940 Manises, Spain; vanessa.huesa@triatlocv.org
* Correspondence: juan.pardo@uchceu.es

Abstract: Triathlon has become increasingly popular in recent years. In this discipline, maximum oxygen consumption (VO$_2$max) is considered the gold standard for determining competition cardiovascular capacity. However, the emergence of wearable sensors (as Stryd) has drastically changed training and races, allowing for the more precise evaluation of athletes and study of many more potential determining variables. Thus, in order to discover factors associated with improved running efficiency, we studied which variables are correlated with increased speed. We then developed a methodology to identify associated running patterns that could allow each individual athlete to improve their performance. To achieve this, we developed a correlation matrix, implemented regression models, and created a heat map using hierarchical cluster analysis. This highlighted relationships between running patterns in groups of young triathlon athletes and several different variables. Among the most important conclusions, we found that high VO$_2$max did not seem to be significantly correlated with faster speed. However, faster individuals did have higher power per kg, horizontal power, stride length, and running effectiveness, and lower ground contact time and form power ratio. VO$_2$max appeared to strongly correlate with power per kg and this seemed to indicate that to run faster, athletes must also correctly manage their power.

Keywords: VO$_2$max; power; running biomechanics; hierarchical cluster analysis; machine learning; triathletes

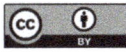

1. Introduction

Triathlon is an increasingly popular sport with broad participation spanning three disciplines (swimming, cycling, and running) in the same event. In recent years in Spain, participation in triathlon has increased by more than 200% among young athletes of school age (Spanish Triathlon Federation) [1]. In this discipline, maximum oxygen consumption (VO$_2$max) is considered the gold standard for determining cardiovascular capacity [2]. Accurate VO$_2$max measurement requires specialised equipment found in exercise physiology laboratories—techniques that are often not available to every professional. In addition, testing an entire team can be time consuming because only one athlete can be evaluated at a time. Therefore, alternative parameters have been developed to predict VO$_2$max that allow several athletes to be tested at the same time without requiring sophisticated laboratory tools [3].

The ability both to maintain a high percentage of VO$_2$max for long periods of time and simultaneously move efficiently, referred to as running effectiveness (RE), comes from a series of physiological attributes that contribute to the success of running performance and help athletes stand out [4]. RE is generally used to refer to steady-state oxygen consumption at a given running speed and expresses the energy expenditure required by individuals to perform at a given intensity [5]. Trained runners have higher REs compared to lesser-trained runners, which indicates that positive adaptations occur in response to regular training. Although a given athlete may be genetically predisposed to having a 'good' RE, various strategies can potentially further enhance an individual's RE by increasing metabolic, cardiorespiratory, biomechanical, and/or neuromuscular responses [4].

Until a few years ago, RE was not considered an important factor in the improvement of athletes' careers. However, this area is now the focus of increasing interest. RE is the result of the interaction between multiple factors. Of these, the most important may be biomechanical factors, neuromuscular variables such as leg stiffness, exposure to training periods at altitude, and anthropometric variables [5]. A good correlation has been observed between RE and oxygen consumption (VO_2) while running. Runners with a good RE use less oxygen than runners with a poor RE at the same speed and under homogeneous conditions [6]. However, it has also been noted that RE can vary by up to 30% between trained runners with a similar VO_2max [7].

In recent years, the advent of portable power estimators has dramatically changed training and competitive running, allowing athletes to be accurately evaluated [8]. Among these systems, Stryd, Boulder, CO, USA (www.stryd.com, accessed on 1 March 2021) pioneered the manufacture of power meters for runners. The Stryd running power meter is a pedometer that attaches to the shoe to measure variables that quantify performance including pace, distance, elevation, power, form power, cadence, ground contact time, vertical oscillation, and leg spring stiffness [9].

This is a relatively new type of instrument, and the validity and reliability of these systems for evaluating power output and space–time parameters have only recently been validated. In this context, the operating power data recorded by Stryd has been successfully used to establish a linear relationship between power and speed to predict power output at different submaximal operating speeds, demonstrating the great potential of this portable equipment for studying efficiency patterns while running. Additionally, a few studies found a positive correlation between Stryd's power data and the operating economy or metabolic demands. Indeed, a recent study by Cerezuela-Espejo et al. determined the correlation between these power meters and oxygen consumption [8]. Moreover, Cartón-Llorente et al. 2021 [10], determined that Stryd could reliably determine the functional threshold power (FTP) of runners.

The detection of running patterns and the variables involved in achieving the maximum possible speed while running has always been the subject of research [11–13]. This allows us to compare which parameters best define running efficiency, meaning that the similarities and discrepancies between athletes who are more or less successful in competitions can be examined. In this sense, the use of objective grouping or classification techniques (which are commonly employed with a variety of goals in different fields such as engineering, science, or technology) is also feasible in sports sciences. Thus, unsupervised classification (commonly known as clustering) is a classical technique used in the area of machine learning [14]. According to Rokach [15], clustering divides data patterns into subsets in such a way that similar patterns are grouped together.

Several studies have focused on gait patterns by using clustering techniques such as hierarchical clustering analysis (HCA). These provide an interpretable analysis of large quantities of data from sensors, as a multivariate problem, to obtain different groups of athletes with similar running gait patterns [16]. The objective of this study was to determine running patterns and variables involved in attaining maximum running speed in young triathletes.

2. Materials and Methods

2.1. Participants

The participants belonged to the high-performance Triathlon Technification Plan based in the Valencian Community in Spain. The study was approved by the Ethics Committee for Biomedical research at the CEU-Cardenal Herrera University, (reference No: CEI18/137) and was registered as a clinical trial (ClinicalTrials.gov registration No: NCT04221698).

Inclusion/Exclusion Criteria

Fifteen healthy triathletes (9 males and 6 females) were enrolled in this study (Table 1):

Table 1. Participant characteristics [a].

	Male ($n = 9$)	Female ($n = 6$)
Age	15 ± 1.5	14 ± 1.0
Weight, kg	56.3 ± 8.9	55.2 ± 3.2
Height, cm	170 ± 7.2	168.5 ± 4.3
Body mass index, kg/m^2	19.4 ± 1.7	19.3 ± 1.2
Years competing	7.8 ± 6.8	6.8 ± 1.0
Training hours per week	19.1 ± 2.8	19.6 ± 2.6

[a] Values are presented as the mean ± SD.

Participants were included if they reported having run a minimum of 2 days per week in the 3 months prior with no reported injuries and with their worst pain rated a minimum of 3 out 10 on a numerical rating scale (NRS) for pain (0 = no pain; 10 = worst possible pain) [17]. Participants were excluded if they reported any previous musculoskeletal surgery, neurological impairment, knee structural deformities, pain caused by trauma or sports activities, having stopped running, or having received additional treatment outside of this study.

2.2. Data Collection

All the participants performed a 5 min warm-up on a treadmill (HP Cosmos Quasar, Nussdorf-Traunstein, Germany) at their preferred speed [17]. The initial running speed was set at 8 km/h with a gradient of 1% [18]. The starting speed was 3 km/h, with speed increments of 1 km/h every 60 s. The subjects walked the first three steps (up to 7 km/h), and continued running from 8 km/h, until volitional exhaustion. After exhaustion, the athletes underwent a 5-min recovery protocol during which the speed was decreased each minute from 100% to 60%, 55%, 50%, 45%, and 40% of the maximal achieved speed [19].

Expired gas was sampled continuously and O_2 and CO_2 concentration in expired gas were determined using the Ultima™ CardiO2® gas exchange analysis system ((MGC Diagnostics Corporation, St Paul, MN, USA, https://mgcdiagnostics.com, accessed on 1 March 2021). Heart rate (HR) was collected using a telemetric heart rate monitor (Polar Electro, Kempele, Finland), and stored in PC memory. The thresholds assessed were Aerobic and Anaerobic Ventilatory Thresholds (VT1 and VT2), identified by different ventilatory criteria, such as: VSlope (VO_2 and VCO_2), Ventilatory Equivalents (EqO_2 and $EqCO_2$), Ventilation (VE), Pressures at the end of each expiration (Pet O_2 and Pet CO_2), and Respiratory Quotient (RER).

The Stryd sensor, paired with a Garmin Forerunner 935 watch, was used to determine running power and recording was started and stopped at the same time as the stress test. As shown in Figure 1, the powers at each threshold were recorded at the same time the ventilation thresholds 1 and 2 (VT1 and VT2) and maximal aerobic power (MAP) occurred, with these physiological variables also being defined.

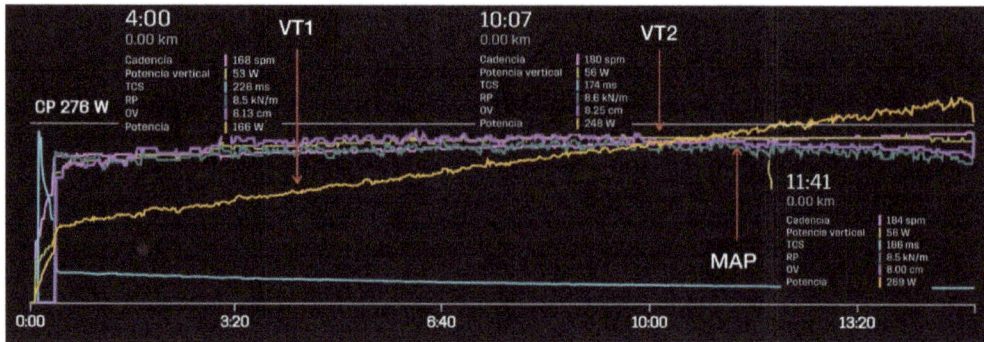

Figure 1. Determination of the ventilation thresholds 1 and 2 (VT1 and VT2) and maximal aerobic power (MAP) with the corresponding power at each physiological threshold.

Once the participant data were acquired, a raw data set was constructed for the purpose of this study. We then assessed and cleaned the database to correct possible errors in the data, e.g., missing values or extreme values gathered from the overall system. Then the data was arranged in "csv" format to be treated by the statistical program RStudio [20]. Finally, the experimental data set was structured with 14 columns referring to the measured variables for each participant and 15 rows corresponding to each athlete.

Variables Analysed

To determine athlete running power, we used a Stryd sensor (Stryd power meter; Stryd, Inc., Boulder, CO, USA, https://www.stryd.com, accessed on 1 March 2021) a relatively new device, which estimates power in watts. Stryd is a carbon fibre-reinforced foot pod that attaches to the shoe and weighs 9.1 g. The sensor is based on a 6-axis inertial motion sensor (3-axis gyroscope and 3-axis accelerometer). We analysed the following variables: power (W), leg spring stiffness (LSS), leg spring stiffness per kg (LSS/kg), vertical oscillation (VO), power per kg (W/kg), horizontal power (HW), speed (SPD), cadence (CAD), ground contact time (GCT), vertical ratio (VR), stride length (SL), running effectiveness (RE), form power ratio (FPR), and maximum oxygen consumption (VO_2max). To determine the VO_2max, the Ultima™ CardiO2® gas exchange analysis system (MGC Diagnostics Corporation, St Paul, MN, USA was used.

2.3. Data Analysis

We used different statistical and artificial intelligence data analysis techniques to examine the data we collected. Our objective was to understand which variables most influence running efficiency. Thus, we studied which factors were related to each other based on their linear correlations and tried to understand how some characteristics influence others with the goal of obtaining clues that could explain different running patterns in young triathletes.

Clustering techniques were used to obtain running patterns that would allow us to visually generate groups of individuals with similar running characteristics [14]. These groups were formed based on the data collected and extracted from the Stryd sensor. Thus, each runner had their own colour pattern which we could use to identify the variables each individual should work on to improve both their speed and efficiency. We performed all of the calculations with RStudio desktop software for macOS (version 1.3.1073, 'Giant Goldenrod' release) [20]. In the following section, we detailed the techniques we used to understand the interpretation of the results.

2.3.1. Linear Correlations

Linear correlation and simple linear regression are statistical methods that study the linear relationship between two variables. Correlation quantifies how related two variables are, while linear regression consists of generating an equation (model) that, based on the relationship between two variables, allows the value of one to be predicted based on the other. Thus, variables X and Y are said to be positively correlated if high values of X are associated with high values of Y, and low values of X are associated with low values of Y. In contrast, if high values of X are associated with low values of Y, and vice versa, the variables are negatively correlated [21]. Correlation coefficients range from −1 (for a negative correlation) to +1 (for a positive correlation)—correlations close to 0 indicate the absence of a linear correlation between two variables [22].

As a general rule, linear correlation studies precede the generation of linear regression models, after the confirmation of a correlation between variables. The difference is that while correlation measures the strength of an association between two variables, regression quantifies the nature of the relationship [21]. Therefore, it is useful to calculate a correlation matrix showing all the variables in rows and columns, in which the intersection values quantify the correlation between them. This matrix can then be used to calculate a 'correlation map' that highlights which variables were linearly related to each other at a statistical given significance level (p-value), in our case, $p = 0.05$.

Thus, we were able to quickly render a colour map that quantified the significance and direction of the relationship between two variables, therefore enabling us to choose which ones merited further study. We mainly focused on the speed variable in this current work, although we did study other possible correlations that (through other measurements) could help explain what influences running efficiency. The correlation map also gave us a much better understanding of running patterns.

2.3.2. Hierarchical Clustering Analysis

The term clustering refers to a wide range of unsupervised techniques from machine learning fields whose purpose is to find patterns or groups of similar objects (known as clusters) within a set of observations [23]. Clustering is one of the most important data mining methods for discovering patterns in multidimensional data. The partitions are established such that observations within the same group are similar to each other and different from the observations of other groups. Thus, unsupervised learning can be viewed as an extension of exploratory data analysis to gain insights into a set of data and how the different variables relate to each other. Additionally, clustering provides tools to analyse these variables and discover relationships and patterns within them [23].

An excellent review of clustering techniques can be found in [14] which also describes a common clustering technique taxonomy proposed by Fraley and Raftery [24]. They suggested dividing these techniques into two different groups: hierarchical and partitioning methods. After testing different techniques in this work, we focused on HCA. Although other techniques with different advantages and disadvantages are available, we considered this technique to be best suited to our data set.

HCA is an alternative to the common K-means technique and is more flexible and better able to discover outlying groups or records. This type of clustering also lends itself to intuitive graphical display, leading to easier cluster interpretation. HCA methods form clusters by iteratively dividing patterns using a top–down or bottom–up approach. Hierarchical clustering methods may be agglomerative or divisive. The former follows the bottom–up approach to build clusters starting with a single object and then merging these atomic clusters groups of increasing size until all of the objects are finally lying in a single cluster or certain termination conditions are satisfied. The latter is a top–down approach which breaks a cluster containing all objects into smaller groups, until each object forms an independent cluster or the termination conditions are satisfied. The hierarchical methods usually lead to the formation of dendrograms that allow the resulting groupings to be visualised.

3. Results

First, we studied the reliability of the Stryd sensor against the gold standard measured in the laboratory by calculating the correlation of the values obtained with the sensor and the standard at each of the three thresholds. Our data demonstrated the reliability of the Stryd compared to laboratory systems, as also shown in some recent studies [8,25] and so we used this data in the subsequent detection of running patterns. Thus, as shown in Table 2, we compared the speed obtained in the laboratory system with the values for W, W/kg, HW, and FPR obtained by the Stryd device. In addition, these data were also compared with VO_2 (mL/kg/min) measured in the laboratory so we could find the variables that best correlated with speed.

Table 2. Correlation between power per kilogram (W/kg), horizontal power (HW), and the form power ratio (FPR) with athlete speed at each running threshold, as well as between VO_2max and the velocity at each threshold. Note: (ST) refers to the measurement made with the Stryd system.

Threshold	Gold Standard	Variables	Pearson's Coefficient (r)
VT1	Speed (km/h)	W/kg (ST)	0.97
	Speed (km/h)	HW (ST)	0.82
	Speed (km/h)	VO_2 (mL/kg/min)	0.22
	Speed (km/h)	FPR (ST)	−0.82
VT2	Speed (km/h)	W/kg (ST)	0.98
	Speed (km/h)	HW (ST)	0.92
	Speed (km/h)	VO_2 (mL/kg/min)	0.38
	Speed (km/h)	FPR (ST)	−0.92
MAP	Speed (km/h)	W/kg (ST)	0.94
	Speed (km/h)	HW (ST)	0.91
	Speed (km/h)	VO_2 (mL/kg/min)	0.67
	Speed (km/h)	FPR (ST)	−0.91

The strongest correlations with speed at each threshold were W/kg, HW, and FPR; on the contrary VO_2max was not significantly correlated with speed at any of the thresholds.

Figure 2 shows the graphs corresponding to the regression models calculated to compare W/kg and VO_2max for each of the three thresholds. This allowed us to identify which variable best explained the dependent variable of speed. In this case, the regression models highlighted two variables as explanatory factors for the speed reached by the study participants.

Power, but not VO_2max, perfectly explained speed for each of the thresholds. As shown in Table 2, there was an exceptionally strong (near 100%) correlation between power and speed, which was also observed in the regression model with an R^2 remarkably close to 1. This indicated that variability in speed could be explained very well by the power of the athlete. Moreover, the regression model indicated how much power would be required to acquire a determined speed at each threshold. On the contrary, this effect was not observed for VO_2max, and the corresponding regression models could not explain the increase or decrease in speed based on this parameter. There was no evidence to indicate a linear relationship between VO_2max and speed.

3.1. Correlations Map

We carried out both Pearson's r analysis (the most commonly used method to assess correlations) and Kendall and Spearman correlations as non-parametric methods commonly used to perform rank-based correlation analysis [23]. Nevertheless, the significant correlations remained the same in both cases and so we used Pearson's correlation coefficient (r) to calculate the correlation matrix to highlight the most pertinent variables to study. As shown in Figure 3. The dots in red tones referred to negative correlations. For example, as the HW variable increased, the FPR decreased, in a significant and quite strong linear correlation remarkably close to −1. In addition, as FPR decreased, GCT decreased, and

SPD, W/kg, HW, W, and LSS increased. Furthermore, as GCT decreased, LSS/kg, VO$_2$max, SPD, W/kg, and HW increased. Finally, as RE increased, SPD and SL also increased.

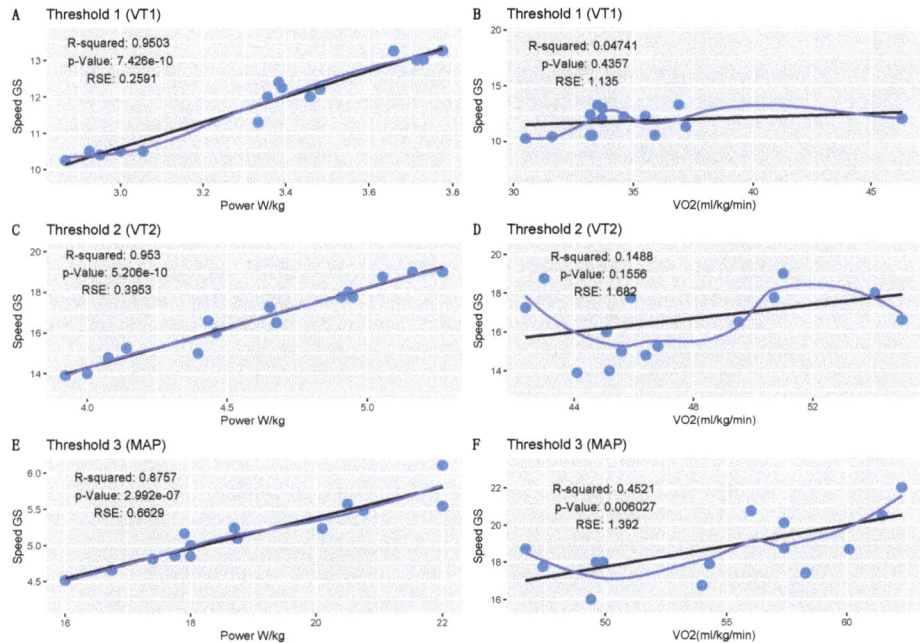

Figure 2. Regression models for power (W) and maximum oxygen consumption (VO$_2$max) with respect to speed. The regression models compared power and VO$_2$max with speed at ventilation threshold 1 (VT1; **A**,**B**), ventilation threshold 2 (VT2; **C**,**D**), and at the maximal aerobic power (MAP) threshold (**E**,**F**).

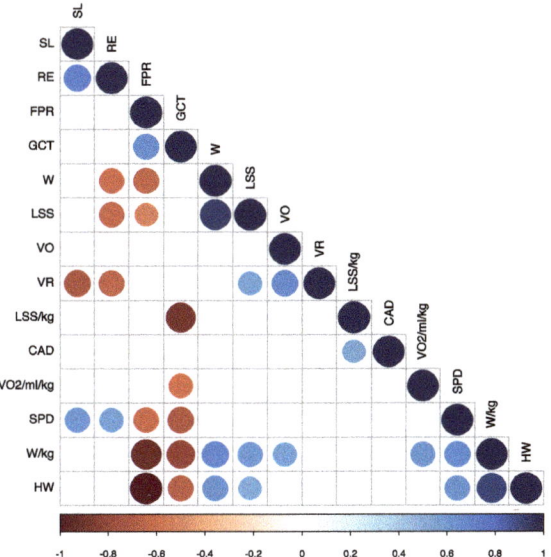

Figure 3. Correlations map representing only the significant ($p < 0.05$) variables. Power (W), leg spring stiffness (LSS), vertical oscillation (VO), power per kilogram (W/kg), speed (SPD), cadence (CAD), ground contact time (GCT), and the form power ratio (FPR).

Dots in blue tones referred to positive correlations such as the reasonable correlation between SPD and W/kg and significant correlation between SPD and HW. This means that the more W/kg and HW, the higher the SPD runners attained—a clear indicator of running pattern. When LSS/kg increased, CAD also increased and the increase in VO$_2$max correlated with the increase in W/kg. As SPD increased, W/kg and HW also increased; increased W/kg produced increased HW, VO, W, and LSS; as HW increased, W and LSS increased; and increased W resulted in increased LSS.

In contrast, some variables were not significantly correlated and when we cross-referenced these there was only one gap in the matrix. For example, our data indicated that a higher running cadence did not mean that the athlete would run faster. Indeed, this variable did not show a significant linear correlation, meaning that, a priori, it was unlikely to be an important factor in the generation of more speed. In contrast, there was no correlation between athletes with a high VO$_2$max and faster speed, as we previously observed in our regression models. However, faster athletes had a higher W/kg and HW, and a lower FPR. VO$_2$max strongly correlated with W/kg and this seemed to indicate that to run fast, athletes must also correctly manage their power.

3.2. Clustering Heat Map

Finally, we decided to study the patterns of each runner by generating a heat map using HCA. First the data was scaled to standardise the variables and minimise the impact of the different magnitudes. Thus, the data were normalised to have zero mean and unit variance. When the data were scaled, the Euclidean distance of the z-scores was the same as the correlation distance. On the other hand, a connectivity-based clustering or HCA approach was used to identify homogeneous gait patterns in the entire participant group by creating a cluster tree or dendrogram. To perform the HCA, we used the R package 'pheatmap' library (Version 1.0.12) [26]. This allowed us to generate clusters of similar runners based on the variables extracted from the Stryd data and to construct a heat map to observe these patterns according to assigned colours.

The procedure for performing agglomerative HCA on the data set consisted of three steps: calculation of the distance matrix between participants, computation of a linkage function, and definition of clusters. In brief, first the Euclidean distance between every pair of athletes was calculated for an M-dimensional space. Second, individual participants were paired into binary clusters based on the distance information using the Ward D2 linkage method [27]. Third, newly formed clusters were grouped into larger clusters until the dendrogram was formed [16,24]. The Ward minimum variance method was used to minimise the total within-cluster variance. At each step, the cluster pair with a minimum between-cluster distance was merged.

Finally, we visually inspected the dendrogram and decided to separate the clusters into three groups based on our knowledge of the athletes. Thus, the K parameter was established at 3. As shown in Figure 4, we represented the result of the clustering as a heat map.

As shown on the heat map, three clusters of athletes with similar characteristics to each other were identified. The reference group was cluster two (athletes S7 and S13), representing the two individuals with the best competitive results. As shown, the SPD variable for these two athletes corresponded to the highest values, highlighted in warmer colours (red tones). In contrast, the participants with SPD marked in cooler colours (blue tones) were the slowest from among the cohort. The colour scale was established by columns, with red being representing the individual with the highest value in each of the variables.

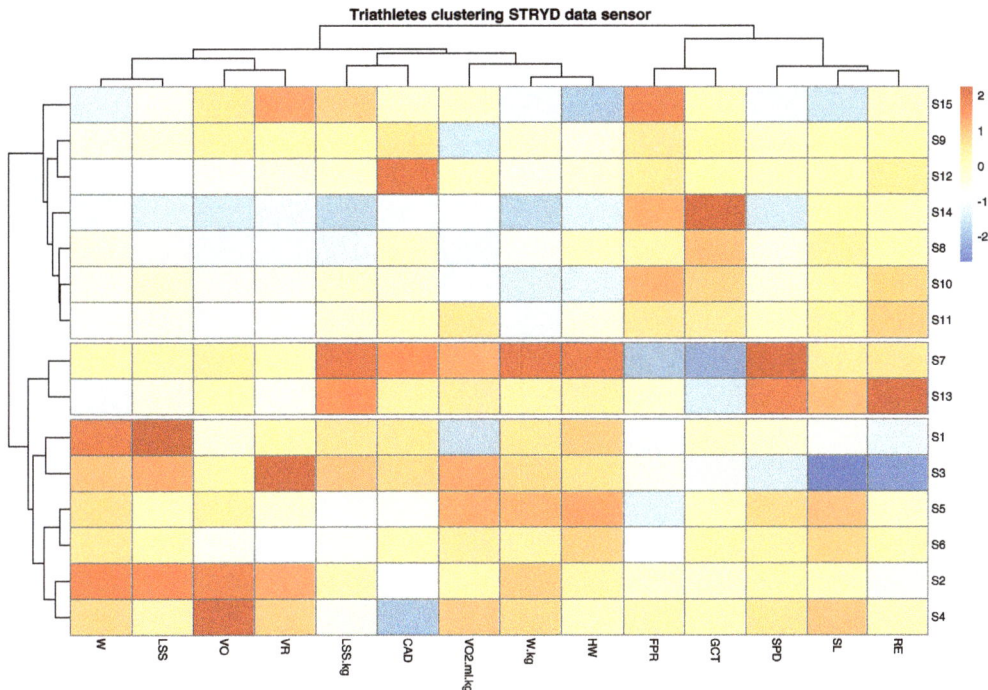

Figure 4. Heat map of the clustering of athletes. The participants distributed into cluster 1 (S1, S2, S3, S4, S5, and S6), cluster 2 (S7 and S13), and cluster 3 (S8, S9, S10, S11, S12, S14, and S15).

Thus, a colour pattern could be observed for each individual with respect to the reference group by noting the variables for which warmer or cooler colours were obtained. For example, participant S14 obtained low SPD, VO_2max consumption, HW, and W/kg values and high values for FPR and GCT, indicating the aspects of their running technique they should work on to increase their RE or running speed. In contrast, athlete S2 had high W/kg, LSS, W, and VO values and low CAD values with respect to the reference participants, even though their running speed was normal. This was probably because of the strong correlation between SPD and W/kg and weak correlation between SPD and the other variables.

Based on these data, we carried out a detailed analysis of which characteristics in each athlete were increased or reduced compared to those who had obtained better results. Moreover, by examining certain reference variables such as RE, we observed differences between the participants. Figure 5 shows a graphical representation of the relationship between speed and the variables that best correlated with it, also separating the individuals by each of the cluster groups. These graphs allowed us to better understand the differences between athletes who run faster and who better manage their performance power compared to those who run slower, according to these groups. Group two was used as the reference and was shown in green.

Thus, the fastest runners had a decreased FPR (A) and GCT (B), and an increased W/kg (C), HW (D), SL (E), and RE (F). Based on these results, it appears that power management and running dynamics play a more important role than VO_2max in athletes who run faster.

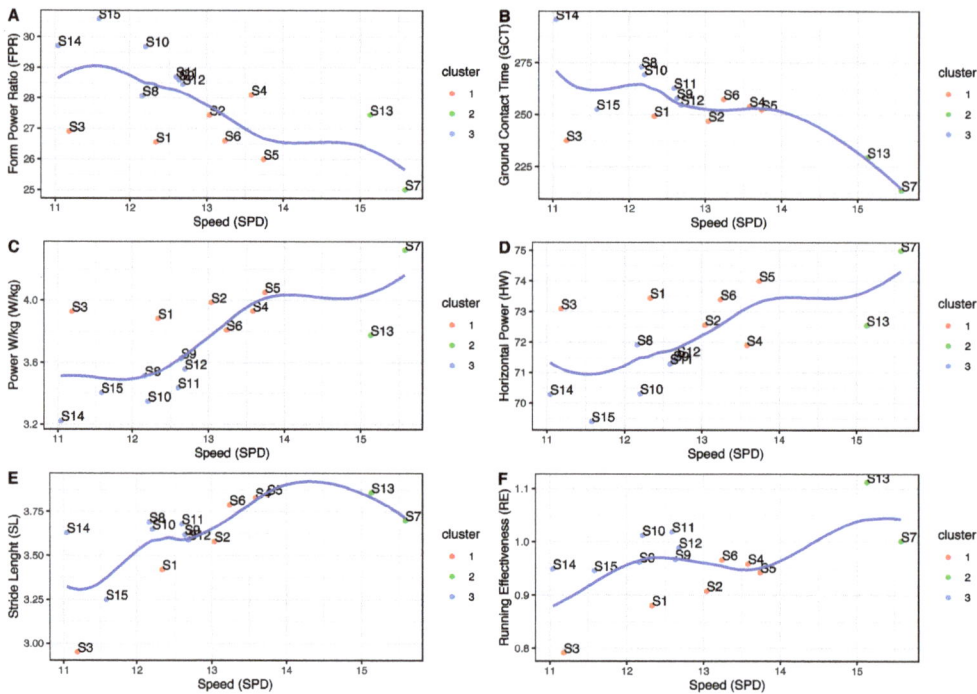

Figure 5. The relationship between speed and the variables that best correlated with it. (**A**) Form power ratio (FPR), (**B**) ground contact time (GCT), (**C**) power per kilogram (W/kg), (**D**) horizontal power (HW), (**E**) stride length (SL), and (**F**) running effectiveness (RE).

4. Discussion

The objective of this study was to determine the running patterns and variables involved in the maximum running speed of young triathletes. We observed that there was a pattern of decreased FPR and GCT, and increased W/kg, HW, SL, and RE among faster athletes. Based on these results, it appears that power management and running dynamics play a more important role than VO_2max in athletes who run faster. Various studies have demonstrated the reliability and validity of portable systems such as Stryd for measuring running power [9,28,29]. Additionally, running power is a more sensitive measure of exercise intensity than other internal and external parameters, such as heart rate or speed [28].

Calculation of the linear correlations for each of the variables we collected in this study was an easy and fast method to understand which factors or characteristics were related to each other. This allowed us to quickly find indications about the influence of some of these variables with respect to others in order to obtain the most important power parameters for running. We observed that the Stryd device data correlated well with VO_2max laboratory equipment data. This added confidence to our study of the interrelation of variables and subsequently, to our comparisons between athletes to reliably apply grouping techniques to search for patterns representative of RE. It was also interesting to see that certain variables did not linearly influence RE and so, could be discarded for the purposes of this work, or studied using other distribution models.

In addition, we consider the clustering techniques represented by heat maps to constitute an especially useful tool for quickly explaining the differences between different runners. The colour codes allowed us to find similar patterns for each variable collected during the test, which corresponded to the patterns of each competitor. The ability to group athletes by these colour patterns represents RE patterns either based on the reference of athletes who obtained the best competitive results or simply on a pre-determined set of variables. This will allow us to extrapolate these findings to techniques for other sports in which different characteristics are measured.

Limitations of the Study and Future Activities

One of the limitations of this work was its sample size because it was only sufficient to allow us to obtain preliminary results related to our research topic. However, this work is encouraging and we believe that future work in this area seems very promising. We must also consider that obtaining data for high-performance athletes is quite difficult because they are a very small population and therefore the sample will never be large. Nevertheless, although our sample cohort was small and homogeneous, we would need a larger number of subjects to have sufficient strength of these results to be able to generalise them with confidence to other athletes with similar characteristics. Additionally, for future research, the variable sex should be considered, as it could be a confusing factor when studying the RE.

Finally, the sample size made it difficult to fully utilise the potential of the some of the artificial intelligence techniques available to us. Future work should be directed towards the application of these results in the training of young triathletes to help improve their performance and to determine biomechanical running patterns that complement the present power study using the Stryd sensor in young athletes.

5. Conclusions

In this work, we studied how to identify running patterns among young athletes based on data from wearable sensors (such as Stryd) as compared to laboratory equipment results. Our findings indicate that power management was key to maximising running speed. VO_2max strongly correlated with W/kg, indicating that to run faster, athletes must also correctly manage their power. We used different techniques to identify the relationship between strength and some of the other variables in our data set. Thus, we were able to establish which parameters each athlete should work on to enhance their running form. Heat maps were a tool that also allowed us to quickly group runners with similar characteristics, defining colour patterns to characterise them. Furthermore, by comparing each athlete's performance with the other competitors, we were able to work with individual runners to set target parameters for their improvement. Given that the data was obtained from measurement sensors, we consider it to be very valuable and totally objective information that could perhaps lead to the modification of certain methodologies or training techniques. This work opens the door for future work with other types of variables, such as biomechanics obtained from other sensors, which will broaden the spectrum of factors that can be studied.

Author Contributions: Conceptualization, J.M.-G. and J.P.A.; methodology, J.M.-G. and I.N.M.; machine learning models, J.P.A. and M.M.-J.; validation, J.P.A. and J.M.-G.; formal analysis, I.N.M.; investigation, J.M.-G., M.M.-J., and J.P.A.; resources, V.H.M.; data curation, M.M.-J.; writing—original draft preparation, J.P.A., M.M.-J., and J.M.-G.; writing—review and editing, J.P.A., M.M.-J., and J.M.-G.; visualization, J.P.A. and M.M.-J.; supervision, J.M.-G. and J.P.A.; project administration J.M.-G. All authors have read and agreed to the published version of the manuscript.

Funding: This research received no external funding.

Institutional Review Board Statement: The study was conducted according to the guidelines of the Declaration of Helsinki and approved by the Institutional Review Board (or Ethics Committee) of University CEU Cardenal Herrera (protocol code CEI18/137 and November 2018).

Informed Consent Statement: Informed consent was obtained from all subjects involved in the study.

Data Availability Statement: The data presented in this study are available on request from the corresponding author. The data are not publicly available due to privacy restrictions.

Acknowledgments: We appreciate the voluntary participation of young athletes from the High-Performance Triathlon Technification Plan based in the Valencian Community in Spain.

Conflicts of Interest: The authors declare no conflict of interest.

References

1. Martínez-Gramage, J.; Albiach, J.P.; Moltó, I.N.; Amer-Cuenca, J.J.; Moreno, V.H.; Segura-Ortí, E. A Random Forest Machine Learning Framework to Reduce Running Injuries in Young Triathletes. *Sensors* **2020**, *20*, 6388. [CrossRef]
2. Dolezal, B.A.; Barr, D.; Boland, D.M.; Smith, D.L.; Cooper, C.B. Validation of the firefighter WFI treadmill protocol for predicting VO2max. *Occup. Med.* **2015**, *65*, 143–146. [CrossRef] [PubMed]
3. Green, M.S.; Esco, M.R.; Martin, T.D.; Pritchett, R.C.; McHugh, A.N.; Williford, H.N. Crossvalidation of Two 20-M Shuttle-Run Tests for Predicting V[Combining Dot Above]O2max in Female Collegiate Soccer Players. *J. Strength Cond. Res.* **2013**, *27*, 1520–1528. [CrossRef]
4. Barnes, K.R.; Kilding, A.E. Strategies to Improve Running Economy. *Sports Med.* **2014**, *45*, 37–56. [CrossRef] [PubMed]
5. Mayoralas, F.G.M.; Díaz, J.F.J.; Santos-García, D.J.; Castellanos, R.B.; Yustres, I.; González-Rave, J.M.A. Running economy and performance. High and low intensity efforts during training and warm-up. A bibliographic review. *Arch. Med. Deporte* **2018**, *35*, 108–116.
6. Saunders, P.U.; Pyne, D.B.; Telford, R.D.; Hawley, J.A. Factors Affecting Running Economy in Trained Distance Runners. *Sports Med.* **2004**, *34*, 465–485. [CrossRef]
7. Barnes, K.R.; Kilding, A.E. Running economy: Measurement, norms, and determining factors. *Sports Med. Open* **2015**, *1*, 1–15. [CrossRef] [PubMed]
8. Cartón-Llorente, A.; Roche-Seruendo, L.E.; Jaén-Carrillo, D.; Marcen-Cinca, N.; García-Pinillos, F. Absolute reliability and agreement between Stryd and RunScribe systems for the assessment of running power. *Proc. Inst. Mech. Eng. Part P J. Sports Eng. Technol.* **2021**. [CrossRef]
9. García-Pinillos, F.; Roche-Seruendo, L.E.; Marcén-Cinca, N.; Marco-Contreras, L.A.; Latorre-Román, P.A. Absolute Reliability and Concurrent Validity of the Stryd System for the Assessment of Running Stride Kinematics at Different Velocities. *J. Strength Cond. Res.* **2021**, *35*, 78–84. [CrossRef] [PubMed]
10. Cartón-Llorente, A.; García-Pinillos, F.; Royo-Borruel, J.; Rubio-Peirotén, A.; Jaén-Carrillo, D.; Roche-Seruendo, L.E. Estimating Functional Threshold Power in Endurance Running from Shorter Time Trials Using a 6-Axis Inertial Measurement Sensor. *Sensors* **2021**, *21*, 582. [CrossRef] [PubMed]
11. Ahamed, N.U.; Kobsar, D.; Benson, L.; Clermont, C.; Kohrs, R.; Osis, S.T.; Ferber, R. Using wearable sensors to classify subject-specific running biomechanical gait patterns based on changes in environmental weather conditions. *PLoS ONE* **2018**, *13*, e0203839. [CrossRef] [PubMed]
12. Ahamed, N.U.; Kobsar, D.; Benson, L.C.; Clermont, C.A.; Osis, S.T.; Ferber, R. Subject-specific and group-based running pattern classification using a single wearable sensor. *J. Biomech.* **2019**, *84*, 227–233. [CrossRef] [PubMed]
13. Clermont, C.A.; Benson, L.C.; Osis, S.T.; Kobsar, D.; Ferber, R. Running patterns for male and female competitive and recreational runners based on accelerometer data. *J. Sports Sci.* **2019**, *37*, 204–211. [CrossRef] [PubMed]
14. Saxena, A.; Prasad, M.; Gupta, A.; Bharill, N.; Patel, O.P.; Tiwari, A.; Er, M.J.; Ding, W.; Lin, C.-T. A review of clustering techniques and developments. *Neurocomputing* **2017**, *267*, 664–681. [CrossRef]
15. Rokach, L. A survey of Clustering Algorithms. In *Data Mining and Knowledge Discovery Handbook*; Springer International Publishing: Cham, Switzerland, 2009; pp. 269–298.
16. Phinyomark, A.; Osis, S.T.; Hettinga, B.A.; Ferber, R. Kinematic gait patterns in healthy runners: A hierarchical cluster analysis. *J. Biomech.* **2015**, *48*, 3897–3904. [CrossRef] [PubMed]
17. Bramah, C.; Preece, S.J.; Gill, N.; Herrington, L. A 10% Increase in Step Rate Improves Running Kinematics and Clinical Outcomes in Runners With Patellofemoral Pain at 4 Weeks and 3 Months. *Am. J. Sports Med.* **2019**, *47*, 3406–3413. [CrossRef]
18. Jones, A.M.; Doust, J.H. A 1% treadmill grade most accurately reflects the energetic cost of outdoor running. *J. Sports Sci.* **1996**, *14*, 321–327. [CrossRef]
19. Lourenço, T.F.; Martins, L.E.B.; Tessutti, L.S.; Brenzikofer, R.; Macedo, D.V. Reproducibility of an Incremental Treadmill Vo2max Test with Gas Exchange Analysis for Runners. *J. Strength Cond. Res.* **2011**, *25*, 1994–1999. [CrossRef]
20. RStudio. Open Source & Professional Software for Data Science Teams—RStudio. Available online: https://rstudio.com/ (accessed on 13 February 2021).
21. Bruce, P.; Bruce, A. *Pratical Statistics*; O'Reilly Media: Newton, MA, USA, 2017; pp. 29–32.
22. Deisenroth. *Mathematics for ML*; Cambridge University Press: Cambridge, UK, 2020; pp. 191–196. Available online: http://www.maa.org/external_archive/QL/pgs75_89.pdf (accessed on 1 March 2021).
23. Kassambara, A. *Multivariate Analysis 1: Practical Guide to Cluster Analysis in R*; Taylor & Francis Group: Oxfordshire, UK, 2015; pp. 1–187.
24. Fraley, C. How Many Clusters? Which Clustering Method? Answers via Model-Based Cluster Analysis. *Comput. J.* **1998**, *41*, 578–588. [CrossRef]

25. Jaén-Carrillo, D.; Roche-Seruendo, L.E.; Cartón-Llorente, A.; Ramírez-Campillo, R.; García-Pinillos, F. Mechanical Power in Endurance Running: A Scoping Review on Sensors for Power Output Estimation during Running. *Sensors* **2020**, *20*, 6482. [CrossRef]
26. Kolde, R. Package 'Pheatmap': Pretty Heat Map. 2019, pp. 1–8 . Available online: https://cran.r-project.org/web/packages/pheatmap/index.html (accessed on 1 March 2021).
27. Ward, J.H. Hierarchical Grouping to Optimize an Objective Function. *J. Am. Stat. Assoc.* **1963**, *58*, 236–244. [CrossRef]
28. Cerezuela-Espejo, V.; Hernández-Belmonte, A.; Courel-Ibáñez, J.; Conesa-Ros, E.; Mora-Rodríguez, R.; Pallarés, J.G. Are we ready to measure running power? Repeatability and concurrent validity of five commercial technologies. *Eur. J. Sport Sci.* **2020**, *1391*, 1–10. [CrossRef]
29. Navalta, J.W.; Montes, J.; Bodell, N.G.; Aguilar, C.D.; Radzak, K.; Manning, J.W.; DeBeliso, M. Reliability of Trail Walking and Running Tasks Using the Stryd Power Meter. *Int. J. Sports Med.* **2019**, *40*, 498–502. [CrossRef] [PubMed]

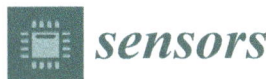

Article

The Use of Infrared Thermography to Develop and Assess a Wearable Sock and Monitor Foot Temperature in Diabetic Subjects

José Torreblanca González [1], Beatriz Gómez-Martín [2], Ascensión Hernández Encinas [3], Jesús Martín-Vaquero [1,*], Araceli Queiruga-Dios [1] and Alfonso Martínez-Nova [2]

1. School of Industrial Engineering, University of Salamanca, E37700 Salamanca, Spain; torre@usal.es (J.T.G.); queirugadios@usal.es (A.Q.-D.)
2. Department of Nursing, Centro Universitario de Plasencia, University of Extremadura, E10600 Plasencia, Spain; bgm@unex.es (B.G.-M.); podoalf@unex.es (A.M.-N.)
3. Faculty of Sciences, University of Salamanca, E37008 Salamanca, Spain; ascen@usal.es
* Correspondence: jesmarva@usal.es

Citation: Torreblanca González, J.; Gómez-Martín, B.; Hernández Encinas, A.; Martín-Vaquero, J.; Queiruga-Dios, A.; Martínez-Nova, A. The Use of Infrared Thermography to Develop and Assess a Wearable Sock and Monitor Foot Temperature in Diabetic Subjects. *Sensors* **2021**, *21*, 1821. https://doi.org/10.3390/s21051821

Received: 14 December 2020
Accepted: 21 February 2021
Published: 5 March 2021

Publisher's Note: MDPI stays neutral with regard to jurisdictional claims in published maps and institutional affiliations.

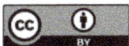

Copyright: © 2021 by the authors. Licensee MDPI, Basel, Switzerland. This article is an open access article distributed under the terms and conditions of the Creative Commons Attribution (CC BY) license (https://creativecommons.org/licenses/by/4.0/).

Abstract: One important health problem that could affect diabetics is diabetic foot syndrome, as risk of ulceration, neuropathy, ischemia and infection. Unnoticed minor injuries, subsequent infection and ulceration may end in a foot amputation. Preliminary studies have shown a relationship between increased skin temperature and asymmetries between the same regions of both feet. In the preulceration phase, to develop a smart device able to control the temperature of these types of patients to avoid this risk might be very useful. A statistical analysis has been carried out with a sample of foot temperature data obtained from 93 individuals, of whom 44 are diabetics and 49 nondiabetics and among them 43% are men and 57% are women. Data obtained with a thermographic camera has been successful in providing a set of regions of interest, where the temperature could influence the individual, and the behavior of several variables that could affect these subjects provides a mathematical model. Finally, an in-depth analysis of existing sensors situated in those positions, namely, heel, medial midfoot, first metatarsal head, fifth metatarsal head, and first toe has allowed for the development of a smart sock to store temperatures obtained every few minutes in a mobile device.

Keywords: diabetic foot; gait; monitoring foot temperature; smart wearable

1. Introduction

1.1. Diabetic Foot

Diabetic foot syndrome is defined as the infection, ulceration or destruction of the deep tissues of the foot, associated with neuropathy and/or peripheral vascular disease of different magnitude, in the lower extremities of patients with diabetes mellitus [1]. The incidence of foot ulcers in diabetics rounds between 15 and 25% [2] and is a frequent cause of hospitalization and could lead to major complications, like lower limb amputations [3]. Actually, it is estimated that about 85% of diabetics suffering from amputations have previously had an ulcer [4]. The mortality rate in subjects with diabetic foot syndrome is more than twice as high than an average population [5].

1.2. The Role Temperature, Pressure Points and Activity on Diabetic Foot

The human being is homeothermic, that is, it maintains the central body temperature constant (oscillating between 36.5 °C and 37.2 °C) despite the variations of ambient temperature. Human beings control their temperature by thermoregulation, where the skin, as the body's largest organ, is a key factor in this process [6]. Skin temperature, in the normal human being, is controlled through many different mechanisms; especially in the extremities (fingers and toes) microcirculatory vasomotion is a crucial determinant of heath preservation of release (not sweating as stated, although being just another way—ischemia and necrosis does not result from sweat gland impairment), and, also, it is normally dependent of the room conditions.

During an activity such as walking, an increase in internal heat is generated, which is manifested in a similar way in the increase in temperature of the skin of the feet [7]. In addition, these are integrated into a complex sports sock-shoe that makes it difficult to transpire properly and evacuate the temperature generated. Thus, socks, together with footwear, become an important element, not only to protect the skin from injury but also to control thermal conditions [8]. In the same way, there are fundamental pieces in the control of moisture (as it will act in the transport of heat in the skin) and therefore in ensuring a correct hydration of the foot [9].

Hence, the evaluation of the pruning temperature helps one to know the internal conditions, which could help to prevent lesions associated with the temperature during gait, or that manifest with changes of the same. An increase of the foot temperature would generate an excess of transpiration in addition to generate changes in the pH of the skin that can turn the foot into the breeding ground for bacterial infections. Similarly, a sudden increase in temperature of an area relative to its contralateral may be indicative of a high risk of injury development, although a reduction may indicate a risk of ischemia. These alterations could lead to further complications, such as pain during gait and development of ulcers, that can become a serious problem in diabetic subjects, with a serious risk of amputation.

Thermographic evaluation of the sole surface of the foot is particularly important in the studies of pathologies associated with the foot at risk, either from neuropathy or from peripheral vasculopathy. Thus, it has been possible to determine certain asymmetries, such as an increase in temperature of 2.2 °C in an area relative to its contralateral, which indicates an underlying subclinical inflammation without apparent signs [10]. This could be a determinant of the risk of ulceration in this area. The sole thermographic evaluation is carried out in different regions of interest (ROIs), being very variable in number and location. The choice of areas of interest can be of great importance, as it could relate the increase or decrease in temperature to the risk of injury in that area, such as a plantar ulcer. However, the literature offers numerous studies, with disparity in number, location and reasoning for choosing ROIs. Recent literature has found studies that analyze from 4 [11,12] to 12 [10] zones, with a number of 5–6 being the most common.

The researchers seem to agree on the study of four specific areas: heel, inner forefoot, fifth metatarsal head and first finger. However, there are important differences, Astasio-Picado et al. [11] analyzed the first metatarsal head, while Chatchawan et al. [13] and Bagavathiappan et al. [14] extended the area to include also the second head. Other researchers focused their attention on five forefoot areas, namely 1st, 3rd and 5th metatarsal heads and 1st and 4th toes [15]. Similarly, Gatt et al. conducted a study in 8 forefoot, medial, lateral, central and the toes [16].

However, other studies do not specify the exact number of regions or their location [17,18], where there is no clear consensus on the criteria for choosing the areas studied, since the studies do not specify this criterion. Thus, it appears that the choice of these areas may be related to areas of frequent ulcer occurrence [11], but in others, the criteria are not specified either. Thus, in neuropathic feet, the highest prevalence was found in the fingers (40.4%) and in the metatarsal area (39.1%), while the ischemic foot group is the most frequent area in the fingers, up to 63.6%. On the other hand, the neuro-ischemic foot group (frequent alteration in diabetic feet of time of evolution) the distribution of ulcers was 51.8% in the area in the inner metatarsal area and the fingers, mainly the first [19].

It seems that the inclusion of the areas of first metatarsal head and first finger is highly recommended, for around 50% of combined prevalence of ulcer appearance. However, the other 50% occur in different areas of the foot, with a significantly lower prevalence, so monitoring other areas becomes a necessity. Choosing areas that are representative of the risk of injury but also able to discriminate between homogeneous temperature zones and provide data on the whole foot without subdividing it into too many regions would be of great importance for rapid realization, simple and reliable podiatric screenings that evaluate the risk of a diabetic foot.

1.3. The Utility of Wearables in Detecting Temperature and Aims of the Study

The proposal of this research is to develop a system, a smart sock, capable of measuring temperature at various points on the foot, to record these measurements during gait by using a smartphone and finally to analyze the data and alert the patient where necessary, i.e., a remote health monitoring system [20,21].

The first step was to make a prediction model so that when any of the measurements exceeds a certain value, the smart sock will send an alert to the telephone and the patient will know that he/she should stop because there is a problem. To develop the mathematical model, data have been collected from a group of diabetic and nondiabetic individuals and a statistical analysis has been developed.

The objective of this work is to analyze and provide good reasons about the number and location of ROIs, which are necessary to perform a good screening of the diabetic foot and to be able to optimize the study, adding necessary areas or eliminating others that offer redundant results. Moreover, a detailed description of the sensors that will be used to measure foot temperate is also included in this study. Thus, the layout of the paper is as follows: A brief overview of the most common sensors employed to measure the temperature is given in Section 2 and their main features in relation to the main goal of the paper are analyzed. In Section 3, a survey that conducted to study the most important variables to study the temperature in both feet is described. A basic statistical analysis of the data is provided and several graphs of feet temperature to determine the most important ROIs are showed. Through further analysis of the sample, a relation of the feet temperature with some of the other variables was found, which allows to develop the corresponding model. The main part of this work is described in Section 4, where a new prototype for a smart sock is described. This smart sock is able to continuously obtain temperatures at several points of the foot, this leaves open the possibility of advancing the study of this disease in the near future. Finally, some conclusions and goals are given in Section 5.

2. Types of Sensors to Monitor Temperatures

Temperature can be defined as a physical quantity that shows the amount of heat in a body. Its perception is linked to the notion of cold and heat.

Its measurement is carried out using a temperature sensor, an instrument that collects the temperature data from a certain source and converts it into information that is understandable by a device or an observer. As the Electronics Tutorials website points out, temperature sensors can be classified into two main groups [22]:

1. Contact sensors, which must physically touch the object, using conductivity to measure changes.
2. Noncontact sensors, which use convection and radiation to warn of a change in temperature.

Of these two types of sensors, the most interesting in this research are the first ones in which there is contact with the object or patient to be measured. The temperature of the human body has been measured and taken into account from the very beginning of medicine. Things related to the change in temperature in different areas of the body have been discovered and have come to the study of numerous diseases.

Measurement taking of this variable is, currently, very well resolved for measurements in industrial processes and for many areas in the human body, but perhaps it is not as well resolved for measurement on the sole of the foot. Some authors have developed an insole [12,23], but our goal is to define the characteristics of a sock that will help to reliably control foot temperature.

Focusing on the contact sensors and, in addition, that they must be small to prevent injuries, the following possibilities were found [24]: Thermocouples, thermoresistances, thermistors, diodes and programmable electronic devices. Detailed information about these electrical devices can be found in [25].

Other sensors are not adequate because it is complicated to obtain a magnitude (temperature) every few minutes when a reliable value is needed. So, infrared, mechanical, color change sensors, etc., are the most suitable for the purposes of this study.

One type of devices that has been tested were thermocouples. Due to its characteristics related to cost, size and temperature range, between others, thermocouples are considered the workhorse of devices capable of measure temperature. A detailed description of different type of thermocouples could be found in [26,27].

Thermoresistances work by varying its resistance with temperature. Their sensitive elements, based on metallic conductors, change their electrical resistance depending on the temperature. The most common devices (called PT100, PT1000, etc.) are built with a platinum resistance. These resistance temperature detector works over a range that varies between $-200°$ and $800°$ with only a single calibration point, and it is considered the best accuracy tool [28].

Thermistors are much more sensitive [29], made up of a synthesized mixture of metal oxides. They are essentially semiconductors that behave like "thermal resistors". They can be found on the market with the denomination NTC (negative temperature coefficient, i.e., the resistance decreases with temperature) and PTC (positive temperature coefficient, i.e., it increases resistance with temperature). They are much easier to measure than thermocouples and thermoresistances, as a simple voltage divider is enough to get the temperature [30,31].

Finally, diodes base their operation on the voltage variation in their terminals since it depends on both the current flowing through it and the temperature at which the diode is located; this variation occurs at the PN junction, very sensitive to temperature changes depending on the internal doping they have. This internal doping makes the internal resistance of the PN junction vary as a function of temperature, which causes the current to increase or decrease and by Ohm's law the same occurs with the voltage at the semiconductor ends. There are a wide variety of devices to measure temperature, from those that vary its voltage (diodes), those that give gradual values of voltage as a function of temperature (analog integrated circuits) to those that are programmed and give a sequence of bits to obtain the value of the temperature (digital integrated circuits). LM35 is an example of analog integrated circuit [32].

The latest generation of sensors for temperature measurement are integrated circuits that, in addition to measuring temperature, can communicate with microcontrollers. The temperature variation is done electronically, as diodes, by variation of voltage and current in the PN junction of the semiconductors. Some examples of these sensors are the MAX30205, the Si7006, etc. [33–36].

From all these sensors, the ideal ones are the programmable electronic devices in integrated circuits, due to their great versatility in being able to program. In addition, their electrical connection is easier by having compatible communication lines between all the sensors that are connected at the same time, such as the I2C communication. Another advantage is the two-way communication possibility in such a way that the temperature value can be obtained directly, and it is not necessary to carry out operations with the values read from the device. The electrical connection of these devices can be very simple with three or four wires at most. Its biggest drawback is electrical welding as they must be made with special materials and equipment, due to the small size of the electrical connections, which are often in the order of 200 microns.

Another very interesting choice are thermistors, since they are small devices, with less rigidity than the previous ones and they are probably better to be included in a sock. Its biggest drawback as with the previous ones are the electrical connections. At this point, they have a certain advantage over the rest of devices, since being less rigid, they can be welded and arranged in a better way. Another disadvantage compared to the previous ones is that the obtained temperature signal must be treated to finally obtain the temperature value, which makes the entire signal acquisition system more complex.

As for the other sensors, the same problems as with programmable electronic devices and thermistors must be addressed. The first ones, being programmable, they already do everything that is needed, i.e., to acquire the signal and transform it to an understandable temperature value for the user, while the seconds may be easier to handle for electrical mounting but worse for acquiring the signal and transforming it to a value understandable by the user.

In any case, and depending on the type of sensor, it could be complicated to place many sensors (not more than 4 or 5), especially if we also want to measure other variables such as pressure or humidity, which are not in the scope of this paper. Hence, it is necessary to know the most important points where temperatures should be calculated.

3. Data Analysis

The goal of this study is to select the positions for sensors to measure the foot temperature and thereby preventing the occurrence of ulcers in diabetic patients. With the aim of analyzing the best position for those sensors, we obtained foot temperatures measured by infrared thermography. A survey with diabetic and nondiabetic individuals was conducted to collect and compare several variables, not only temperatures.

3.1. Data Collection

The sample consisted of 93 subjects. All were patients of the CPUEX Clinic of the University of Extremadura. Since CPUEX Clinic is not large, it is considered that they are a good representation of this institution since the number of male and female patients is similar, also the people with and without diabetes. This analysis is expected to continue with more patients from other institutions. In this way, it will be easier to follow the standards suggested in works such as [37], for example, in the number of subjects and the way to choose them. The thermal images of patients that participate in this research were taken with a FLIR E60bx Infrared camera.

The measure of foot temperature was taken before and after a 100 m walk. In this study patients of different ages were considered, some of them elders, and they cannot walk long distances. Moreover, they should not go outside because the measures could be affected by ambient temperature. A 100 m walk was sufficient to cause a change in temperature by activation. In the future, to study how walking longer distances may affect diabetic patients could be considered.

Although some studies attempt to define the most critical ROIs and thus more likely to suffer serious injuries, there is no final decision about that. This is the reason why a total of 17 temperature measurements from 17 ROIs were collected, from the plant and dorsal areas (9 form the plant and 8 form the dorsal), from both feet. These 17 ROIs were selected following anatomical and functional criteria (i.e., importance in gait, blood flow and risk of ulceration). Plantar measurements included the heel, being not included it in dorsal vision. Measures (indices) that have been selected were: from heel (I_1), medial midfoot (I_2), lateral midfoot (I_3), first metatarsal head (I_4), central metatarsal heads (I_5), fifth metatarsal head (I_6), first toe (I_7), central toes (I_8) and fifth toe (I_9), and the same areas in the dorsal (I_{10}–I_{17}) [38].

Data collection was made using a survey that includes 11 sections:

1. General data about the individual, such as gender, age, weight, height, blood type, and the use of high heels; data specific for diabetes patients: type of diabetes, treatment, control of their diabetes; individuals suffering neuropathy disability; results of the modified Edinburgh questionnaire to diagnose arterial claudication; ankle-brachial index (ABI) and measurement of glycosylated hemoglobin.

2. Habits: Way of life (sedentary lifestyle or practicing a sport); type of feeding (healthy diet or not); alcohol consumption; smoker or nonsmoker; any regular medication; and dominant foot.
3. Comfort: Recent activity with current shoes; intensity of the most recent activity (no activity, walking, running, etc. during the last 30 min); comfort level with the current footwear (during the last 30 min) by means of a 1 to 5 Likert scale, being 1 "very comfortable" and 5 "very uncomfortable"; and the type of footwear that they usually use.
4. Blood pressure and central temperature: data of systolic blood pressure (high), diastolic blood pressure (low), and central temperature (thermometer).
5. Climate data (season data) including date, and number of photos from the foot (sole and dorsal from both feet).
6. Temperature measurements (prewalk right foot data) were performed with a thermal camera FLIR E60bx, with an infrared resolution of 320 × 240 pixels, a sensitivity of 0.05 °C and a precision of ±2%. Thermal picture were taken 1 m far from a foot covered in black cardboard. A total of 17 data average temperatures (9 plantar and 8 dorsal) of each participant were collected and stored using the The Flir Tools® software (Similar to Figure 1). This number of ROIs has been used previously in thermographyc assessments [38–40] (see Figure 2). Room humidity (%) and temperature (°C) were also measured with a Flir MR 77 device.
7. Temperature measurements (prewalk left foot data).
8. Temperature measurements (postwalk right foot data). After the 100 m walking, the temperature was recorded in the same way as in point 6.
9. Temperature measurements (postwalk left foot data).
10. Foot Posture. Scores of Foot Posture Index (FPI) for left and right foot were assessed following standard procedure [41], subjects in their relaxed stance position, both limb support, arms relaxed and looking straight ahead; foot posture classification was found to be neutral when the score was between 0 to 5, supinated from −1 to −12 and pronated from 6 to 12 [42]; presence of plantar hyperkeratosis at any zone of the foot was also recorded.
11. Final comments and remarks.

Each measurement take the research team a set-up of 20 min for each participant.

A study with a sample of 93 individuals was carried out, of whom 44 are diabetics and 49 nondiabetics and among them 43% are men and 57% are women. Figure 3 left shows that in both cases (diabetics and nondiabetics, and men and women) the percentage is quite similar, the data is similarly distributed. Histograms of age, weight, height and body mass index (BMI) have also been represented in the right part of Figure 3. The weight basically is between 60 and 90 kg and the height between 1.60 and 1.70 m. The largest number of individuals corresponds to an age between 70 and 80 years since the patients who go to the consultation are older people who have problems for their basic care and the body mass index is between 20 and 35.

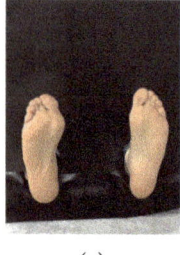 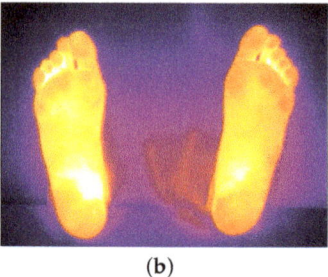 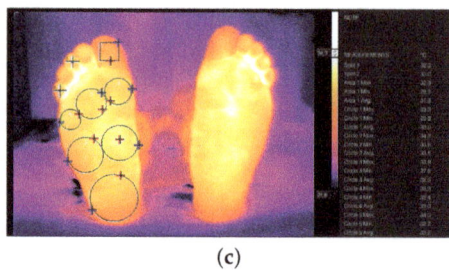

(a)　　　　　　　　　　(b)　　　　　　　　　　(c)

Figure 1. (**a**) Feet covered with a black cardboard prior to the thermal picture, (**b**) Thermographic picture obtained and (**c**) Taking data temperatures of the nine regions of the foot (with Spanish format, where the comma indicates decimal point).

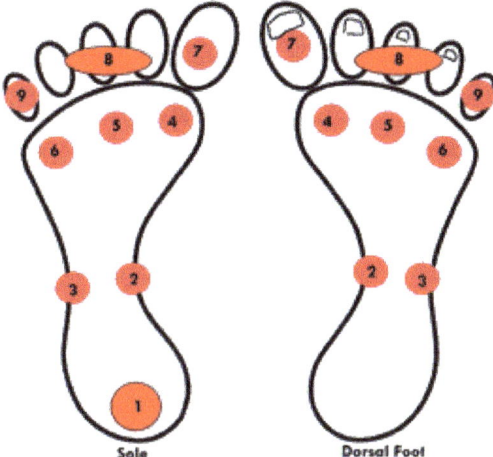

Figure 2. Feet regions where temperature data is collected.

The study was conducted in accordance with the Declaration of Helsinki, and the experiment developed for this paper received a positive report from the bioethics and biosafety commission of the University of Extremadura (with Ref. 04/2018). It follows Spanish and European legislation, and all the people who participated in the survey gave their consent for research purposes.

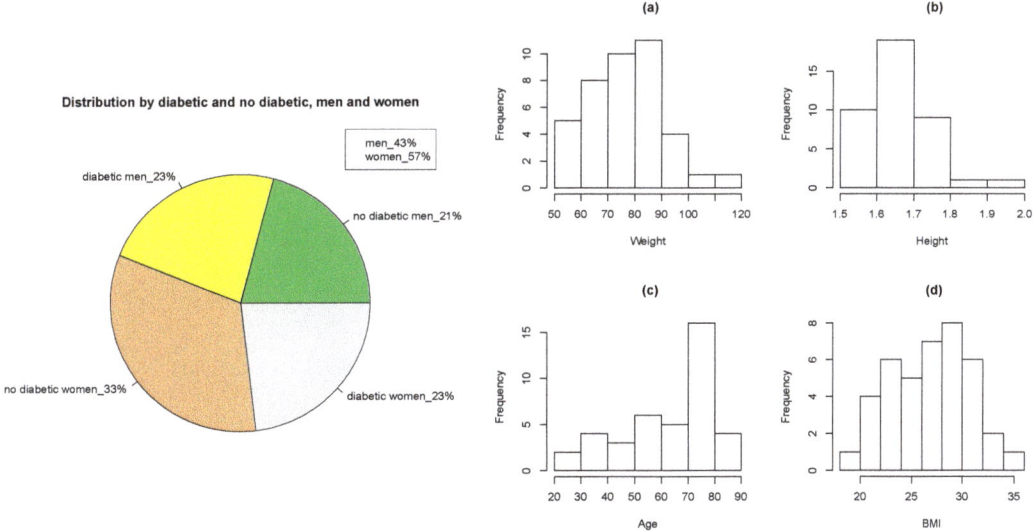

Figure 3. Data distribution (**left**) and Histograms for different variables (**right**): (**a**) Weight, (**b**) Height, (**c**) Age, and (**d**) BMI.

3.2. Statistical Data Analysis

Correlation shows the relationship between two variables, whilst regression analysis generates a mathematical equation that serves to predict the behavior of the process output by changing its inputs. Correlation is usually the first analysis carried out since you want to check if there is a relationship between the variables, and, the regression analysis usually takes data in order to find a relationship that provides for the output of the process by changing the data that affect this. In this work these two statistical procedures were used and also dendograms to determine which are the locations where sensors should be placed.

A correlation higher than 0.8 between sole and dorsal indices at the same position was established in [38], so sole data have only been considered (from I_1 to I_9 from sole) before and after a 100 m walk. This walk was performed to determine if the diabetic feet, after the walk, show any difference with the nondiabetic feet. To do this different measures were taken, which will allow developing a model with the aim of predicting the temperature in some points of the foot and check if they are within "normal" values or if there is any deviation.

Specifically, the data obtained from the survey detailed in Section 3.1 have been considered.

Dendograms were represented for diabetic and nondiabetic individuals to determine if there is a difference between them and also what are the most influential indices (to select these points as the places to put sensors on the socks). In all dendrograms, the most significant points are I_1 I_2, I_3 or I_7, and points I_4, I_5 and I_6 related to each other, as can be seen in Figure 4 for the right floor of diabetic patients (left) and nondiabetics (right) before the walk.

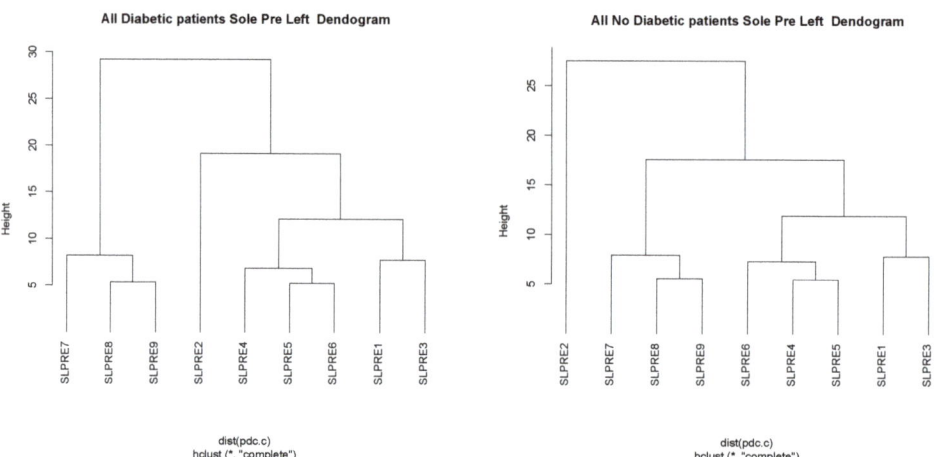

Figure 4. Dendograms of the right sole after the walk: Diabetics (**left**) and nondiabetics (**right**). SLPRE$_i$ represents the temperature for left sole before the walk for index i.

According to the literature, the points where the most ulcers appear are in the metatarsal area of the foot, i.e., indices I_4, I_5, and I_6 from Figure 2a, and index I_7 (30% of the ulcers according to [39] in the fingers. The dendrogram indicates that there is a relation between those three metatarsal points. Consequently, indices I_4 and I_6 have been chosen because they have a higher percentage, 22% and 11%. Thus, considering points I_4 and I_6, all the variability of the upper metatarsal part were obtained.

On the other hand, the index I_1 was also selected because there is a relation between and there are usually more difficult problems. Apart from that it seems reasonable to consider I_1, as a greater force is applied to this area when walking and it is a point of greater probability of ulcer. Point I_7 was also chosen as it is an area not related to the previous ones and presents a probability of ulceration of 30%. The dendrogram also indicates that I_2 is totally different from the rest. The area of I_2 carries irrigation to the metatarsal head and the first toe. This is an interesting area since if it cools, the front side will also cools and no blood will go there, with the risk of ulcer. Moreover, this point receives less friction from the footwear, with a difference in relation to the other points where we measure the temperature. That is why we decided to include it as it is a singular point, totally different from the others but where practically no ulcers appear. In this way there is an element of control of the other areas that will be considered for the smart sock.

In summary, the points that will be studied are I_j with $j \in \{1, 2, 4, 6, 7\}$.

For this study a pool of candidate variables have been considered, in addition to the temperature. This allowed the possibility of discarding the variables that do not affect diabetic foot. After a stepwise regression, a prediction model has been developed for all the data, in which the following variables are included: AGE, SEX, BMI, DB (Nondiabetic = 1, diabetic = 2), TNMX (Systolic Blood Pressure), TNMN (Diastolic Blood Pressure), TC (central temperature), TEXT (outside temperature), TPRE (air temperature of the room before the walk), HPRE (humidity of the room (in%) before the walk). The coefficients that have been obtained for the different models are shown in Table 1. The model only considering the variables that influence is calculated with the command *Stepwise* provided by the R program.

Table 1. Coefficients that have been obtained with the model. SRPREi represents the temperature for right (R) sole (S) before (PRE) the walk for index i, SLPOSTi represents the temperature for left (L) sole (S) after (POST) the walk for index i, and SRPOSTi represents the temperature for right sole after the walk for index i. Where I can be 1, 2, 4, 6 and 7 indicating the region where the index is considered.

CAT	CTE	AGE	BMI	DB	TNMX	TNMN	TC	TEXT	TPRE	HPRE
SRPRE1	8.78695	0.03		−0.91140	0.04171	−0.05392			0.56426	0.12670
SRPRE2	17.94235	0.01558		−1.47390	0.03612	−0.03644			0.38426	0.07408
SRPRE4	−20.96860	0.02549	0.10193	−1.36591		−0.04557	0.82781		0.67369	0.13880
SRPRE6	−26.14073		0.13748	−1.02450	0.04952	−0.09264	0.79693		0.74866	0.18130
SRPRE7	−38.27672	0.03712	0.11602	−1.28288		−0.05528	1.14328		0.81583	0.15686
SLPRE1	−14.00475	0.03628		−0.84698	0.04798	−0.05280	0.61893		0.53951	0.11614
SLPRE2	15.65169			−0.74912	0.04795	−0.04274			0.39359	0.09685
SLPRE4	−31.30703		0.11339	−1.42929	0.06371	−0.08094	0.93555		0.72724	0.16288
SLPRE6	−32.83695	0.02528	0.09846	−1.33277	0.05504	−0.07547	0.92974		0.76525	0.15994
SLPRE7	−39.72836	0.04965		−1.20896			1.11495		0.84074	0.14443
SRPOST1	−7.01999	0.04641		−0.93266			0.48558		0.64667	
SRPOST2	−3.44379		0.10557	−1.33277	0.06073	−0.04858	0.56932	0.07686	0.27156	
SRPOST4	−15.45718	0.02753		−1.63835	0.04549	−0.05258	0.67605		0.73318	
SRPOST6	−20.78108		0.11620	−1.07018	0.05828	−0.08463	0.65984		0.79016	0.08394
SRPOST7	−24.79945	0.03964		−1.35335			0.88517		0.78046	
SLPOST1	−12.99850	0.03859		−1.03925	0.05417	−0.04706	0.58444		0.63557	
SLPOST2	15.67648	0.02831		−1.21562	0.03380				0.39475	
SLPOST4	−15.34189	0.02699		−1.32829	0.04989	−0.05053	0.62868		0.74446	
SLPOST6	−20.94168	0.02664		−1.15666	0.05514	−0.04966	0.73794		0.76450	
SLPOST7	−29.61293	0.04579		−1.07319			0.96990		0.81785	

There are variables that do not influence the model, such as SEX and TEXT, and there are other variables that have little influence, such as BMI. In addition, the HPRE practically only influences before the walk. As it can be observed, being diabetic or not does influence the model, therefore data have been separated in diabetic and nondiabetic people and since sex does not influence the sample was not separated by sex. In Figure 5 the graph of the data for the coefficient SRPRE1 (black, solid line) of the sole before the walk for the complete sample is represented, and a comparison with the complete model (with all the variables, in red, dashed line), and the model with the variables given in the legend (blue, dash-dot line). This model suggests that some of the variables in this study have small influence in the temperatures.

Figure 5 shows the sample data in black color; the blue graph corresponds to the calculated model only considering the variables that influence; finally, the red line is the model when all variables are taken into account. The correlation coefficients obtained correspond to the correlation between the calculated model and the real values (blue $r = 0.628$), between the complete model, considering all the variables and the real values (red $r = 0.638$) and between the blue model and the red model ($r = 0.985$). A confidence interval of 95% was considered for this study. It can be appreciated that both models are very well correlated, so it is not worth using all the variables, only the ones in Table 1. Moreover, the correlation coefficients are not much improved by choosing more variables and it is more realistic to choose only those that influence.

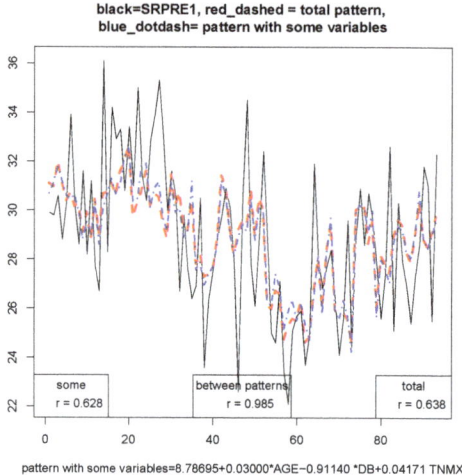

Figure 5. Pattern for the sole of the index 1, right foot before the walk.

A Bland Altman plot of the model is presented in Figure 6 comparing the two measurements in the index 1 before the walk: the sample data and the model only considering the variables that influence, calculated with the command *Stepwise* provided by R. In other indices, we see similar results. The proposed model is not predictive and the approximation is not quite good, because we have found outliers for both the lower and upper values. The multiple regression coefficient between the real values (SRPRE1) and the model is $R^2 = 0.3948$. As was mentioned in Section 3.1, the study was carried out with all diabetic patients from the podiatry clinic with the goal of selecting the variables that could influence the values of the defined indices and to improve the measurement of these variables.

The goal of this study is the proposal of socks capable to send a signal to a mobile telephone when a difference of temperature is detected, of more than 2 degrees (hyperthermia) or less than 2 degrees (ischemia) between the same indices of the two feet. For doing this the difference of the indices in the sole in the 5 points ($I_j, j \in \{1, 2, 4, 6, 7\}$) was calculated and a basic statistical study was developed for all of them starting with all sample data and later on for individuals when diabetics from nondiabetics are separated, and before and after the walk.

As an example, Table 2 shows the data for nondiabetic patients before the walk for the sole of the right foot. In this case the index with the highest coefficient of variation is I_6, followed by I_7, in which the interquartile range is also the highest of all. Indices I_1, I_4 and I_6 have a negative skewness and are the ones with the highest kurtosis, while I_2 and I_7 have a skewness close to zero and a kurtosis that is also very small.

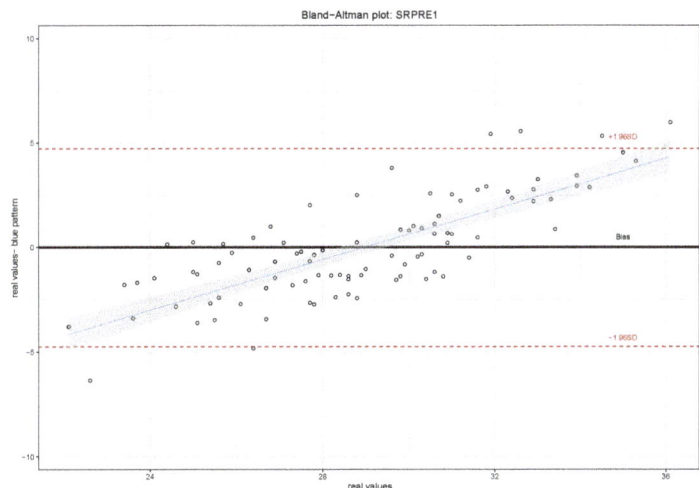

Figure 6. Bland Altman plot, for the sole of the index 1, right foot before the walk, comparing the two measurements: the sample data given by the survey and the model only considering the variables that influence (see Table 1).

Table 2. Difference between the indices on the two sole (left and right) for nondiabetic people before the walk in the regions 1, 2, 4, 6 and 7 (see Figure 1). Here we can see the most important statistic of then like mean, the standard deviation (sd), the standard error of the mean (sem), interquartile range (IQR), the coefficient of variation (cv), the degree of distortion from the symmetrical bell curve or the normal distribution or the measure of symmetry (Skewness), the measure of whether the data are heavy-tailed or light-tailed relative to a normal distribution (Kurtosis), and the quartiles.

DSPRE	Mean	sd	se(mean)	IQR	cv	Skewness	Kurtosis	0%	25%	50%	75%	100%
DSPRE1	0.0938	0.8234	0.1176	0.7	8.7716	−1.7464	7.6044	−3.6	−0.2	0.1	0.5	1.7
DSPRE2	0.4326	0.5550	0.0792	0.6	1.2828	0.2910	0.9031	−0.9	0.1	0.4	0.7	2.0
DSPRE4	0.2081	1.2282	0.1754	0.9	5.9005	−1.1939	3.8264	−3.9	−0.1	0.3	0.8	3.1
DSPRE6	0.0551	0.9757	0.1393	1.1	17.7082	−1.2871	5.0223	−4.0	−0.5	0.1	0.6	1.8
DSPRE7	0.1163	1.1422	0.1631	1.1	9.8193	0.25053	0.3911	−2.7	−0.5	0.0	0.6	3.0

For the indices I_j, $j \in \{1,2,4,6,7\}$, a violin graph with a boxplot with a mustache inside is represented in Figure 7. It can be appreciated that there is an overlap between the mean (red dot) and the median (middle straight line of the boxplot with a mustache).

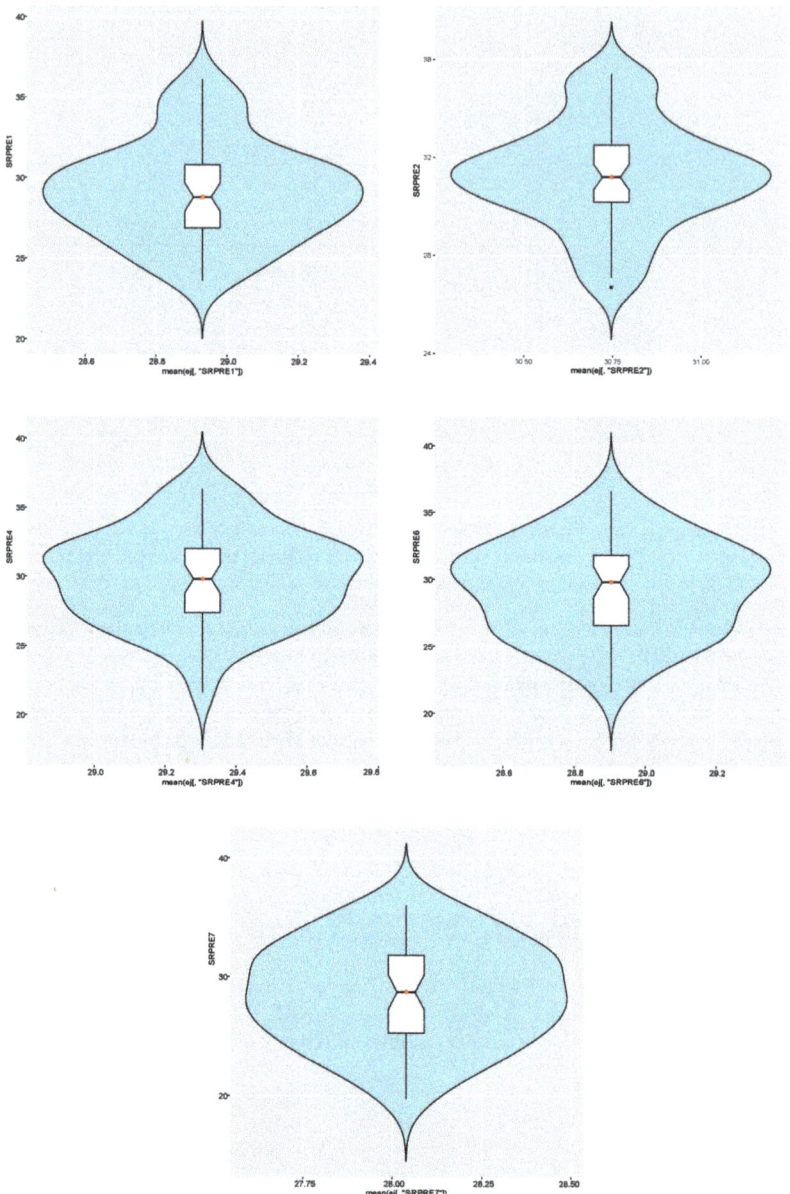

Figure 7. Violin plot for indices I_j, $j \in \{1,2,4,6,7\}$.

4. A Prototype of a Smart Sock

4.1. Introduction

As was mentioned before, the goal of this research is to get a smart sock, capable of measuring temperature in diabetic foot. Some examples of prototypes of socks appear in [43,44] but sensors there are large, so they are not the better option for diabetic patients. The proposed system will be composed of several sensors located in predefined ROIs, these sensors will be managed by an Arduino board, which will send the collected data to a smartphone that will be able to create an alarm in case of needed. A block diagram of the proposed structure is shown in Figure 8.

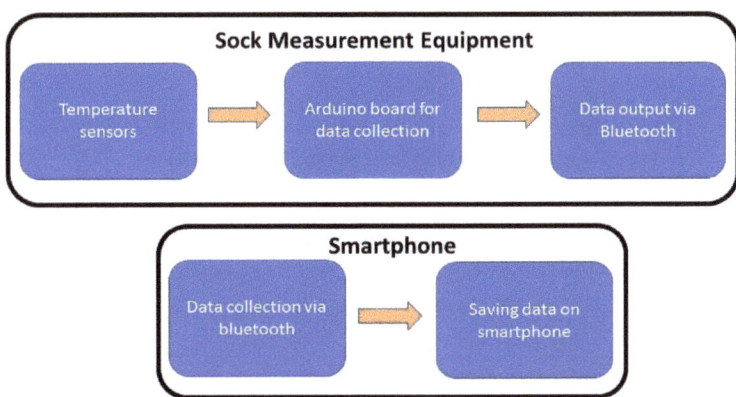

Figure 8. Block diagram of the proposed system that will be able to measure temperature, analyze it and send an alarm to the smartphone when needed.

4.2. NTC TTF 103 Thermistor

In Section 3 the areas of the feet to place the sensors for measure the temperature were selected. The next step is to think about which sensor that could be used to measure the temperature because it is a very delicate situation, since they should not disturb when walking. Thermistors were considered the best option, since they are very sensitive. As was mentioned in Section 2, they can be found on the market with the denomination NTC and PTC.

For the device proposed in this study, the NTC TTF 103 thermistor with 10 kΩ will be used. This sensor has very small dimensions, 25 mm long, 3.8 mm wide and 0.4 mm high, which makes it ideal to avoid disturbing the foot. Moreover, the manufacturer provides tables with the resistive values and their corresponding temperatures. Although data table from the manufacturer is available, they have been calibrated using the Steinhart–Hart equation and their coefficients A, B and C were obtaining.

The Steinhart–Hart equation is an empirical expression that has been determined to be the best mathematical expression for the resistance temperature ratio of NTC thermistors and NTC probe sets. The most common equation is:

$$T_i = \frac{1}{A + B \ln(R_i) + C \ln^3(R_i)}, \tag{1}$$

where T_i is measured in degrees Kelvin, and A, B and C are calculated following these steps: first of all the thermistor at three different temperatures is measure, and then this values are used to solve the resulting simultaneous equations, considering

$$L_i = \ln(R_i), \quad Y_i = \frac{1}{T_i}, \quad \gamma_2 = \frac{Y_2 - Y_1}{L_2 - L_1}, \quad \gamma_3 = \frac{Y_3 - Y_1}{L_3 - L_1}.$$

Finally, the parameters are obtained taking the following expressions for A, B and C:

$$C = \frac{\gamma_3 - \gamma_2}{L_3 - L_2}(L_1 + L_2 + L_3)^{-1}, \quad B = \gamma_2 - C(L_1^2 + L_1 L_2 + L_2^2), \quad A = Y_1 - L_1(B + CL_1^2). \tag{2}$$

These coefficients are used from three measurements in real conditions. With these three parameters and obtaining the resistance, value the temperature is obtained with the NTC thermistors. It is also possible to obtain that value using the website of Thermistor Calculator for Laser Diode and TEC Controllers. [45].

The six NTC sensors were calibrated (an extra sensor calibration is included, just in case one fail later). As Figure 9 shows, both the resistences that will be placed in series with the NTC thermistor and the thermistor itself are numbered, so considering each resistance together with its NTC, they will always form the same voltage divider.

To carry out the measurements, units calibrated have been used to take the temperature and to measure the resistance. These units are shown in Figure 9. The RS1314 unit has been used for temperature, capable of measuring very precise temperatures with thermocouples. This unit is equipped with two thermocouples that measure the temperature at the same time, and thus they take the values when both measures are the same. To measure the electrical resistance a FLUKE 87 was taken. This device is able to measure various parameters such as resistance, voltage, electric current and it is even possible to measure the temperature with a type K thermocouple.

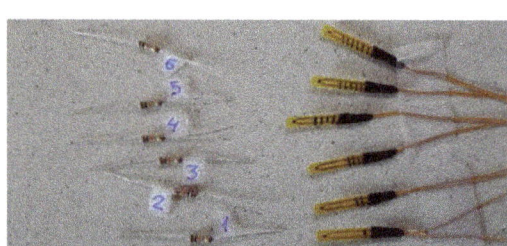
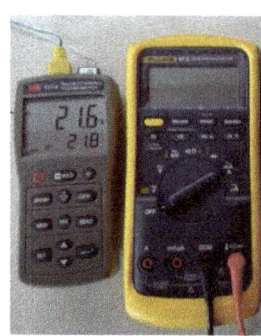

Resistences and thermistors *Units*

Figure 9. Units calibrated to take the temperature and measure the resistance.

The measurements have been made in four temperature ranges, the first with water almost at 0 °C, specifically at 1.6 °C, the next measurement around 29 °C, and finally the temperature has risen to around 43 °C (we also calculated data at 21.6 °C to check the function given by Equation (1)). We found that 1.6 °C and 29 °C temperatures were more stable, and 43 °C temperature had some small variations. When we measured both resistance and temperature, these variations have been taken into account when entering data on the website to calculate the parameters of the Steinhart–Hart equation.

The way to obtain these temperatures has been through ice water and waiting about 20 min to stabilize the temperature, then it has been heated with a microwave and cold water has been added to obtain 43 °C and 29 °C. This is shown in Figure 10.

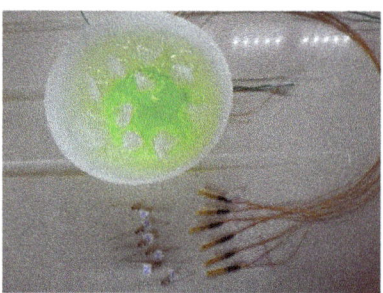
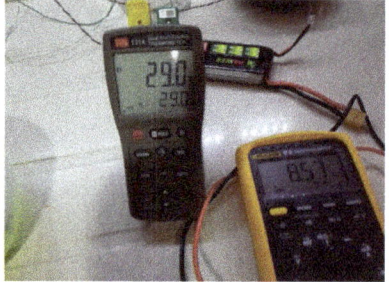

Temperature at 1.6 °C *Temperature at 29 °C*

Figure 10. Calculating the parameters of the Steinhart–Hart equation.

All six NTC sensors have been calibrated. The obtained values of resistance (Res i) and temperature (Temp i) are shown in Table 3.

Table 3. Data of resistances (Res 1 to 6) and temperatures (Temp 1 to 6) taken by the six NTC sensors.

Resistence/Thermistor	Res 1	Temp 1	Res 2	Temp 2	Res 3	Temp 3	Res 4	Temp 4
R1/NTC1	9.80 kΩ	21.6 °C	24.88 kΩ	1.6 °C	8.31 kΩ	29.7 °C	5.02 kΩ	43.5 °C
R2/NTC2	9.83 kΩ	21.6 °C	24.33 kΩ	1.6 °C	8.38 kΩ	29.7 °C	5.20 kΩ	43.5 °C
R3/NTC3	9.82 kΩ	21.6 °C	24.19 kΩ	1.6 °C	8.30 kΩ	29.6 °C	5.15 kΩ	43.3 °C
R4/NTC4	9.85 kΩ	21.6 °C	24.50 kΩ	1.6 °C	8.34 kΩ	29.4 °C	5.19 kΩ	43.2 °C
R5/NTC5	9.79 kΩ	21.6 °C	25.12 kΩ	1.6 °C	8.34 kΩ	29.4 °C	5.26 kΩ	42.8 °C
R6/NTC6	9.84 kΩ	21.6 °C	25.21 kΩ	1.6 °C	8.47 kΩ	29.3 °C	5.47 kΩ	42.0 °C

Once measurements were taken, the parameters for each thermistor are obtained (see Table 4).

Table 4. Parameters of the Steinhart–Hart equation for the six NTC sensors. These parameters A, B and C are constants that are obtained for the equation that defines the resistance variation of the sensors. B were multiplied times 10^3, B times 10^4 and C times 10^7.

Thermistor	$A \cdot 10^3$	$B \cdot 10^4$	$C \cdot 10^7$
NTC1	1.409294790	1.684156947	5.069508025
NTC2	1.149226326	2.051360360	4.064329590
NTC3	1.076255140	2.180997134	3.519982960
NTC4	0.762209845	2.695628622	1.483573950
NTC5	1.300653498	1.843001087	4.536745780
NTC6	0.579418628	2.997765865	0.2115108092

4.3. Arduino

The next step is to establish the element for obtaining the measures to dump them on the smartphone. For reading the sensors we started with ARDUINO board (https://www.arduino.cc/, accessed on 13 January 2021).

As is well known, Arduino is a platform of electronics prototypes based on flexible and easy-to-use hardware and open-source software. It is intended for artists, designers, as a hobby and for anyone interested in creating interactive objects or environments.

For this study, an Arduino Nano has been used to collect the data. It is a reduced version of Arduino UNO, although with some differences. Arduino Nano minimizes the energy demand that it consumes and moreover, less space is needed to host the board, making it ideal for this project as it has to be worn as an ankle strap. This Arduino board is a small, flexible and easy-to-use microcontroller. It is based on the ATmega328 microcontroller. It works at a frequency of 16 Mhz. The memory consists of 32 KB of flash memory. It has a 5 V supply voltage, but the input voltage can vary from 7 to 12 V. It has 14 digital pins, 8 analog pins, 2 reset pins and 6 power pins (Vcc and GND). In the case of analogs, they allow a 10-bit resolution from 0 to 5 V. It uses a standard miniUSB for connecting with the computer for programming or power it. Its power consumption is 19 mA. Printed circuit board size is 18 × 45 mm weighing only 7 g.

Arduino microcontrollers have multichannel analog-digital converters. The converter has a resolution of 10 bits, i.e., it takes values between 0 and 1023. Thus, if the resolution is maximum, that is, 5 V, the converter will give an integer value of 1023, if the measured voltage is intermediate, for example 2.5 V, the converter will store an integer value equal to 512, and if the voltage is zero (0 V), then the converter will give an integer value of 0. The Arduino resolution is calculated as the quotient between the reference voltage and $2^N - 1$. The reference voltage is the maximum voltage that is applied to the converter, normally it is the supply voltage, then 5 V, although it can be modified and changed to a smaller value, thereby increasing resolution. It is not possible to set higher values than the power supply, and lower values can be increased to a certain value threshold set by the manufacturer of the microcontrollers. The exponent N refers to the bits resolution of the converter, in this case, 10.

Therefore, the resolution that we have calculated for our device is 4.88 mV.

4.4. Smartphone Application

A mobile phone application has been developed to collect and analyze data. This application takes the data from the sensors and transmit them by a Bluetooth connection that is paired with the smartphone. The data transmission is made through the HC-06 Bluetooth module, which only needs to be paired with the mobile in order to receive data. This module only has four terminals, two for power, one to transmit the signal and the last one to receive it, which means that communication can be bidirectional, although in our case we only use unidirectional communication, from the measuring system to the smartphone.

The smartphone stores the data in real time on a plain text file (.csv file) that can then be processed. The phone application has been implemented with App Inventor 2 software. This is developed from a web page available to everyone (https://appinventor.mit.edu/, accessed on 13 Januray 2021).

When building the Android applications we work with two tools: App Inventor Designer and App Inventor Blocks Editor. In Designer environment we build the user interface, choosing and placing the elements with which the user will interact and the components that the application will use. In the Blocks Editor we define the behavior of the components of the application.

In Figure 11 some images of the smart sock working connected to the smartphone application are shown. A set of sensors have been placed in the ROIs established in Section 3, after measuring the temperature data from these regions, they are submitted to the mobile device and stored in a spreadsheet.

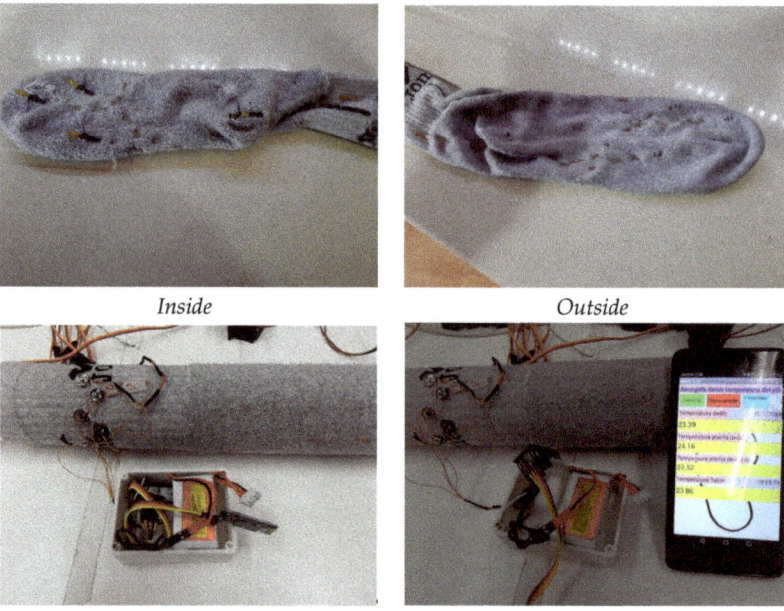

Inside *Outside*

Resistors and thermistors *Units*

Figure 11. Smart sock working. In the top part we show details of one of the socks with the sensors. In the bottom, readers can see the smart sock working connected to the cell phone application.

On the other hand, a battery called LIPO has been used. It is composed of lithium and polymer, which is a battery widely used due to the large amount of current that it can give at a certain moment, but it is adequate for this proposal because it can be used for a long time without recharging. Nickel-Cadmium batteries and even Nickel-Metal Hydride could be used.

5. Conclusions and Future Work

Foot pathologies result directly from several diseases, mainly related with gait, and they are among the most serious and costly complications that affect diabetes mellitus patients. To monitor these patients, their gait and quality care will avoid the increase of costs, patients' consultation or centers overcrowding. The proposal of this study is to develop a smart sock to monitor diabetic patients' foot temperature.

We had to solve the following obstacles before this could be achieved:

(i) The first one was that several different papers do not agree about how many sensors are necessary and where they should be placed. To select the ROIs we have analyzed temperature data obtained with an infrared camera from 93 individuals with the purpose of finding the optimal position for temperature sensors. To analyze if this condition affects temperature results, the data was obtained before and after a 100 m walk. After a statistical analysis, the model inferred from it lead us to define five specific areas where the temperature must be measure: heel, medial midfoot, first metatarsal head, fifth metatarsal head and first toe.

(ii) After that, the best type of sensor was also analyzed, since many of them are not adequate for a diabetic foot.

A prototype of a smart sock was developed, with NTC sensors situated in those positions. This device gather a large amount of data with the support of an Arduino board, and then they are transferred and stored in a mobile device for subsequent processing.

After a description of the different types of sensors, the NTC sensor has seemed very good to us to make the prototype. This sensor is characterized by being very small, easy to take measurements, easy to attach to the sock and being the least annoying as it is the smallest. This sensor has many advantages over the others, perhaps the only drawback is its precision, but the precision in this study is not very relevant since we only need to check if the temperature varies in the area of the foot that we are measuring. It could become annoying if the sock used is very thin but being a medium sock there are no discomforts, since the sensor and the threads are integrated with the fibers of the sock. The effects of foot moisture are not taken into account in this first prototype; we are already seeing if significant temperature variations can be seen in the foot.

The development of a sock to measure the temperature of different parts of the foot has been carried out on the basis of a commercial sock, in which electrical wires of a very small section have been inserted so that they will not disturb when the user is moving. The threads are braided with the sock, that is, they are sewn so that they do not move, finally the sensor is also sewn and glued to the sock fabric. The sensors were welded to the electric wire and the weld was covered with shrink material to avoid damaging the foot as much as possible, an objective achieved by this method. All of this gives the prototype a long-lasting consistency and hold so it can be used in data collection sessions. Some tests have already been done, and the data collection has been acquired during one or two hours depending on the disposition of the individuals. Although the sock has worked properly during these sessions, there were some first measurements in which we had to make corrections in the hold of the threads and sensors, but once corrected, the sock measured perfectly. One thing that has not been taken into account was the possibility that foot sweated influenced the measurement; this was discarded since it is not necessary to have a good temperature measurement but to obtain a slight variation in temperature in the areas of the foot studied. For the purposes of this device, a degree or two more or less in the temperature measurement do not influence the results, but what is needed is the appreciation of a temperature change in those points, for this reason the measurements must not be exactly precise either, and hence we have used those tiny sensors that do not harm the patient when they are walking.

The present study has some limitations: (1) The temperature evaluation in this study was recorded only after a 100 m walk, being a short-term assess. It is necessary to re-evaluate the data in a longer walk, to assess its reliability in an activity similar to that of daily life; (2) the solution was tested indoors, so the results (where environmental temperature can affect the body temperature) cannot be extrapolated to outdoors conditions; and (3) the comfort of these smart socks (thinner sensors and wires) to be used by elders in a normal activity in daily life wear must be improved. This issues will be taken into account in future research, where the prototype will be tested in different conditions, looking for better solutions in order to achieve the best wearable to continually assess foot temperature and try to identify early disorders that could avoid infections, plantar ulcers and further amputations in diabetics.

Author Contributions: Conceptualization, J.M.-V., A.M.-N. and A.H.E.; methodology, A.M.-N. and J.M.-V.; software, J.T.G. and J.T.G.; validation, A.Q.-D., B.G.-M. and J.M.-V.; investigation, B.G.-M., J.T.G. and A.H.E.; resources, B.G.-M. and A.M.-N.; writing—original draft preparation, B.G.-M., A.M.-N. and A.H.E.; writing—review and editing, J.M.-V., A.M.-N. and A.Q.-D.; funding acquisition, J.T.G. All authors have read and agreed to the published version of the manuscript.

Funding: This research was funded by Fundación Samuel Solórzano grant number FS/18-2018 and authors acknowledge Programa V by Universidad de Salamanca.

Institutional Review Board Statement: Not applicable.

Informed Consent Statement: Not applicable.

Data Availability Statement: Not applicable.

Acknowledgments: This research was funded by Fundación Samuel Solórzano grant number FS/18-2018 and authors acknowledge Programa V by Universidad de Salamanca.

Conflicts of Interest: The authors declare no conflict of interest.

References

1. Dounis, E.; Makrilakis, K.; Tentolouris, N.; Tsapogas, P. *Atlas of the Diabetic Foot*; John Wiley & Sons: Hoboken, NJ, USA, 2010.
2. Singh, N.; Armstrong, D.G.; Lipsky, B.A. Preventing foot ulcers in patients with diabetes. *JAMA* **2005**, *293*, 217–228. [CrossRef]
3. Litzelman, D.K.; Marriott, D.J.; Vinicor, F. Independent physiological predictors of foot lesions in patients with NIDDM. *Diabetes Care* **1997**, *20*, 1273–1278. [CrossRef]
4. National Diabetes Data Group (U.S.); National Institute of Diabetes and Digestive and Kidney Diseases (U.S.); National Institutes of Health (U.S.). *Diabetes in America*; NIH Publication: Washington, DC, USA, 1995.
5. Karrer, S. Diabetisches Fußsyndrom. *Der Hautarzt* **2011**, *62*, 493–503. [CrossRef] [PubMed]
6. Lahiri, B.; Bagavathiappan, S.; Jayakumar, T.; Philip, J. Medical applications of infrared thermography: A review. *Infrared Phys. Technol.* **2012**, *55*, 221–235. [CrossRef]
7. Akimov, E.; Son'kin, V. Skin temperature and lactate threshold during muscle work in athletes. *Hum. Physiol.* **2011**, *37*, 621. [CrossRef]
8. Purvis, A.; Tunstall, H. Effects of sock type on foot skin temperature and thermal demand during exercise. *Ergonomics* **2004**, *47*, 1657–1668. [CrossRef] [PubMed]
9. McLellan, K.; Petrofsky, J.S.; Bains, G.; Zimmerman, G.; Prowse, M.; Lee, S. The effects of skin moisture and subcutaneous fat thickness on the ability of the skin to dissipate heat in young and old subjects, with and without diabetes, at three environmental room temperatures. *Med. Eng. Phys.* **2009**, *31*, 165–172. [CrossRef]
10. Macdonald, A.; Petrova, N.L.; Ainarkar, S.; Allen, J.; Plassmann, P.; Whittam, A.; Bevans, J.T.; Ring, F.; Kluwe, B.; Simpson, R.M.; et al. Thermal symmetry of healthy feet: A precursor to a thermal study of diabetic feet prior to skin breakdown. *Physiol. Meas.* **2017**, *38*, 33–44. [CrossRef] [PubMed]
11. Astasio-Picado, A.; Martínez, E.E.; Nova, A.M.; Rodríguez, R.S.; Gómez–Martín, B. Thermal map of the diabetic foot using infrared thermography. *Infrared Phys. Technol.* **2018**, *93*, 59–62. [CrossRef]
12. Rodríguez-Sáenz, S.D.; Franco-Pérez, S.S.; Espinoza-Valdez, A.; Salido-Ruiz, R.A.; Curiel-López, F.B. Instrumented Footwear for Diabetic Foot Monitoring: Foot Sole Temperature Measurement. In Proceedings of the Latin American Conference on Biomedical Engineering, Cancún, Mexico, 2–5 October 2019; Springer: Cham, Switzerland, 2019; pp. 501–507.
13. Chatchawan, U.; Narkto, P.; Damri, T.; Yamauchi, J. An exploration of the relationship between foot skin temperature and blood flow in type 2 diabetes mellitus patients: A cross-sectional study. *J. Phys. Ther. Sci.* **2018**, *30*, 1359–1363. [CrossRef]

14. Bagavathiappan, S.; Philip, J.; Jayakumar, T.; Raj, B.; Rao, P.N.S.; Varalakshmi, M.; Mohan, V. Correlation between Plantar Foot Temperature and Diabetic Neuropathy: A Case Study by Using an Infrared Thermal Imaging Technique. *J. Diabetes Sci. Technol.* **2010**, *4*, 1386–1392. [CrossRef] [PubMed]
15. Petrova, N.L.; Whittam, A.; MacDonald, A.; Ainarkar, S.; Donaldson, A.N.; Bevans, J.; Allen, J.; Plassmann, P.; Kluwe, B.; Ring, F.; et al. Reliability of a novel thermal imaging system for temperature assessment of healthy feet. *J. Foot Ankle Res.* **2018**, *11*, 1–22. [CrossRef] [PubMed]
16. Gatt, A.; Falzon, O.; Cassar, K.; Ellul, C.; Camilleri, K.P.; Gauci, J.; Mizzi, S.; Mizzi, A.; Sturgeon, C.; Camilleri, L.; et al. Establishing Differences in Thermographic Patterns between the Various Complications in Diabetic Foot Disease. *Int. J. Endocrinol.* **2018**, *2018*, 9808295. [CrossRef] [PubMed]
17. Gatt, A.; Falzon, O.; Cassar, K.; Camilleri, K.P.; Gauci, J.; Ellul, C.; Mizzi, S.; Mizzi, A.; Papanas, N.; Sturgeon, C.; et al. The Application of Medical Thermography to Discriminate Neuroischemic Toe Ulceration in the Diabetic Foot. *Int. J. Low. Extrem. Wounds* **2018**, *17*, 102–105. [CrossRef] [PubMed]
18. Skafjeld, A.; Iversen, M.; Holme, I.; Ribu, L.; Hvaal, K.; Kilhovd, B. A pilot study testing the feasibility of skin temperature monitoring to reduce recurrent foot ulcers in patients with diabetes—A randomized controlled trial. *BMC Endocr. Disord.* **2015**, *15*, 55. [CrossRef] [PubMed]
19. Pit'hová, P.; Patkova, H.; Galandakova, I.; Dolezalova, L.; Kvapil, M. Differences in ulcer location in diabetic foot syndrome. *Vnitr. Lek.* **2007**, *53*, 1278–1285.
20. Mansor, H.; Shukor, M.H.A.; Meskam, S.S.; Rusli, N.Q.A.M.; Zamery, N.S. Body temperature measurement for remote health monitoring system. In Proceedings of the 2013 IEEE International Conference on Smart Instrumentation, Measurement and Applications (ICSIMA), Kuala Lumpur, Malaysia, 25–27 November 2013; IEEE: Piscataway, NJ, USA, 2013; pp. 1–5.
21. Majumder, S.; Mondal, T.; Deen, M.J. Wearable sensors for remote health monitoring. *Sensors* **2017**, *17*, 130. [CrossRef]
22. Electronics Tutorials (s.f.). Temperature Sensors. Available online: https://www.electronics-tutorials.ws/io/io_3.html (accessed on 13 January 2021).
23. Reddy, P.N.; Cooper, G.; Weightman, A.; Hodson-Tole, E.; Reeves, N. An in-shoe temperature measurement system for studying diabetic foot ulceration etiology: Preliminary results with healthy participants. *Procedia CIRP* **2016**, *49*, 153–156. [CrossRef]
24. Recreational Physics (Spanish). Available online: https://www.fisicarecreativa.com/guias/sensorestemp.pdf (accessed on 13 January 2021).
25. Martín-Vaquero, J.; Hernández Encinas, A.; Queiruga-Dios, A.; José Bullón, J.; Martínez-Nova, A.; Torreblanca González, J.; Bullón-Carbajo, C. Review on wearables to monitor foot temperature in diabetic patients. *Sensors* **2019**, *19*, 776. [CrossRef] [PubMed]
26. Childs, P.R.; Greenwood, J.; Long, C. Review of temperature measurement. *Rev. Sci. Instrum.* **2000**, *71*, 2959–2978. [CrossRef]
27. González, J.T.; Nova, A.M.; Encinas, A.; Martín-Vaquero, J.; Queiruga-Dios, A. Statistical Analysis to Control Foot Temperature for Diabetic People. In Proceedings of the World Conference on Information Systems and Technologies, Budva, Montenegro, 7–10 April 2020; Springer: Cham, Switzerland, 2020; pp. 295–306.
28. Nath, J.K.; Sharma, S.; Sarma, K.C. A Comparative Study of Accuracy Improvement of Temperature Measurement with PT100 and PT1000 for Wider Range. *Int. J. Electron. Eng. Res.* **2017**, *9*, 735–743.
29. Classification of Thermoresistances (Spanish). Available online: http://server-die.alc.upv.es/asignaturas/lsed/2003-04/0.Sens_Temp/Clasify/Termorresistencias.htm (accessed on 13 January 2021).
30. NTC Thermistor. Available online: http://www.resistorguide.com/ntc-thermistor/ (accessed on 13 January 2021).
31. PTC Thermistor. Available online: http://www.resistorguide.com/ptc-thermistor/ (accessed on 13 January 2021).
32. Carr, J.J. *Sensors and Circuits: Sensors, Transducers, and Supporting Circuits for Electronic Instrumentation, Measurement, and Control*; PTR Prentice Hall: Englewood Cliffs, NJ, USA, 1993.
33. Sudha, S.; Shruthi, P.; Sharanya, M. IOT Based Measurement of Body Temperature using MAX30205. *Int. Res. J. Eng. Technol.* **2018**, *5*, 3913–3915.
34. MAX30205 Temperature Sensor. Available online: https://datasheets.maximintegrated.com/en/ds/MAX30205.pdf (accessed on 13 January 2021).
35. Si7006-A20. Available online: https://www.silabs.com/documents/public/data-sheets/Si7006-A20.pdf (accessed on 13 January 2021).
36. AD590 Temperature Transducer. Available online: http://www.analog.com/media/en/technical-documentation/data-sheets/AD590.pdf (accessed on 13 January 2021).
37. Bossuyt, P.M.; Reitsma, J.B.; Reitsma, J.B.; Bruns, D.E.; Gatsonis, C.A.; Glasziou, P.P.; Irwig, L.M.; Moher, D.; Rennie, D.; de Vet, H.C.W.; et al. The STARD statement for reporting studies of diagnostic accuracy: Explanation and elaboration. *Ann. Intern. Med.* **2003**, *138*, 1–12. [CrossRef] [PubMed]
38. Queiruga-Dios, A.; Pérez, J.B.; Encinas, A.H.; Martín-Vaquero, J.; Nova, A.M.; González, J.T. Skin Temperature Monitoring to Avoid Foot Lesions in Diabetic Patients. In Proceedings of the International Conference on Practical Applications of Computational Biology & Bioinformatics, Porto, Portugal, 21–23 June 2017; Springer: Cham, Switzerland, 2017; pp. 110–117.
39. Armstrong, D.G.; Lavery, L.A.; Harkless, L.B. Validation of a Diabetic Wound Classification System: The contribution of depth, infection, and ischemia to risk of amputation. *Diabetes Care* **1998**, *21*, 855–859. [CrossRef] [PubMed]

40. Escamilla-Martínez, E.; Gómez-Martín, B.; Sánchez-Rodríguez, R.; Fernández-Seguín, L.M.; Pérez-Soriano, P.; Martínez-Nova, A. Running thermoregulation effects using bioceramics versus polyester fibres socks. *J. Ind. Text.* **2020**. [CrossRef]
41. Pascual-Huerta, J.; Arcas Lorente, C.; Trincado Villa, L.; García Carmona, F.; Fernández Morato, D. Relationship between foot posture index and plantar pressure distribution in patients with limb length inequality: A case series study. *Rev. Esp. Podol.* **2018**, *29*, 21–26.
42. Sánchez-Rodríguez, R.; Valle-Estévez, S.; Fraile-García, P.; Martínez-Nova, A.; Gómez-Martín, B.; Escamilla-Martínez, E. Modification of Pronated Foot Posture after a Program of Therapeutic Exercises. *Int. J. Environ. Res. Public Health* **2020**, *17*, 8406. [CrossRef]
43. Hughes-Riley, T.; Lugoda, P.; Dias, T.; Trabi, C.L.; Morris, R.H. A Study of thermistor performance within a textile structure. *Sensors* **2017**, *17*, 1804. [CrossRef] [PubMed]
44. Hatamie, A.; Angizi, S.; Kumar, S.; Pandey, C.M.; Simchi, A.; Willander, M.; Malhotra, B.D. Textile based chemical and physical sensors for healthcare monitoring. *J. Electrochem. Soc.* **2020**, *167*, 037546. [CrossRef]
45. Thermistor Calculator V1.1. Available online: https://www.thinksrs.com/downloads/programs/Therm%20Calc/NTCCalibrator/NTCcalculator.htm (accessed on 13 January 2021).

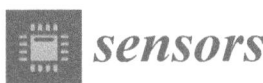

Article

Estimating Functional Threshold Power in Endurance Running from Shorter Time Trials Using a 6-Axis Inertial Measurement Sensor

Antonio Cartón-Llorente [1], Felipe García-Pinillos [2,3], Jorge Royo-Borruel [1], Alberto Rubio-Peirotén [1], Diego Jaén-Carrillo [1,*] and Luis E. Roche-Seruendo [1]

[1] Health Sciences Faculty, Universidad San Jorge, 50830 Zaragoza, Spain; acarton@usj.es (A.C.-L.); royojorge@gmail.com (J.R.-B.); arubio@usj.es (A.R.-P.); leroche@usj.es (L.E.R.-S.)
[2] Department of Sports and Physical Education, University of Granada, 18071 Granada, Spain; fegarpi@gmail.com
[3] Department of Physical Education, Sports and Recreation, Universidad de La Frontera, Temuco 14811, Chile
* Correspondence: djaen@usj.es; Tel.: +34-615-635-708

Citation: Cartón-Llorente, A.; García-Pinillos, F.; Royo-Borruel, J.; Rubio-Peirotén, A.; Jaén-Carrillo, D.; Roche-Seruendo, L.E. Estimating Functional Threshold Power in Endurance Running from Shorter Time Trials Using a 6-Axis Inertial Measurement Sensor. *Sensors* **2021**, *21*, 582. https://doi.org/10.3390/s21020582

Received: 11 November 2020
Accepted: 12 January 2021
Published: 15 January 2021

Publisher's Note: MDPI stays neutral with regard to jurisdictional claims in published maps and institutional affiliations.

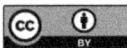

Copyright: © 2021 by the authors. Licensee MDPI, Basel, Switzerland. This article is an open access article distributed under the terms and conditions of the Creative Commons Attribution (CC BY) license (https://creativecommons.org/licenses/by/4.0/).

Abstract: Wearable technology has allowed for the real-time assessment of mechanical work employed in several sporting activities. Through novel power metrics, Functional Threshold Power have shown a reliable indicator of training intensities. This study aims to determine the relationship between mean power output (MPO) values obtained during three submaximal running time trials (i.e., 10 min, 20 min, and 30 min) and the functional threshold power (FTP). Twenty-two recreationally trained male endurance runners completed four submaximal running time trials of 10, 20, 30, and 60 min, trying to cover the longest possible distance on a motorized treadmill. Absolute MPO (W), normalized MPO (W/kg) and standard deviation (SD) were calculated for each time trial with a power meter device attached to the shoelaces. All simplified FTP trials analyzed (i.e., FTP10, FTP20, and FTP30) showed a significant association with the calculated FTP ($p < 0.001$) for both MPO and normalized MPO, whereas stronger correlations were found with longer time trials. Individual correction factors (ICF% = FTP60/FTPn) of ~90% for FTP10, ~94% for FTP20, and ~96% for FTP30 were obtained. The present study procures important practical applications for coaches and athletes as it provides a more accurate estimation of FTP in endurance running through less fatiguing, reproducible tests.

Keywords: aerobic; assessment; performance; physiology; technology; training; wearable

1. Introduction

Monitoring workload is a milestone for endurance sports athletes and coaches for training prescription and competition. A wide array of physiological parameters has been targeted in search for a single biomarker truly coupled to the current intensity of the effort which, at the same time, was easy to track. These psychophysiological responses are classified as internal workload measures and mainly include the evaluation of heart rate (HR) and its derivatives (e.g., heart rate variability), blood lactate concentration, muscle oxygen saturation, and rate of perceived exertion (RPE). To date, none of them have turned out to be sensitive or handy enough to instantly quantify the athlete's response to training stimuli [1], and multiple external (often called objective) workload metrics needed to be added to assess in-field racing intensity [2].

The development of portable global positioning system technologies (GPS) allowed the use of external metrics, such as distance and velocity, and so controlling the training pace and observing the internal responses to it became widely used as one of the best methods to assess current training stress. Unfortunately, pace is highly dependent on external conditions, such as wind, terrain, or slope, and therefore its use for quantifying intensity in the field provides results that are imprecise and is not repeatable enough. In this context, new technologies were developed in a search for an objective workload metric, giving rise to the era of mechanical power assessment.

Power output refers to the product of force and velocity, so once you are able to calculate the instant force applied to a given activity, you can accurately measure the actual workload your body is putting out. The huge step forward came when comparing power output´s instantaneous response to an increase or decrease of intensity with other traditional metrics such as heart rate, which take their time to respond. Actually, mean power output (MPO) (i.e., the averaged power output during a given time period) has proven to be more reliable and sensitive to little changes in exercise intensity than other internal and external commonly used workload indicators [3].

Accordingly, the use of power meters in cycling increased exponentially due to their capacity to assess workload considering external conditions such as wind, drafting, slope or terrain. New racing strategies (e.g., uphill pacing) emerged and power-related data also became widely used to inform decisions relating to cycling position, technique and equipment selection [4]. Through strain gauges located in the pedals, crank, or rear hub, the quantity and direction of the force applied by the cyclist, as well as the instant angular velocity, can be obtained. Therefore, power output in cycling is calculated based on the torque applied multiplied by cadence.

Analogously, running mechanical power could be quantified using force instrumented treadmills [5] which reflects forward, vertical and lateral forces applied to the integrated force plate at any given velocity. Of note, the actual external mechanical work of the foot against the ground is negligible, so the term power output in running represents an abstraction of the mechanical power theoretically applied to the runner´s centre of mass. Despite its accuracy, force instrumented treadmills are not usable for an in-field evaluation, thus, some commercial companies started to develop wearable power meters for running. These novel devices can estimate the force applied by the subjects derived from their height, body mass, and velocity, using GPS technology in outdoor environments and IMUs when indoors [6]. In fact, a model proposed recently by Jenny and Jenny [7] supports that the mechanical energy for steady flat running could be expressed as the sum of the energy employed to counteract aerodynamic drag and the energy dissipated to produce vertical oscillation and braking.

In the aforementioned mathematical approach [7] the rate of mechanical energy (i.e., the power output) dissipated to break through the air can be estimated knowing both the runner and the wind´s velocity, and the runner and the air´s density. Energy dissipation due to braking ground reaction forces may be estimated assuming the sine wave movement described by the runner's centre of mass, following the spring-mass model presented by Blickhan [8]. Finally, dissipation in vertical oscillation is calculated based on spatiotemporal parameters (speed, step rate, ground contact time) and a potential energy recovery factor. This factor depends on the athlete´s ability to reuse the elastic energy stored during the braking phase, into kinetic energy during the propulsion phase. As this condition is highly variable between individuals, it represents the main concern within the entire model.

Given the complexity of testing the validity of wearable running power meters against a gold standard method (i.e., instrumented treadmill), a recent study from Cerezuela-Espejo [9] compared PO obtained with five commercially available portable devices and two of the mathematical models applied to theoretically calculate running power. The results showed the closest agreement corresponded to the Stryd^{TM} system among all investigated devices.

Regarding the agreement between mechanical and metabolic power, another published comparison between five portable devices [10] showed a promising correlation ($r^3 = 0.911$, SEE = 7.3%) between power output data obtained with the Stryd^{TM} foot pod and oxygen consumption as a measure of energy expenditure, both in laboratory (i.e., treadmill running) and the in-field conditions, even when changes in body mass and slope were applied [10]. Table 1 summarizes the scientific evidence found on the use of the main commercially available power meters, and further information is available in a recently published scoping review on sensors for running power output assessment [11].

Table 1. Studies (n = 5) evaluating the use of wearable power meters or using their power output data during running protocols.

	System Used	Device & Location	Aim	Results
Cerezuela-Espejo et al. (2020) [10]	RunScribe	Attached to shoelaces and paired to a Garmin Forerunner 235	To compare 4 power meter devices in terms of repeatability and concurrent validity between P data and oxygen consumption (VO_2).	Fair repeatability indoor: SEM $\geq$ 30.1 W, CV $\geq$ 7.4%, ICC $\leq$ 0.709, and SEM $\geq$ 59.3 W, CV $\geq$ 14.8%, ICC $\leq$ 0.563. Low correlation between P and VO_2 (r $\geq$ 0.582, SEE $\leq$ 13.7%)
	Garmin Running Power	Garmin TRI^{TM} heart rate (chest) monitor band and Garmin Forerunner 935 watch Kansas, USA		Low repeatability indoor: SEM $\geq$ 47.0 W, CV $\geq$ 9.4%, ICC $\leq$ 0.495, fair repeatability outdoor: SEM $\geq$ 24.5 W, CV $\geq$ 7.7%, ICC = 0.823. Low correlation between P and VO_2 (r $\geq$ 0.539, SEE $\leq$ 17.5%)
	Polar Vantage V	Sport watch on the wrist. GPS and barometer sensors		Low repeatability outdoor: SEM $\geq$ 40.6 W, CV $\geq$ 14.5%, ICC = 0.487. Good correlation between P and VO_2 (r = 0.841, SEE = 9.7%)
	Stryd (foot pod)	Attached to shoelaces and paired to a Garmin Forerunner 235 or a mobile phone		Best repeatability values both indoor: SEM $\leq$ 7.4 W, CV $\leq$ 2.8%, ICC $\geq$ 0.980, and outdoor: SEM $\leq$ 12.5 W, CV $\leq$ 4.3%, ICC $\geq$ 0.989. High correlation between P and VO_2 ($r^3 \geq$ 0.911, SEE $\leq$ 7.3%)
García-Pinillos et al. (2019) [12]	Stryd (foot pod)	Attached to shoelaces and paired to a mobile phone	To evaluate the stability of power output data while running at a constant comfortable velocity on a motorized treadmill.	P running at an easy pace is a stable metric with negligible differences, between intervals ranging from 10 to 180 s.
García-Pinillos et al. (2019) [13]	Stryd (foot pod)	Attached to shoelaces and paired to a mobile phone	To confirm the linear P-V relationship in endurance runners at submaximal velocities, and to predict P values with the "two-point method".	Two distant velocities were able to provide P with the same accuracy than the multiple-point method.
Austin et al. (2018) [14]	Stryd (foot pod)	Attached to shoelaces and paired to a Garmin Fenix 3 watch	To determine the correlations between P and running economy at LT pace.	RE is positively correlated with Stryd's power output data, however it may not be precise enough to notice changes in running economy
Aubry et al. (2018) [15]	Stryd (chest strap)	Stryd Pioneer 3-axial accelerometer chest band in conjunction with a mobile phone (with GPS).	To assess if running power could be a valid surrogate of metabolic demand (VO_2) in a population of different level of training runners.	Running power is not a valid surrogate of the energy cost of running in a mixed ability population of runners.

LT: blood lactate thresholds; VO2: oxygen uptake; P: power; V: velocity; SEM: standard error of measurement; CV: coefficient of variation; ICC: intraclass correlation coefficient; RE: running economy.

Regarding the application of power output data to determine training stress and intensity zones, Allen and Cogan [16] proposed a performance index known as the Functional Threshold Power (FTP). It refers to the highest MPO maintained in a quasi-steady state for 60 min (FTP_{60}) without the onset of fatigue [16]. FTP has demonstrated its validity as a surrogate for lactate threshold (LT) [17] and maximum lactate steady state (MLSS) [18,19]. LT is defined as the maximum intensity preceding an exponential rise in blood lactate values during an incremental test [20], being addressed that during a continuous effort at LT blood lactate concentration steadily rises [17]. However, MLSS refers to the maximum workload that can be maintained over time without continual blood lactate accumulation (i.e., 45–70 min) [18,21]. Additionally, MLSS demonstrated to better predict endurance performance than maximum oxygen uptake (VO2max) in trained athletes [20]. Thus, FTP is considered a good indicator of the main physiological events of the aerobic-anaerobic transition for endurance activities and therefore it has been commonly used lately to determine training intensities (i.e., training zones) and quantify athletes' responses to training stimuli.

Although FTP_{60} is a highly reproducible and widely accepted method to assess aerobic condition [11], less time-consuming time trials (TT) are demanded for in-season regular evaluations. The 20-min TT (FTP_{20}) has become the most popular simplified test to predict FTP_{60} [22,23]. Allen and Cogan [16] set 95% of the MPO obtained in FTP20 as a predictive value for FTP_{60} in cycling. Thereafter, a few studies [23–25] confirmed this 95% individual correction factor (ICF% = FTP_{60}/FTP_{20}) between both TTs, whereas some others [26–28] found stronger associations between FTP_{20} and MLSS subtracting ~10% to the MPO achieved during the TT, instead of 5%. Furthermore, other TTs ranging from 3 to 30 min were proposed as MLSS predictors of FTP_{60} [24,29]. Despite an overall moderate to high level of agreement between these simplified TTs and FTP_{60}, most referred to cycling.

The advent of wearable running power meters allows the transfer of knowledge (and the FTP60 assessment) from cycling to running. Unlike other parameters such as HR, VO2max or RPE, the physiological response of blood lactate showed no differences between cycling and running at constant submaximal velocities [30]. Therefore, the determination of FTP_{60} as a valid substitute of MLSS would be a key point for endurance running. Unfortunately, knowledge about the level of agreement and correction factor between simplified TTs and FTP_{60} in running is unknown. Nevertheless, the development of novel technologies, such as running power meters, may help evaluate athletes' functional performance and monitor changes over time. A recent study confirmed a linear power–velocity relationship in running for maximal and submaximal protocols [13]. This enables the prediction of MPO at different submaximal running velocities using the two-point method, underlining the need to accurately determine the relationship between simplified FTP tests and FTP_{60} method.

Up to date, there are no studies which investigate the validity of simplified running test to predict FTP_{60}. Consequently, this study aims to analyse the level of agreement between mean power values during three different running TTs (10-, 20- and 30-min) compared to a 60-min TT, and to establish the correction factor for each simplified FTP running test. Considering the high concordance reported in cycling, we hypothesized that the 10-, 20-, and 30-min TTs (i.e., FTP_{10}, FTP_{20} and FTP_{30}) would have a good level of agreement with FTP_{60} in running, and they could be valid substitutes of the FTP_{60}.

2. Materials and Methods

2.1. Participants

Twenty-two recreationally trained male endurance runners (age: 34.0 ± 7.5 years; height: 1.76 ± 0.04 m; body mass: 71.1 ± 5.8 kg; BMI: 22.9 ± 1.5 kg/m^2) voluntarily participated in this study. All participants met the inclusion criteria: older than 18 years old, able to run 10 km under 40 min, used to running treadmill, and free from injuries the last 6 months before data collection. After receiving detailed information of the study, participants signed an informed consent form, complied with the ethical standards of the

World Medical Association's Declaration of Helsinki (2013), prior to participation. It was made clear that participants were free to leave the study at any point. The study was approved by the local Ethics Committee.

2.2. Procedures

The study protocol was executed between March and June 2019 in the laboratory of biomechanics of the founding institution. Participants were asked to complete four submaximal time trials (10, 20, 30, and 60 min) attempting to cover the longest distance they could on a motorized treadmill (HP cosmos Pulsar 4P; HP cosmos Sports & Medical, Gmbh, Nußdorf, Germany). During all tests slope was maintained at 0° and ventilation was assured using two industrial fans located laterally at 2 m distance from both sides of the treadmill. Fluid intake was ad libitum while temperature and humidity were controlled with a wireless weather station (Ea2 LABS DE903) and kept between 18 and 20 °C and 50–60%, respectively.

Participants were encouraged to maintain their normal dietary pattern and to avoid ergogenic aids and severe physical activity for 48 h before the tests, which were scheduled at the same time of the day and performed within a 1-week separation interval. Trial order was randomly set, and participants wore their usual running shoes during the entire protocol to reproduce their usual performance.

2.3. Materials and Testing

Body height (cm) and mass (kg) were measured at the beginning of the first testing session using a precision stadiometer and weighing scale (SECA 222 and 634, respectively, SECA Corp., Hamburg, Germany). Additionally, personal best time in a 10-km race within the last 6 months were recorded and all the athletes were instructed on the use of the RPE scale [31].

Before each time trial, participants' body mass was re-evaluated to adjust the power data collected. A standardized 8-min protocol (4-min at self-selected velocity and 4-min approaching their expected velocity for the trial) was completed for avoiding the accommodation effect of treadmill running [32].

During the tests, participants received verbal encouragement from the same researcher to complete the longest distance they can, and slight velocity variations were allowed along the entire protocol. HR was continuously monitored using a chest belt (Polar, FS2c, Kempele, Finland), and RPE was assessed every 5 min until the end of the test. MPO (in W) was calculated using the Stryd™ power meter (Stryd Power meter, Stryd Inc. Boulder, CO, USA) attached to the shoelaces.

After each test, maximum HR and total distance covered was recorded and mean velocity calculated. Data from Stryd™ power meter were obtained from their website (https://www.stryd.com/powercenter/analysis) into .fit file. Then, data were analyzed using a free-license software (Golden Cheetah, version 3.4) and exported as .csl file into Excel® (2016, Microsoft, Inc., Redmond, WA, USA). Absolute MPO (W), normalized MPO (W/kg), and standard deviation (SD) were calculated for each time trial.

2.4. Stryd™ System

This device is a lightweight (9.1 g) carbon fibre-reinforced foot pod that includes a 6-axis inertial motion sensor (3-axis gyroscope, 3-axis accelerometer). With a sampling rate of 1000 Hz, the 6-degrees-of-freedom device senses forward, vertical and lateral accelerations and angular velocities of rolling, pitching and yawing, to infer ground reaction forces and orientation. Integrating accelerations, the sensor gets velocities, and doble integrating it gets positions. Assuming the lateral motion as negligible in running, inverse dynamics might be applied to model vertical and horizontal forces from the positional and velocity changes of the device in each step.

As it has been roughly explained by the Stryd™ team in a recent white paper on their web site (https://blog.stryd.com/tag/validation-white-papers/), accounting vertical decelerations and accelerations, the height and body mass of the runner, and the flight time between steps, an algorithm estimates the vertical displacement of the runner´s center of mass, and thus, its potential energy variation is available to calculate vertical power (named as form power by the Stryd^{TM} manufacturers). While moving forward, a runner losses momentum on foot impact and gains it during take-off. The change in kinetic energy between events is given by the difference between the minimum and maximum instant velocities and the body mass of the runner, allowing forward power calculation. Finally, external PO is the time derivative of the summation of changes in potential and kinetic energy.

As a result, this wearable power meter additionally provides real time measures of vertical oscillation, elevation, distance and ground contact time, and interesting power-related metrics (i.e., averaged elapsed power, maximal power, form power, leg spring stiffness and running effectiveness). Of note, the presented model does not account for the internal power the runner needs to relocate the limbs in relation to the center of mass. However, the manufacturers presume the newest version of the product include a sensor to detect wind force and direction that might allow a better estimation of these internal forces.

Although the actual strategy Stryd^{TM} use to isolate the sensor to avoid measurement noise, and the algorithmic computation to process raw data still undisclosed by the company as part of their knowhow, this system has demonstrated reliable to assess running spatiotemporal parameters in indoor setting compared to 3D motion analysis [33] and the OptoGait infrared system [13]. Furthermore, this sensor has shown moderate to excellent intra-system reliability for all measures through trail running bouts [34].

Presumably, the algorithm employed by the company to calculate power output might be based on the model proposed by Jenny and Jenny [7] and assumes certain controversial simplifications related to the athletes´ individual energy recovery factor. However, a recent study [10] evaluated the agreement between energy expenditure (i.e., oxygen consumption) and Stryd´s PO data under different conditions (i.e., athletic track, flat, and inclined treadmill running) showing strong correlations between variables in all conditions ($r \geq 0.911$, SEE $\leq 7.3\%$).

2.5. Statistical Analysis

Descriptive statistics are represented as mean ($\pm$SD). Before analysis, normal distribution and homogeneity were confirmed through the Shapiro-Wilk and Levene's test, respectively. A repeated measures analysis of variance (ANOVA), with post-hoc Bonferroni test, was conducted to compare the acute response (i.e., running speed, MPO and RPE) to the different time trials conditions (i.e., 10, 20, 30 and 60 min). Additionally, the level of agreement between MPO reported during shorter time trials (i.e., 10-min, 20-min and 30-min) and the reference trial (i.e., 60-min) was examined. Therefore, a Pearson correlation analysis was performed and intra-class correlation coefficients (ICC) with 95% confidence interval (CI) were calculated (i.e., 10-min, 20-min and 30-min vs. 60-min). The following criteria were adopted to interpret the correlations magnitude between variables: <0.1 (trivial), 0.1–0.3 (small), 0.3–0.5 (moderate), 0.5–0.7 (large), 0.7–0.9 (very large) and 0.9–1.0 (almost perfect) [35]. Based on the characteristics of this experimental design and following the guidelines reported by Koo and Li [36], the authors decided to conduct a "two-way random-effects" model (ICC [2,k]), "mean of measurements" type, and "absolute" definition for the ICC measurement. The interpretation of the ICC was based on the benchmarks reported by a previous study [37]: ICC < 0 (poor), 0–0.20 (slight), 0.21–0.40 (fair), 0.41–0.60 (moderate), 0.61–0.80 (substantial), and >0.81 (almost perfect). Finally, a linear regression analysis was conducted between 60-min MPO and MPO during shorter trials. The level of significance used was $p < 0.05$. Data analysis was performed using SPSS (version 23, SPSS Inc., Chicago, IL, USA).

3. Results

Table 2 shows the acute response of the examined variables to the different running protocols. The repeated measures ANOVA reported significant differences between tests in running speed ($p < 0.001$), MPO in absolute and relative values ($p < 0.001$) and RPE ($p = 0.011$). After post-hoc testing, differences between each test were found in all variables, apart from RPE, with the 30-min trial showing lower values than the rest of trials. The individual average running speed and MPO for each time trial are shown in Figures 1 and 2, respectively.

Table 2. Acute response (mean, SD) to the different running time trials.

	10-min Trial	20-min Trial	30-min Trial	60-min Trial	Main Effect of Test p-Value
Running speed (km/h^{-1})	17.16 (0.65) [b,c,d]	16.33 (0.53) [a,c,d]	15.88 (0.50) [a,b,d]	15.12 (0.56) [a,b,c]	<0.001
Mean power output (W)	341.73 (27.19) [b,c,d]	326.90 (26.97) [a,c,d]	320.63 (25.51) [a,b,d]	306.15 (25.33) [a,b,c]	<0.001
Normalized mean power output (W/kg^{-1})	4.78 (0.15) [b,c,d]	4.58 (0.15) [a,c,d]	4.47 (0.15) [a,b,d]	4.29 (0.13) [a,b,c]	<0.001
RPE (6–20)	19.27 (0.83) [c]	18.95 (0.84)	18.64 (0.73) [a,d]	19.27 (0.88) [c]	0.011

[a] indicates significant differences regarding 10-min trial after post-hoc testing; [b] indicates significant differences regarding 20-min trial after post-hoc testing; [c] indicates significant differences regarding 30-min trial after post-hoc testing; [d] indicates significant differences regarding 60-min trial after post-hoc testing.

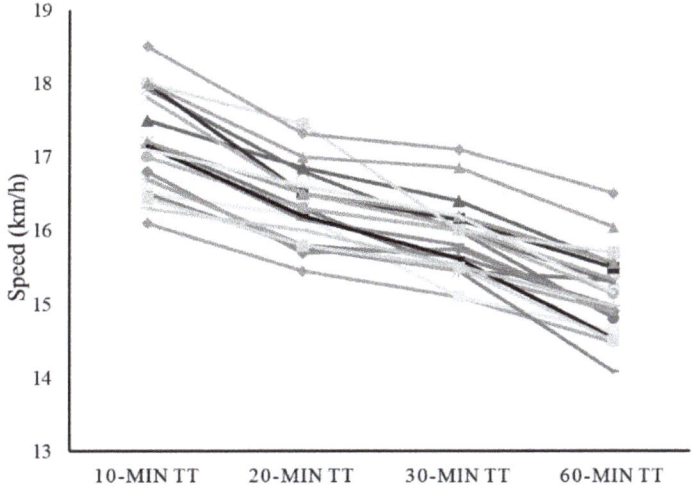

Figure 1. Individual average running speed for each time trial (i.e., 10 min, 20 min, 30 min and 60 min). Each athlete's speed mean values are represented in a different color line.

The level of agreement of power values obtained during running protocols with different durations, as compared to 60-min time trial, was examined (Table 2). For mean power values (W), all the durations (i.e., 10, 20, and 30 min) showed an almost perfect correlation ($r > 0.9$), whereas the ICC was moderate with data obtained from the 10-min trial (ICC = 0.647), and very large with 20-min and 30-min trials (ICCs = 0.839 and 0.899, respectively). Regarding the normalized mean power values (W/kg), the correlation with data reported during the 60-min trial was very large ($r = 0.720$ for 10-min trial, 0.868 for 20-min trial and 0.859 for 30-min trial) and the ICCs revealed slight (ICC = 0.188), moderate (ICC = 0.432) and substantial (ICC = 0.625) coefficients for 10-min, 20-min and 30-min time trials, respectively, compared to 60-min protocol. Additionally, the ICF% and CI for each TT were calculated for both MPO and normalized MPO (Table 3).

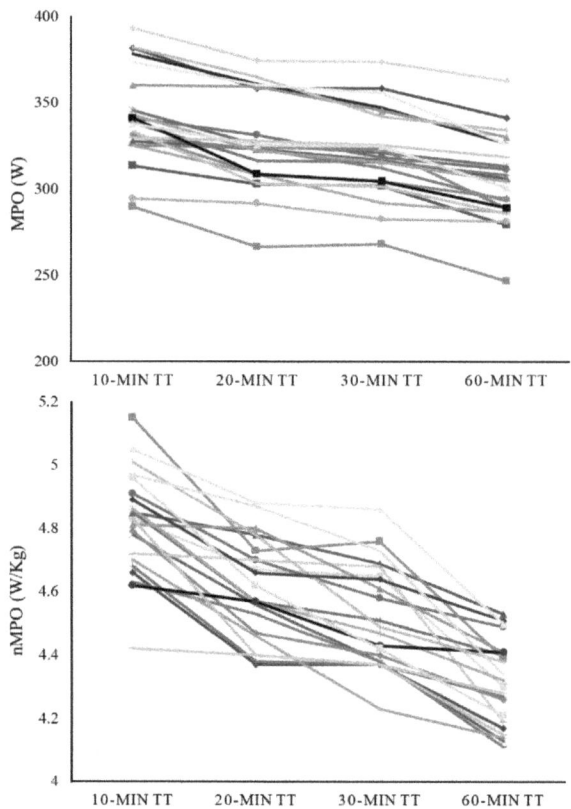

Figure 2. Individual analysis of the power output during running, in absolute (upper panel) and relative values (lower panel) (i.e., 10-min, 20-min, 30-min and 60-min time trials). MPO: mean power output; nMPO: normalized mean power output.

Table 3. Level of agreement between power output obtained during different running based-time trials regarding the reference duration (60-min time trial).

		Mean Power (W)	Normalized Mean Power (W/kg)
10-min vs. 60-min	Correlation (r-coefficient)	0.916 ***	0.720 ***
	ICC (95% CI)	0.647 (−0.084–0.909)	0.188 (−0.046–0.566)
	ICF% (CI)	89.6 (88.2–90.9)	89.8 (88.8–90.7)
20-min vs. 60-min	Correlation (r-coefficient)	0.949 ***	0.868 ***
	ICC (95% CI)	0.839 (−0.120–0.964)	0.432 (−0.061–0.808)
	ICF% (CI)	93.6 (92.5–94.7)	93.7 (93.1–94.4)
30-min vs. 60-min	Correlation (r-coefficient)	0.946 ***	0.859 ***
	ICC (95% CI)	0.899 (−0.089–0.976)	0.625 (−0.152–0.895)
	ICF% (CI)	95.5 (94.3–96.6)	95.9 (95.2–96.6)

*** $p < 0.001$; ICC: intra class correlation coefficient; ICF%: individual correction factor (%); CI: confidence interval.

The regression analysis revealed a significant association ($p < 0.001$) between 60-min MPO and the MPO reported during shorter trials (i.e., 10-, 20- and 30-min) (Figure 3). The 10-min MPO obtained the lowest r^2 ($r^2 = 0.839$) and the greater SEE (10.4 W), whereas almost identical values were obtained in 20- and 30-min ($r^2 = 0.901$, SEE = 8.2 W; $r^2 = 0.895$, SEE = 8.4 W, respectively). Regarding normalized MPO (Figure 1), a significant association ($p < 0001$) was found between 60-min values and those reported during shorter trials (i.e.,

10-, 20- and 30-min), with stronger associations found with longer time trials ($r^2 = 0.519$, SEE = 0.09 W for 10-min; $r^2 = 0.753$, SEE = 0.07 W for 20-min and; $r^2 = 0.720$, SEE = 0.07 W for 30-min).

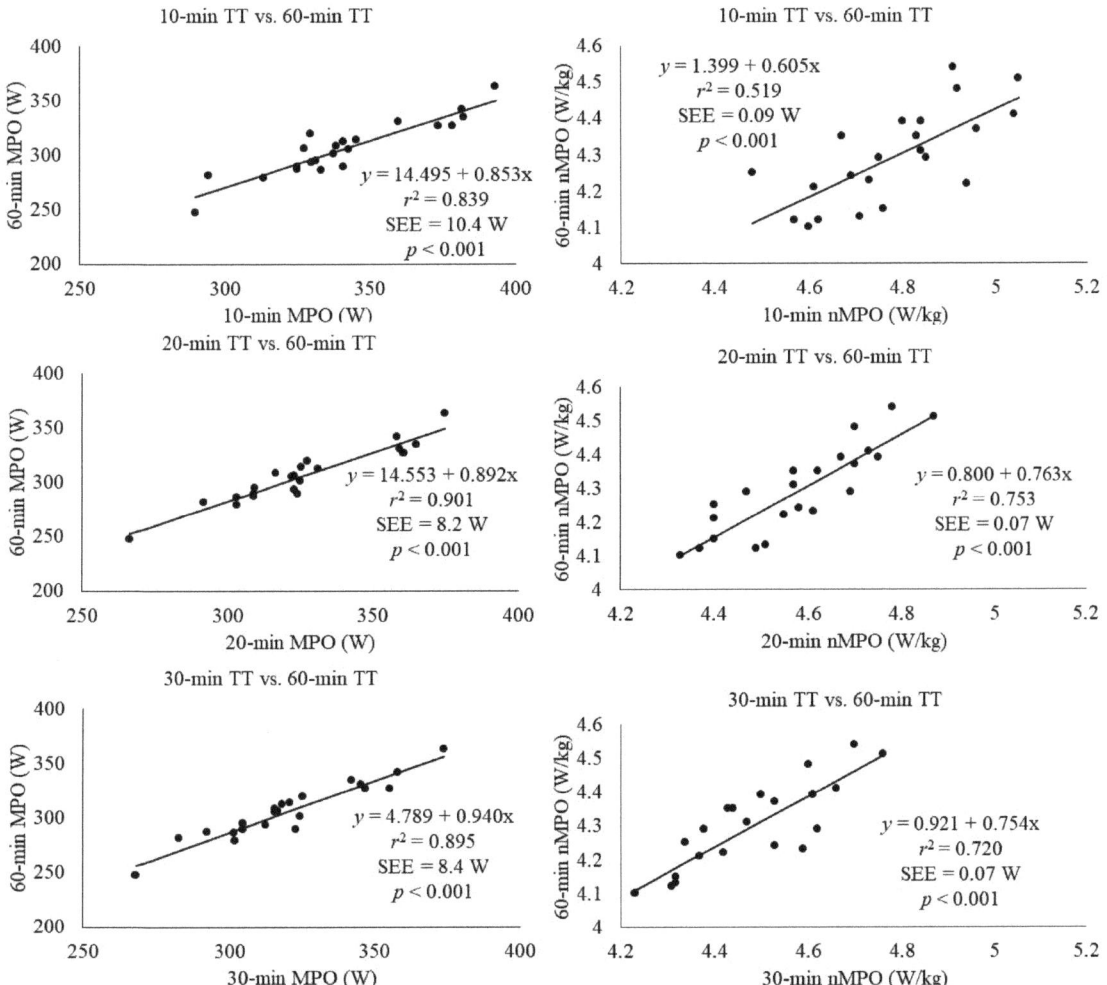

Figure 3. Association between the mean power output achieved during a 60-min time trial (TT) and the MPO achieved during 10-min, 20-min and 30-min TTs in trained endurance runners. (Absolute values in left column and relative values in right column). The average value of each runner was used for each TT. Circles indicate individual data. The solid lines represent the predictive linear regression model between 60-min TT and the shorter TTs. SEE: standard error of estimate; MPO: mean power output; nMPO: normalized mean power output.

4. Discussion

This study sought to analyze the level of agreement between the 60-min TT and three shorter TTs. The main finding of this study is that all simplified FTP trials analyzed (i.e., FTP_{10}, FTP_{20} and FTP_{30}) showed a significant association with the FTP_{60} for both MPO and normalized MPO, exhibiting stronger correlations with longer TTs (i.e., FTP_{20} and FTP_{30}). Moreover, the ICF% determined for each TT were 89.6%, 93.6%, and 95.5% of the

MPO from the FTP_{10}, FTP_{20} and FTP_{30}, respectively; and 89.8%, 93.7%, 95.6% from the aforementioned TTs when MPO was normalized to the daily athletes' body mass.

4.1. FTP_{60}

To the best of the authors' knowledge, this is the first study aimed to establish the relationships between FTP_{60} and shorter TTs based on running power metrics. An average MPO of 306.15 ± 25.33 W was obtained for the FTP60 at a mean speed of 15.12 ± 0.56 km/h in trained endurance runners. This result seems to be in line with a previous study [21] which addressed a MPO of 285.2 ± 25.6 W in a group of trained athletes during a 3-min run at 15 km/h. Considering normalized MPO, our results for the FTP_{60} test showed a mean of 4.29 ± 0.13 W/kg. In a previous study [28], the average normalized MPO reported at their LT pace was 4.4 ± 0.5 W/kg. As the MPO in this study was assessed at their calculated LT pace, comparison between both studies should be cautiously considered as the MPO at MLSS might be considerably lower. Additionally, a normalized MPO of 4.29 W/kg is considered as excellent in cycling [16] and therefore our results are supported by previous studies for this level of endurance athletes [16].

4.2. FTP_{10}

The agreement between FTP60 and FTP10 ranged from very large to almost perfect for relative and absolute power output assessment, respectively. In addition, the ICF% obtained was ~90%, for both MPO and normalized MPO. The average MPO obtained was 341.73 ± 27.19 W, the normalized MPO was 4.78 ± 0.15 W/kg, and the mean velocity of the test was 17.16 ± 0.56 km/h. These results slightly exceed those found in previous studies [13,15], although the speeds are not entirely comparable. Despite the results for FTP10 exhibiting the lowest association with FPT60 within the three TTs tested, previous studies confirmed a good association between short TTs (i.e., ≤10 min) and LT derivatives [22,38,39]. Despite the good association found between FTP_{10} and FTP_{60}, our results were slightly weaker compared with longer TTs (i.e., FTP_{20} and FTP_{30}). Of note, these studies [38,39] also found broader differences between calculated MLSS and FTP estimated with shorter TTs (i.e., ≤10-min) than with longer TTs (i.e., ≥20-min). These discrepancies might partially be explained as a result of differences in the athletes' metabolic profile, as the MPO of shorter TTs is more likely to be achieved with a higher participation of the anaerobic metabolism [40]. Despite these controversial precedents, we found a large association between FTP_{10} and FTP_{60}, and therefore it could be useful for running practitioners aiming to execute a rapid test that fairly identifies training zones and adaptations.

4.3. FTP_{20}

Regarding FTP_{20} association with FTP_{60}, our results showed a very large to almost perfect correlation for both absolute and normalized MPO. The ICF% found was 93.6%, which contradicted the 95% established by Allen and Coggan [16] and supported others [23–25]. Contrary, recent studies [26–28] pointed that the well-accepted rule of subtracting 5% from the FTP_{20} MPO is not a "one-size-fits-all" accurate method for FTP_{60} estimation as it may differ depending on the athlete's level of performance. Our findings support this statement as an overestimating trend would affect our non-elite athletes when 95% of the FTP_{20} is applied. Furthermore, Valenzuela et al. [24] tested two different cyclist groups (i.e., trained and recreational) and claimed that lower fitness status could result in FTP_{60} overestimation as only the trained group matched the 95% adjustment for FTP20. Moreover, MacInnis described an ICF% of 90% for FTP_{20} in 8 well-trained cyclists [39], whereas Lillo-Bevia tested 11 trained cyclist and triathletes finding an ICF% of 91% [27]. It should be considered that the aforementioned studies did not match the 95% adjustment [26–28] followed by a modified warm-up protocol (i.e., ≤15 min at self-selected pace), whereas those that reported a 95% correction between test [23–25] strictly followed the warm-up protocol originally proposed by Allen and Coggan [16] (50 min, including three 1-min accelerations and a 5-min all-out effort). Therefore, it was hypothesized that the type of warm-up selected may explain the differences between studies [25]. As a 50-min warm-up protocol would jeopardize running performance, and the final purpose of a simplified TT is to reduce the duration and fatigue induced by the testing protocol itself, a modified warm-up protocol was adopted [28] seeking for a more practical approach.

The average MPO obtained in our FTP_{20} (326.9 ± 26.97 W) and the normalized MPO (4.58 ± 0.15 W/kg) are similar to those found in previous studies [13,15]. Of note, the recording time in these studies lasted two and three min, respectively. Thus, the minor mean differences found might be attributed to the fatigue induced along the 20-min test.

4.4. FTP_{30}

A strong association was found between FTP_{30} and FTP_{60} with substantial to very large confidence interval for relative and absolute values. Our results also identify an ICF% of ~96%, an MPO of 320.63 ± 25.51 W and a normalized MPO of 4.47 ± 0.15 W/kg. Previous studies [13,15] evaluated absolute MPO and normalized MPO at similar velocities (~16 km/h) showing similar results for same-level trained runners. Unfortunately, to our knowledge there are no previous studies assessing the relationship between both tests. It is worth mentioning that many studies conducted several constant-velocity 30-min TTs as a valid method to determine MLSS [27], nevertheless, it is hard to establish a comparison because in these TTs the participants were not encouraged to cover the longest distance they could but to keep a previously fixed PO. Despite this, our results showed to be consistent and allow an accurate prediction of FTP_{60}. However, as the results found little differences between FTP_{20} and FTP_{30} for their correlation with FTP_{60} (ICCs = 0.839 and 0.899, respectively), it would be advisable to opt for the shortest one to reduce both time needed and stress caused in the athletes.

Although the use of IMU technology for estimating running power is quite recent, its rapid development might be a promising step forward in the field of exercise physiology. Added to heart rate monitors and GPS technology, real-time power output data could help for a better understanding of the cardio-respiratory and skeletal muscle responses to different intensity runs. In order to effectively monitor the physical impact of running through portable running power meters, an accurate determination of the main physiological boundaries is mandatory. Whereas previous works validated the use of power meters in cycling for FTP assessment [22,41], analogous evidence for running devices is lacking. Despite up to date no studies have investigated the concurrent validity of running power meters, Olaya et al. [42] found and almost perfect association between PO (measured with Stryd^{TM} system) and pace data (measured via GPS technology) in their comparison of five methods to determine the FTP during level running. Additionally, in a recent review on sensors for running power [11] it has been stated that the Stryd foot pod has the highest repeatability and agreement with metabolic power among all commercially available portable running power devices. In this context, a broader framework related with the validity and applicability of Stryd^{TM} system is becoming of relevance.

Despite the findings reported here, there are some limitations to consider. First, blood lactate concentration during the tests was not directly assessed. Additionally, the MPO corresponding to the MLSS (i.e., the FTP) was not validated through other calculation methods, assuming that the time-to-exhaustion at their MLSS intensity should be approximately 60 min for a homogenous sample of trained athletes [19]. However, constant-duration time trials were conducted as they have proven to be more reliable than time-to-exhaustion protocols [43]. Additionally, we assessed RPE and HR during all tests in order to control performance intensity. Despite lower mean values for RPE during the 30-min trial, the physiological and perceptual responses to simplified TTs confirmed an intensity above MLSS, whereas most of the FTP_{60} was performed at an intensity equal to or slightly above MLSS. Maximal RPE of every test was ≥18, and HR peak differ ≤5% between tests. Regarding data generalization, only male trained runners participated in the study, preventing the possible sex differences analysis. The sample size was selected by convenience. Nevertheless, a post hoc analysis of the achieved power for this sample was conducted (G*Power software vs. 3.1) revealing a moderate to high power (~0.6). Ultimately, although all participants were familiar with its use, the entire experimental protocol was conducted on a motorised treadmill. Thus, the accuracy of the ICF% could be reduced when applied in field-based conditions. Notwithstanding these limitations, the current study highlights that the 10-, 20-, and 30-min TTs are valid for the estimation of FTP_{60} in trained endurance runners fitting FTP_{20} and FTP_{30} better for this purpose than FTP_{10}.

5. Conclusions

The results obtained here showed that the three simplified TTs (i.e., FTP_{10}, FTP_{20} and FTP_{30}) can provide good estimations of MPO and normalized MPO achieved during a 60-min submaximal TT (i.e., FTP_{60}). Moreover, as FTP_{10} showed a lower correlation, and FTP_{20} and FTP_{30} exhibited similar results, the FTP_{20} would be the preferred simplified TT to assess FTP_{60} in endurance runners, as it is less prone to fatigue. Additionally, an ICF% of ~94% for the FTP_{20} was found to be more compliant with FTP_{60} in recreationally trained runners than the well-accepted 95%.

FTP is an essential parameter in prominent commercially available software such as TrainingPeaks for both determining training intensity (i.e., intensity factor) and monitoring training load (i.e., training stress score). Moreover, the ICF% revealed for each test (~90% for FTP_{10}, ~94% for FTP_{20} and ~96% for FTP_{30}) may lead practitioners to an accurate evaluation of FTP through less fatiguing, more easily reproducible tests. However, the predictive value of the simplified TTs reported here might differ between laboratory and on-field conditions.

Future research should focus on the on-field repeatability of the algorithms reported hereabouts in order to incorporate them to the endurance runners´ performance assessment. Once validated it might lead coaches and athletes' decisions for training and racing, as it happens before with cycling. Additionally, shorter TT may be also included for a better understanding of the individual aerobic–anaerobic profile of the athletes. Finally, the response of female athletes as well as different levels of performance runners should be evaluated, for a better adjustment of the aforementioned algorithms.

Author Contributions: Conceptualization, A.C.-L., L.E.R.-S., and F.G.-P.; methodology, L.E.R.-S., F.G.-P., and D.J.-C.; software, A.C.-L. and L.E.R.-S.; validation, L.E.R.-S., F.G.-P., and A.C.-L.; formal analysis, A.C.-L. and F.G.-P.; investigation, A.C.-L., D.J.-C., J.R.-B., and A.R.-P.; resources, L.E.R.-S.; data curation, L.E.R.-S. and F.G.-P.; writing—original draft preparation, A.C.-L., D.J.-C., J.R.-B., and A.R.-P.; writing—review and editing, A.C.-L. and D.J.-C.; visualization, L.E.R.-S., F.G.-P., and A.R.-P.; supervision, L.E.R.-S., F.G.-P., and A.C.-L.; project administration, A.C.-L. and L.E.R.-S. All authors have read and agreed to the published version of the manuscript.

Funding: This research received no external funding.

Institutional Review Board Statement: The study was conducted according to the guidelines of the Declaration of Helsinki, and approved by the Institutional Ethics Committee of Universidad San Jorge (protocol code: 009-18/19, date of approval: 06 March 2019).

Informed Consent Statement: Informed consent was obtained from all subjects involved in the study.

Data Availability Statement: The data presented in this study are available on request from the corresponding author. The data are not publicly available due to authors preferences.

Acknowledgments: The authors would like to thank to all the participants.

Conflicts of Interest: The authors declare no conflict of interest.

References

1. Mujika, I. Quantification of Training and Competition Loads in Endurance Sports: Methods and Applications. *Int. J. Sports Physiol. Perform.* **2017**, *12* (Suppl. 2), S29–S217. [CrossRef]
2. Borresen, J.; Lambert, M.I. The quantification of training load, the training response and the effect on performance. *Sports Med.* **2009**, *39*, 779–795. [CrossRef] [PubMed]

3. Sanders, D.; Myers, T.; Akubat, I. Training-Intensity Distribution in Road Cyclists: Objective Versus Subjective Measures. *Int. J. Sports Physiol. Perform.* **2017**, *12*, 1232–1237. [CrossRef] [PubMed]
4. Passfield, L.; Hopker, J.G.; Jobson, S.; Friel, D.; Zabala, M. Knowledge is power: Issues of measuring training and performance in cycling. *J. Sports Sci.* **2017**, *35*, 1426–1434. [CrossRef] [PubMed]
5. Kram, R.; Griffin, T.M.; Donelan, J.M.; Chang, Y.H. Force treadmill for measuring vertical and horizontal ground reaction forces. *J. Appl. Physiol.* **1998**, *85*, 764–769. [CrossRef]
6. Norris, M.; Anderson, R.; Kenny, I.C. Method analysis of accelerometers and gyroscopes in running gait: A systematic review. *Proc. Inst. Mech. Eng. Part P-J. Sports Eng. Technol.* **2014**, *228*, 3–15. [CrossRef]
7. Jenny, D.F.; Jenny, P. On the mechanical power output required for human running—Insight from an analytical model. *J. Biomech.* **2020**, *110*, 109948. [CrossRef]
8. Blickhan, R. The spring-mass model for running and hopping. *J. Biomech.* **1989**, *22*, 1217–1227. [CrossRef]
9. Cerezuela-Espejo, V.; Hernández-Belmonte, A.; Courel-Ibáñez, J.; Conesa-Ros, E.; Martínez-Cava, A.; Pallarés, J.G. Running power meters and theoretical models based on laws of physics: Effects of environments and running conditions. *Physiol. Behav.* **2020**, *223*, 112972. [CrossRef]
10. Cerezuela-Espejo, V.; Hernandez-Belmonte, A.; Courel-Ibanez, J.; Conesa-Ros, E.; Mora-Rodriguez, R.; Pallares, J.G. Are we ready to measure running power? Repeatability and concurrent validity of five commercial technologies. *Eur. J. Sport Sci.* **2020**, 1–10. [CrossRef]
11. Jaén-Carrillo, D.; Roche-Seruendo, L.E.; Cartón-Llorente, A.; Ramírez-Campillo, R.; García-Pinillos, F. Mechanical Power in Endurance Running: A Scoping Review on Sensors for Power Output Estimation during Running. *Sensors* **2020**, *20*, 6482. [CrossRef]
12. García-Pinillos, F.; Soto-Hermoso, V.M.; Latorre-Román, P.; Párraga-Montilla, J.A.; Roche-Seruendo, L.E. How Does Power During Running Change when Measured at Different Time Intervals? *Int. J. Sports Med.* **2019**, *40*, 609–613. [CrossRef]
13. García-Pinillos, F.; Latorre-Román, P.; Roche-Seruendo, L.E.; García-Ramos, A. Prediction of power output at different running velocities through the two-point method with the Stryd(TM) power meter. *Gait Posture* **2019**, *68*, 238–243. [CrossRef]
14. Austin, C.L.; Hokanson, J.F.; McGinnis, P.M.; Patrick, S. The Relationship between Running Power and Running Economy in Well-Trained Distance Runners. *Sports* **2018**, *6*, 142. [CrossRef]
15. Aubry, R.L.; Power, G.A.; Burr, J.F. An Assessment of Running Power as a Training Metric for Elite and Recreational Runners. *J. Strength Cond. Res.* **2018**, *32*, 2258–2264. [CrossRef]
16. Allen, H.; Coggan, A. *Training and Racing with a Power Meter*, 2nd ed.; Velopress: Boulder, CO, USA, 2006.
17. Coyle, E.F.; Coggan, A.R.; Hopper, M.K.; Walters, T.J. Determinants of endurance in well-trained cyclists. *J. Appl. Physiol.* **1988**, *64*, 2622–2630. [CrossRef]
18. McGrath, E.; Mahony, N.; Fleming, N.; Donne, B. Is the FTP Test a Reliable, Reproducible and Functional Assessment Tool in Highly-Trained Athletes? *Int. J. Exerc. Sci.* **2019**, *12*, 1334–1345.
19. Lajoie, C.; Laurencelle, L.; Trudeau, F. Physiological responses to cycling for 60 minutes at maximal lactate steady state. *Can. J. Appl. Physiol.* **2000**, *25*, 250–261. [CrossRef]
20. Faude, O.; Kindermann, W.; Meyer, T. Lactate threshold concepts: How valid are they? *Sports Med.* **2009**, *39*, 469–490. [CrossRef]
21. Cerezuela-Espejo, V.; Courel-Ibáñez, J.; Morán-Navarro, R.; Martínez-Cava, A.; Pallarés, J.G. The Relationship Between Lactate and Ventilatory Thresholds in Runners: Validity and Reliability of Exercise Test Performance Parameters. *Front. Physiol.* **2018**, *9*, 1320. [CrossRef]
22. Sanders, D.; Taylor, R.J.; Myers, T.; Akubat, I. A field-based cycling test to assess predictors of endurance performance and establishing training zones. *J. Strength Cond. Res.* **2020**, *34*, 3482–3488. [CrossRef]
23. Borszcz, F.K.; Tramontin, A.F.; Bossi, A.H.; Carminatti, L.J.; Costa, V.P. Functional Threshold Power in Cyclists: Validity of the Concept and Physiological Responses. *Int. J. Sports Med.* **2018**, *39*, 737–742. [CrossRef]
24. Valenzuela, P.L.; Morales, J.S.; Foster, C.; Lucia, A.; de la Villa, P. Is the Functional Threshold Power a Valid Surrogate of the Lactate Threshold? *Int. J. Sports Physiol. Perform.* **2018**, *13*, 1293–1298. [CrossRef]
25. Klitzke Borszcz, F.; Tramontin, A.F.; Costa, V.P. Reliability of the Functional Threshold Power in Competitive Cyclists. *Int. J. Sports Med.* **2020**, *41*, 175–181. [CrossRef]
26. Jeffries, O.; Simmons, R.; Patterson, S.D.; Waldron, M. Functional Threshold Power Is Not Equivalent to Lactate Parameters in Trained Cyclists. *J. Strength Cond. Res.* **2019**. [CrossRef]
27. Lillo-Beviá, J.R.; Courel-Ibáñez, J.; Cerezuela-Espejo, V.; Morán-Navarro, R.; Martínez-Cava, A.; Pallarés, J.G. Is the Functional Threshold Power a Valid Metric to Estimate the Maximal Lactate Steady State in Cyclists? *J. Strength Cond. Res.* **2019**. [CrossRef]
28. Inglis, E.C.; Iannetta, D.; Passfield, L.; Murias, J.M. Maximal Lactate Steady State Versus the 20-Minute Functional Threshold Power Test in Well-Trained Individuals: "Watts" the Big Deal? *Int. J. Sports Physiol. Perform.* **2019**, *1*, 1–7. [CrossRef]
29. Capostagno, B.; Lambert, M.I.; Lamberts, R.P. A Systematic Review of Submaximal Cycle Tests to Predict, Monitor, and Optimize Cycling Performance. *Int. J. Sports Physiol. Perform.* **2016**, *11*, 707–714. [CrossRef] [PubMed]
30. Fontana, P.; Boutellier, U.; Knöpfli-Lenzin, C. Time to exhaustion at maximal lactate steady state is similar for cycling and running in moderately trained subjects. *Eur. J. Appl. Physiol.* **2009**, *107*, 187–192. [CrossRef] [PubMed]
31. Borg, G. *Borg's Perceived Exertion and Pain Scales*; Human Kinetics Pub Inc.: Champaign, IL, USA, 1998.
32. Schieb, D. Kinematic Accommodation of Novice Treadmill Runners. *Res. Q. Exerc. Sport* **1986**, *57*, 1–7. [CrossRef]

33. Garcia-Pinillos, F.; Latorre-Roman, P.A.; Ramirez-Campillo, R.; Parraga-Montilla, J.A.; Roche-Seruendo, L.E. How does the slope gradient affect spatiotemporal parameters during running? Influence of athletic level and vertical and leg stiffness. *Gait Posture* **2019**, *68*, 72–77. [CrossRef] [PubMed]
34. Navalta, J.W.; Montes, J.; Bodell, N.G.; Aguilar, C.D.; Radzak, K.; Manning, J.W.; DeBeliso, M. Reliability of Trail Walking and Running Tasks Using the Stryd Power Meter. *Int. J. Sports Med.* **2019**, *40*, 498–502. [CrossRef] [PubMed]
35. Hopkins, W.G.; Marshall, S.W.; Batterham, A.M.; Hanin, J. Progressive statistics for studies in sports medicine and exercise science. *Med. Sci. Sports Exerc.* **2009**, *41*, 3–13. [CrossRef] [PubMed]
36. Koo, T.K.; Li, M.Y. A Guideline of Selecting and Reporting Intraclass Correlation Coefficients for Reliability Research. *J. Chiropr. Med.* **2016**, *15*, 155–163. [CrossRef]
37. Landis, J.R.; Koch, G.G. The measurement of observer agreement for categorical data. *Biometrics* **1977**, *33*, 159–174. [CrossRef]
38. Nimmerichter, A.; Williams, C.; Bachl, N.; Eston, R. Evaluation of a field test to assess performance in elite cyclists. *Int. J. Sports Med.* **2010**, *31*, 160–166. [CrossRef]
39. MacInnis, M.J.; Thomas, A.C.Q.; Phillips, S.M. The Reliability of 4-min and 20-min Time Trials and Their Relationships to Functional Threshold Power in Trained Cyclists. *Int. J. Sports Physiol. Perform.* **2018**, *14*, 38–45. [CrossRef]
40. Gastin, P.B. Energy system interaction and relative contribution during maximal exercise. *Sports Med.* **2001**, *31*, 725–741. [CrossRef]
41. Morgan, P.T.; Black, M.I.; Bailey, S.J.; Jones, A.M.; Vanhatalo, A. Road cycle TT performance: Relationship to the power-duration model and association with FTP. *J. Sports Sci.* **2019**, *37*, 902–910. [CrossRef]
42. Olaya Cuartero, J.; Pérez, S.; Ferriz-Valero, A.; Cejuela, R. A comparison between different tests for functional threshold power determination in running. *J. Phys. Educ. Hum. Mov.* **2019**, *1*, 4–15.
43. Currell, K.; Jeukendrup, A.E. Validity, reliability and sensitivity of measures of sporting performance. *Sports Med.* **2008**, *38*, 297–316. [CrossRef] [PubMed]

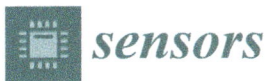 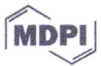

Article

Foot Strike Angle Prediction and Pattern Classification Using Loadsol™ Wearable Sensors: A Comparison of Machine Learning Techniques

Stephanie R. Moore [1], Christina Kranzinger [2], Julian Fritz [3], Thomas Stöggl [1,4], Josef Kröll [1] and Hermann Schwameder [1,*]

1. Department of Sport and Exercise Science, University of Salzburg, Schlossallee 49, 5400 Hallein/Rif, Austria; stephanie.moore@sbg.ac.at (S.R.M.); thomas.stoeggl@sbg.ac.at (T.S.); josef.kroell@sbg.ac.at (J.K.)
2. Salzburg Research Forschungsgesellschaft m.b.H., Jakob-Haringer-Straße 5, 5020 Salzburg, Austria; christina.kranzinger@salzburgresearch.at
3. Adidas AG, Adi-Dassler-Strasse 1, 91074 Herzogenaurach, Germany; julian.fritz@adidas.com
4. Athlete Performance Center, Red Bull Sports, Brunnbachweg 71, 5303 Thalgau, Austria
* Correspondence: hermann.schwameder@sbg.ac.at; Tel.: +43-662-8044-4897

Received: 12 October 2020; Accepted: 21 November 2020; Published: 25 November 2020

Abstract: The foot strike pattern performed during running is an important variable for runners, performance practitioners, and industry specialists. Versatile, wearable sensors may provide foot strike information while encouraging the collection of diverse information during ecological running. The purpose of the current study was to predict foot strike angle and classify foot strike pattern from Loadsol™ wearable pressure insoles using three machine learning techniques (multiple linear regression—MR, conditional inference tree—TREE, and random forest—FRST). Model performance was assessed using three-dimensional kinematics as a ground-truth measure. The prediction-model accuracy was similar for the regression, inference tree, and random forest models (RMSE: MR = 5.16°, TREE = 4.85°, FRST = 3.65°; MAPE: MR = 0.32°, TREE = 0.45°, FRST = 0.33°), though the regression and random forest models boasted lower maximum precision (13.75° and 14.3°, respectively) than the inference tree (19.02°). The classification performance was above 90% for all models (MR = 90.4%, TREE = 93.9%, and FRST = 94.1%). There was an increased tendency to misclassify mid foot strike patterns in all models, which may be improved with the inclusion of more mid foot steps during model training. Ultimately, wearable pressure insoles in combination with simple machine learning techniques can be used to predict and classify a runner's foot strike with sufficient accuracy.

Keywords: decision tree; human running; random forest; regression; wearable devices

1. Introduction

Recreational running is a globally accessible activity due to the limited necessity of sport-essential equipment and facilities. Due to its full-body nature, the human anatomical system has many ways to affect running performance. Some factors of paramount importance are joint angles (which thus affect stride length), flight time, and the minimization of lateral force-dissipation [1,2]. The selection of the running shoe also appears to affect performance [3,4], the subjective experience of comfort [5,6], and the injury risk of runners [3,7]. Equipment-based recommendations should include the consideration of a runner's foot strike pattern (FSP) [8]. A midsole design that facilitates the repetitive and comfortable execution of the preferred FSP (i.e., rear foot (RF), mid foot (MF), or fore foot (FF)) can aid the consumer-based shoe selection and recommendation process [3]. Such a recommendation thus requires a reliable method for the discrete classification of a runner's FSP as a prerequisite.

Some performance-related outcome variables are affected by the FSP used, including the vertical compliance of the anatomical system [9], ankle and knee stiffness [10], vertical impact force [11], and instantaneous loading rates [11]. Importantly, these variables can be measured on a continuous scale and are likely responsive to more sensitive foot strike angle (FSA) measurements. More specifically, the FSA is the angular degree of the foot at the instant of ground contact (often defined by a force or loading rate threshold) [12,13]. Therefore, the ability to detect the degree of foot strike on a continuous level enables greater correlational insights that may be overlooked by a discrete classification-based system [14]. Thus, in addition to the necessity of FSP classification, the continuous-scale identification of a runner's FSA should be accessible for researchers and performance-centered practitioners.

With the growing importance for ecologically valid shoe prescription and scientific investigation of runners, the ability to detect and classify the FSA of a runner using wearable sensors is essential. Inertial measurement units (IMUs) are a viable and validated option for ecological FSA collection [8,15,16], although the calculated angular displacements are prone to poor reliability due to drifts over time which thus affect the integration of the inertial signals in IMU systems [17]. The combination of inertial, gyroscopic, and magnetometer information that an IMU provides helps in the reduction and correction of its measured drift, though the rigidity and alignment of the sensor attachment also directly influence the reliability of the angular measures [17]. Alternative to IMU systems, the holistic pairing of kinetic information with the kinematic measurement of FSA from a single measurement system may enable greater insights about performance and injury indicators in running. Thus, a simple, "low-friction" wearable device that could validly provide this holistic view would be groundbreaking for the running industry.

In an effort to fill this innovative gap, the accelerometer-based Stryd^{TM} foot pod attempts to provide this holistic view of the kinematic and kinetic information by estimating running power [18–20]. However, Stryd^{TM} appears to have limitations when detecting temporal variables [20]. From a methodological context, running power calculations that require both kinetic and kinematic inputs appear to have better prediction performance of a linear power-velocity relationship than those using kinematic data only [21]. Unfortunately, single IMU-based estimations of ground reaction force (GRF) come with substantial limitations; (i) the placement of an IMU can affect GRF estimate accuracy, (ii) magnetic disturbances can affect the orientation of the IMU, and (iii) the existence of kinematic estimate errors would be inherent in subsequent GRF estimates [22,23]. Thus, a wearable kinetic system may be better equipped to provide this holistic view.

The wearable application of pressure insoles already extends to temporal gait events [24,25], therefore they may be a plausible alternative to IMUs to facilitate ecological kinematic estimation while also enabling a valid measurement of vertical force (Fong et al., 2008). Importantly, Loadsol^{TM} wearable insoles can measure vertical force in the rear and fore foot separately; thus the time and force relationships of the fore and aft sensors may provide enough information for FSA prediction and FSP classification [26,27]. Further, the separation of the insole into multiple components is encouraged by the assumption that the foot is not a singularly rigid segment as was traditionally considered [28,29]. The Loadsol^{TM} has been previously validated under running stimulus [13,30,31], therefore it is an appropriate system to establish the potential for the kinematic estimation of FSA and FSP.

Machine learning techniques may enable the estimation of FSA and FSP from pressure sensors; these are practical tools that can be trained and implemented into large-scale problems and data sets, with the inherent goal being to capitalize on the distinctive qualities of the data set [32]. Due to a linear relationship between strike index (the percent of foot length at which the center of pressure exists) and FSA [14,16], the linear approach of a multiple regression may be appropriate for the prediction of FSA [27]. In contrast to linear regression models that are based on numerous assumptions (e.g., normality of residuals, homoscedasticity, etc.) [33], nonparametric models such as conditional inference trees or random forests, need only the assumption that similar inputs lead to similar outputs [32]. The prediction and classification accuracy may thus be greater with nonparametric frameworks. Conditional inference trees are a non-parametric class of regression trees that allow for unbiased variable selection and do not require pruning based on resampling [34]. They are based on conditional inference procedures for testing independence between response and each input variable [34]. Alternatively, robust random forest frameworks encourage accuracy gains with the development of multiple variable-randomized trees [35,36].

Ultimately, to confirm best-practice recommendations, the prediction and classification of foot strike using kinetic sensors should be approached from distinctly different statistical techniques. Thus, the purposes of the current study were to compare the accuracy and precision of i) continuous FSA prediction and ii) FSP classification as calculated from three statistical methodologies (multiple regression, conditional inference tree, and random forest) using independent variables derived from the Loadsol^{TM} pressure insoles.

2. Materials and Methods

2.1. Participants and Experimental Approach

Thirty injury-free recreational male runners (Mean ± SD; 1.79 ± 0.07 m; 80.1 ± 9.6 kg; 34.0 ± 6.9 yr) provided written informed consent approved by the institutional review board to participate in the study. Participants appeared for one testing occasion where they were asked to perform over-ground running using six types of FSPs at a comfortable speed (average velocity = 2.69 ± 0.40 m·s^{-1}). The first condition investigated was their natural running pattern (NA; no constraints), followed by extreme-FF, FF, MF, RF, and extreme-RF in a randomized counterbalanced order. The extreme-FF and extreme-RF conditions were instructed by asking the participants to over-exaggerate their performance of the FF and RF conditions, respectively. Participants were not given any condition-based feedback. All trials were performed with participants running back-and-forth (i.e., shuttle-wise) in a laboratory environment; participants ran a straight distance (5 m) over a force platform located in the center of the straight phase. Participants then quickly changed direction before running the same straight phase. For each participant, 20 non-consecutive left foot-fall instants were recorded per foot strike condition (n = 120 steps). Participants were allowed 5–10 minutes for a self-selected running warm up and familiarization laps were performed before each condition until the participants expressed comfortability with the desired foot strike condition. Importantly, the measured foot falls were labelled as their true pattern or angle, regardless of the condition in which it was performed (see subsequent sections). However, the consistency of participant's performance of the FSA was assessed in a supplementary analysis which boasted generally good consistency [37].

2.2. Measurements

Insole pressure, force plate kinetics, and kinematics were recorded for 3,489 foot falls (originally, 120 steps per participant × 30 participants = 3,600 foot falls; however only 3,489 are reported due to collection error or data loss). The pressure measurements were achieved with a two-sensor (fore-aft) wireless insole (Loadsol^{TM}; Novel GmbH; Munich, Germany) inserted into standardized shoes worn by the participants (Adidas Duramo 6; weight = 280 g., heel drop = 11 mm). The Loadsol^{TM} system was applied over the shoe's insole and recorded at its maximum sampling rate (100 Hz). Kinetic data from a force platform (AMTI; Watertown, MA, USA; BP6001200) and three-dimensional (3D) motion capture was recorded with a Qualysis system (13-camera setup; 2019.3, Göteborg, Sweden) and sampled at 100 Hz to match the maximum sampling rate of the Loadsol^{TM} system. A six-marker anatomical marker set was applied to the left foot segment (over the shoe when necessary); retroreflective markers were secured on the medial and lateral malleoli, the head of the 2nd metatarsal, the heel (placed at the same height as the 2nd metatarsal), the medial side of the 1st metatarsal, and the lateral side of the 5th metatarsal (Figure 1A,B) [38]. The kinematic and Loadsol^{TM} data were synchronized by aligning the peak force of a stomp measured by the AMTI force platform (data logging with Qualysis) and Loadsol^{TM} at the beginning of each trial.

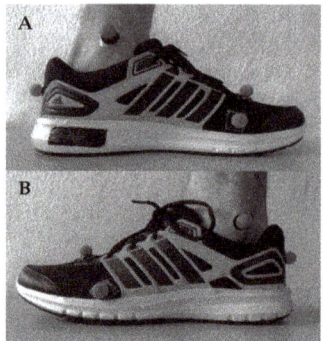

Figure 1. A medial view (**A**) and lateral view (**B**) of the left foot marker placements can be seen on the test shoe.

2.3. Data Processing

Initial contact (IC) and toe off (TO) were identified from the Loadsol™ measurements as the frame in which the loading rate of the pressure insoles was greater than 1500 or −1500 Newtons per second, respectively [13]. Ten force and time related variables were extracted from the measurements. Two parameters were calculated from the first third (IC to 33%) and eight parameters from the entire (IC to TO; 100%) stance phase (Table 1). Finally, the FSA was identified for each IC captured. To achieve this, raw kinematic data were filtered using a low-pass 15 Hz filter. Visual 3D ×64 Professional (v6.03.06; Germantown, MD, USA) was used to model the foot segment so that the shoe-elicited angulation was negated and the subsequent foot segment angle (in relation to the laboratory coordinate system) was reported [39].

Table 1. Ten variables calculated from the Loadsol™ insole measurements are defined with respect to the sensor used and the percentage of the stance phase used in calculation.

Parent Variable	Variable	Definition	Insole Sensor	Stance Phase [%]	Abbreviation
Impulse [N·s]	Impulse Ratio [%]	Impulse ratio between the insole sensor and total foot during the entire or first third of the stance phase	Fore	0–100%	IR_Fore
			Aft	0–100%	IR_Aft
			Fore	0-33%	IR_Fore$_{0-33\%}$
			Aft	0-33%	IR_Aft$_{0-33\%}$
Peak Force [N]	Peak Force Ratio [%]	Ratio of peak force measured from the insole sensor and total foot during the entire stance phase	Fore	0–100%	PF_Fore
			Aft	0–100%	PF_Aft
Peak RFD [N·s^{-1}]	Peak RFD Ratio [%]	Ratio of peak RFD between the insole sensor and total foot	Fore	0–100%	RFD_Fore
			Aft	0–100%	RFD_Aft
	Ln(Peak RFD) [unit]	Natural logarithm of the occurrence of the peak RFD (as a stance phase %)	Fore	% of Stance	Ln(%RFD_Fore)
			Aft	% of Stance	Ln(%RFD_Aft)

RFD = rate of force development; FF = fore foot; RF = rear foot; N = Newton; s = second.

2.4. Modeling Approaches

As a pre-requisite for model development, all variables were assessed for normality (i.e., skewness or kurtosis statistic ≤ 2.58). If the assumption of a normal distribution was not met for any of the variables, a natural logarithm transformation was performed to ensure their use was appropriate for parametric statistics (noted in Table 1). The data was then split record-wise into two sets; one was a training data set (70%; n = 2442 steps) and the other a validation ("test" or "hold out") set (30%; n = 1047 steps). This was done to avoid model under-fitting and high classification errors [40–42].

Three modelling techniques (multiple linear regression, conditional inference tree and random forest) were then trained using the training data set to predict FSA and to classify FSP from the pressure insole data. For the classification of FSP, all models employed the degree-based ranges defined by Altman and Davis [14] to categorize steps into either FF (FSA < −1.6°), MF (−1.6° ≤ FSA ≤ 8.0°), or RF

(FSA > 8.0°). Steps were classified regardless of the trial condition in which they were performed (i.e., the extreme FF and FF conditions were primarily classified as FF strikes, and similarly, extreme RF and RF conditions as RF strikes).

2.5. Model Development

First, a parametric stepwise multiple linear regression (MR) to predict the FSA at IC was modelled using SPSS Statistics (SPSS Inc.; Version 26.0, Chicago, IL, USA). Seven significant (α = 0.05) regression equations were developed (F-to-enter ≤ 0.050, F-to-remove ≥ 0.0100), therefore the Akaike Information Criterion (AIC) and Schwartz-Bayesian Information Criterion (BIC) were calculated for each regression to guide model selection for the subsequent comparisons [43]. The resulting model (Equation (1)) retained the lowest AIC and BIC, and highest model fit (R^2 = 0.914, $R^2_{ADJUSTED}$ = 0.914; p < 0.001; standard error of the estimate = 5.10°; df = 2434). The same MR model was used for classification by categorizing the predicted FSA (calculated from Equation (1)) of the validation set according to the previously mentioned FSP ranges [14].

$$FSA = -89.2 + 94.4\ (IV_1) + 62.3\ (IV_2) + 17.9\ (IV_3) + 8.8\ (IV_4) - 8.4\ (IV_5) + 3.4\ (IV_6) + 1.8\ (IV_7) \quad (1)$$

where IV_1 = IR_Aft, IV_2 = PF_Fore, IV_3 = RFD_Aft, IV_4 = IR_Aft$_{0-33\%}$, IV_5 = PF_Aft, IV_6 = Ln(%RFD_Fore), IV_7 = Ln(%RFD_Aft).

Two conditional inference trees were modeled with the statistical software R ("ctree" function of "partykit" package) [34,44,45]. The two models differed in their outcomes: one model predicted continuous FSA (TREE$_{PRED}$), while the other classified FSP (TREE$_{CLASS}$; defined classes: RF, MF, FF). For both models, the significance level was set to α = 0.01 (minimum splitting criterion = 0.99). A maximum depth of eight was achieved for TREE$_{PRED}$, and TREE$_{CLASS}$ achieved a depth of six.

Finally, two random forest models as developed by Breiman [35] were trained using the statistical software R ("randomForest" package) [44,46]. The first model was trained for the purpose of continuous FSA prediction (FRST$_{PRED}$) and the second for FSP classification (FRST$_{CLASS}$). A large number of trees (n = 500) was selected for the development of the FRST$_{PRED}$ and FRST$_{CLASS}$ models to decrease out-of-bag errors [47]. Variable selection was randomly initialized in order to define candidates for each split. The final models were chosen because they had the lowest root mean squared error (RMSE; FRST$_{PRED}$) and the highest mean accuracy (FRST$_{CLASS}$) in a 5-fold cross-validation comparison of the different parameter settings ("caret" package) [44,48]. The important variables for the FRST$_{PRED}$ and FRST$_{CLASS}$ can be seen in Figure 2, where high "Mean Decrease Gini" is associated with decreased node impurity, and therefore higher variable importance [49].

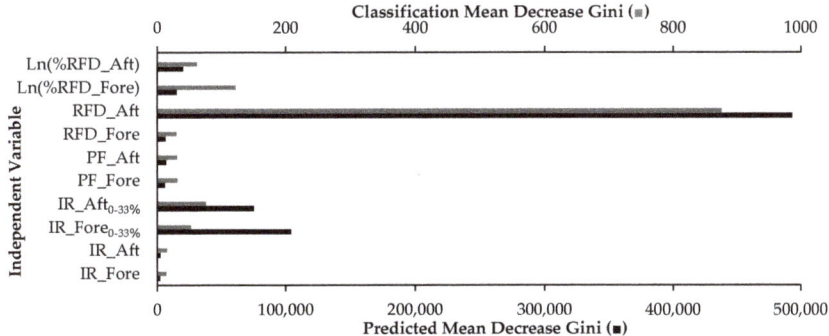

Figure 2. The variable importance for the random forest model of foot strike pattern classification is presented with gray bars (scaled to the secondary *x*-axis), while the foot strike angle prediction is presented in black (primary *x*-axis). The variables of higher importance can be seen with larger "Mean Decrease Gini.".

2.6. Model Accuracy and Precision

The models for FSA (MR, TREE$_{PRED}$, FRST$_{PRED}$) and FSP (MR, TREE$_{CLASS}$, and FRST$_{CLASS}$) were tested with the remaining validation set (n = 1047 steps). Accuracy and precision metrics were calculated for each of the models using the comparison of the true FSA/FSP (measured with 3D kinematics) and the estimated FSA/FSP (i.e., estimated from Loadsol^{TM} metrics).

For model comparison of the three approaches that predicted FSA (MR, TREE$_{PRED}$, and FRST$_{PRED}$), four performance metrics were calculated per recommendations of Galdi and Tagliaferri [50]. These included the mean squared error (MSE), RMSE, mean absolute error (MAE) and mean absolute percentage error (MAPE) of the true versus predicted FSA outcomes. The precision of the prediction models was quantified by calculating the limits of agreement (LoA) and bias of the predicted data set according to Bland and Altman [51]. Specifically, the 95% LoA was calculated using the mean difference (true FSA–predicted FSA) ± 1.96 standard deviations of the differences, and the maximum precision was reported as the difference between the subsequent limits.

Confusion matrices were created for the FSP classification models (MR, TREE$_{CLASS}$, and FRST$_{CLASS}$) utilizing the true classes (measured by kinematic FSA) and the estimated classes (i.e., the class estimated from each model). From these confusion matrices, three metrics were computed as recommended by Galdi and Tagliaferri [50] for model comparison. These included the model accuracy (Equation (2)), classifier recall (Equation (3)), and classifier precision (Equation (4)).

$$model\ accuracy = \frac{total\ correct}{total\ sample\ (n)} \times 100\% \quad (2)$$

$$classifier\ recall = \frac{true\ positives\ of\ a\ true\ class}{total\ sample\ of\ a\ true\ class} \times 100\% \quad (3)$$

$$classifier\ precision = \frac{true\ positives\ of\ a\ estimated\ class}{total\ sample\ of\ a\ estimated\ class} \times 100\% \quad (4)$$

where *total correct* = number of cases correctly classified, *true class* = true positives + false negatives of a classifier, *estimated class* = true positives + false positives of a classifier

3. Results

Descriptive statistics (mean ± standard deviation) are presented in Table 2 for each of the independent variables of each step according to their FSP class (FF, MF, RF).

Table 2. Descriptive statistics (mean ± standard deviation) are presented for each variable used in model development, grouped by FSP (classified by measured kinematic FSA).

Variable	Units	FF	MF	RF
FSA	°	−10.2 ± 6.6	3.0 ± 2.8	24.9 ± 8.0
IR_Fore	%	96.2 ± 5.7	89.3 ± 7.0	65.4 ± 11.5
IR_Aft	%	3.8 ± 5.7	10.6 ± 7.0	34.6 ± 11.5
IR_Fore$_{0-33\%}$	%	92.5 ± 9.8	77.2 ± 12.9	31.7 ± 16.3
IR_Aft$_{0-33\%}$	%	7.5 ± 9.9	22.8 ± 12.9	68.2 ± 16.3
PF_Fore	%	95.8 ± 8.2	93.3 ± 6.1	77.0 ± 11.5
PF_Aft	%	8.1 ± 12.3	22.2 ± 13.4	59.9 ± 15.3
RFD_Fore	%	88.3 ± 12.8	70.0 ± 20.8	49.2 ± 16.2
RFD_Aft	%	14.5 ± 16.5	40.5 ± 22.0	91.2 ± 11.0
Ln(%RFD_Fore)	unit	2.69 ± 0.55	2.27 ± 0.33	2.43 ± 0.23
Ln(%RFD_Aft)	unit	2.72 ± 0.41	2.89 ± 0.35	3.25 ± 0.26

3.1. FSA Prediction

The Bland–Altman Bias and Precision of the FSA prediction models is shown in Figure 3. Further FSA prediction model accuracy can also be seen in Table 3. In general, the FRST$_{PRED}$ performed with greater prediction accuracy than the MR or TREE$_{PRED}$. The MR and FRST$_{PRED}$ had minimal biases (MR = −0.01, FRST$_{PRED}$ = −0.11; Figure 3) and the maximum precision of the two methods was less than 15° (MR = 13.75°, FRST$_{PRED}$ = 14.30°). A larger maximum precision was found for the TREE$_{PRED}$ (19.02°).

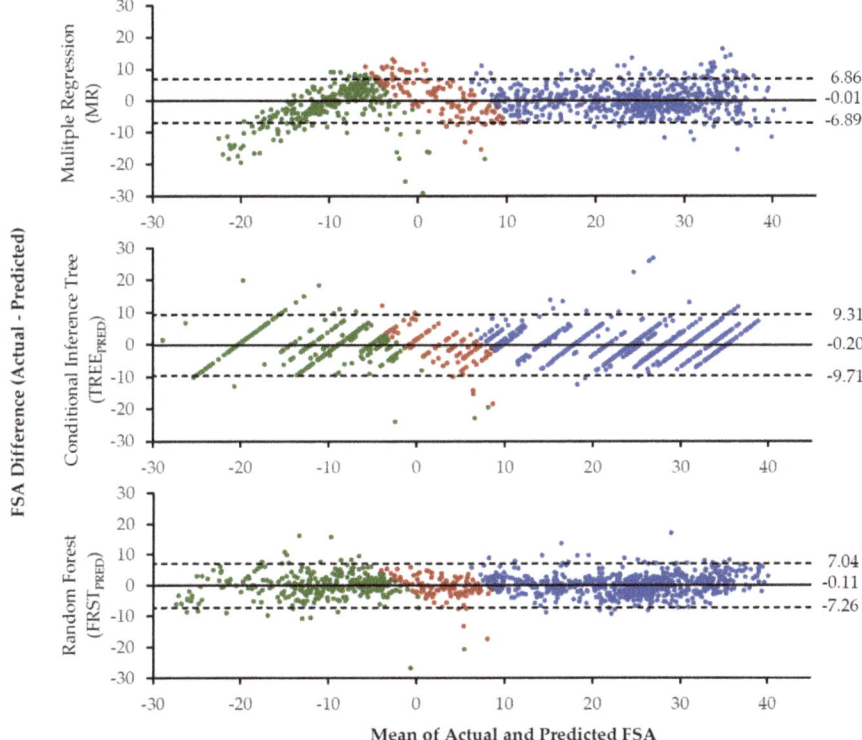

Figure 3. The Bland–Altman bias (solid line) and 95% limits of agreement (dashed lines) are presented for each of the foot strike angle (FSA) prediction methods. Green = rear foot strikes; Red = mid foot strikes; Blue = fore foot strikes; Bias = average of the residuals; Limits of agreement = ± 1.96 standard deviations around the bias.

Table 3. Foot strike angle prediction model performance accuracy is displayed.

	Multiple Regression (MR)	Conditional Inference Tree (TREE$_{PRED}$)	Random Forest (FRST$_{PRED}$)
MSE	26.61	23.57	13.31
RMSE	5.16	4.85	3.65
MAE	3.85	3.51	2.69
MAPE	0.32	0.45	0.33

MSE = mean squared error; RMSE = root mean squared error; MAE = mean absolute error; MAPE = mean absolute percent error.

3.2. FSP Classification

The confusion matrices developed for each FSP classification model (MR, TREE$_{CLASS}$, FRST$_{CLASS}$) are displayed in Table 4A. The associated accuracy (Equation (2)), recall (Equation (3)), and precision (Equation (4)) results are presented in Table 4B. All models yielded classification accuracies larger than 90% (Table 4B). The MF condition had markedly lower recall and precision than its RF and FF counterparts for all models calculated (Table 4B).

Table 4. Confusion matrices are displayed to indicate where correct (white) and incorrect (grey) classifications occurred for three types of classification methods (multiple linear regression, conditional inference tree, and random forest). Matrices are reported for the validation data set that was not included in model training. All models classified foot strikes into three classes: RF = rear foot, MF = mid foot, and FF = fore foot.

A			Multiple Regression (MR)			Conditional Inference Tree (TREE$_{CLASS}$)			Random Forest (FRST$_{CLASS}$)		
		RF	621	13	0	613	21	0	611	23	0
	True MF	26	46	48	14	88	18	16	92	12
		FF	5	8	280	5	6	282	3	8	282
			RF	MF	FF	RF	MF	FF	RF	MF	FF
				Estimated			Estimated			Estimated	

B			MR	TREE$_{CLASS}$	FRST$_{CLASS}$
Accuracy (%)		ALL	90.4	93.9	94.1
Recall (%)		RF	97.9	96.7	96.4
		MF	38.0	73.3	76.7
		FF	95.6	96.3	96.3
Precision (%)		RF	95.2	97.0	97.0
		MF	68.7	76.5	74.8
		FF	85.4	94.0	95.9

4. Discussion

The purposes of the current study were to compare three statistical techniques used to (i) predict FSA and (ii) classify FSP using independent variables derived from the Loadsol^{TM} pressure insoles. Generally, clear differences in the three foot strike styles were noticeable by similarly stratified independent variables (Table 2), with the exception of the variable PF_Fore. For this variable, the differentiation between FF and MF strike types is not clear. This lack of dichotomy may be a result of speed or flight time inconsistencies during MF strike pattern performance, which is supported by the fact that the MF condition was the most difficult condition for participants to perform [37]. However, the apparent stratification of the independent variables for each strike condition thus confirms the applicability of the fore/aft Loadsol^{TM} sensors to estimate FSA and FSP [26,27]. Supporting this, the MR and FRST$_{PRED}$ models developed for the prediction of FSA were both evidently good fits (MR = 91.4% and FRST$_{PRED}$ = 95.42% of variance explained) and the classification accuracy of FSP for all statistical techniques was greater than 90% (Table 4B).

4.1. FSA Prediction

The three models (MR, TREE$_{PRED}$ and FRST$_{PRED}$) assessed for FSA prediction had comparable performance when tested using the validation set (Figure 3 and Table 3). The most important independent variable in the FRST model was RFD_Aft as evidenced by the highest mean decrease in node impurity (Gini; Figure 2). Importantly, RFD_Aft is also a predictor used in the TREE$_{PRED}$ and MR models. However, the specific variable importance of RFD_Aft in the MR (via beta coefficients) cannot be interpreted because the model violated the assumption of collinearity [52]. Collinearity considered, the overall prediction of the model should be unaffected [52].

The linear approach of the MR as suggested by Fritz and colleagues [27] appears to be appropriate to generally explain the variance of the FSA (R^2 = 0.914). In a similar application, a univariate linear regression to determine strike index via the onset time difference of a fore and aft pressure sensor resulted in a lower coefficient of determination (R^2 = 0.836) [26]. Although participants were asked to perform RF, MF, and FF foot strikes, Cheung and colleagues [26] did not carry out further analyses to confirm the performance of the FSPs or if there was a stratified model fit. Importantly, a strong linear relationship between the strike index and 3D FSA kinematics is supported in literature, however the relationship appears to be driven primarily by FF and RF strike types [14,16]. Upon visual inspection, those foot strikes that fell closer to the MF range of FSA had the largest standard errors [16]. A similar visual phenomenon is seen in the current study's data, however the more extreme FF and RF also appear to be indicative of greater prediction errors (Figures 3 and 4). The methodological inclusion of the extreme FF and RF conditions in the current study make it possible to see the potential that there are two linear relationships (Figure 4). Thus, greater accuracy in FSA prediction using MR may be gained from developing a model for the RF and FF FSPs independently.

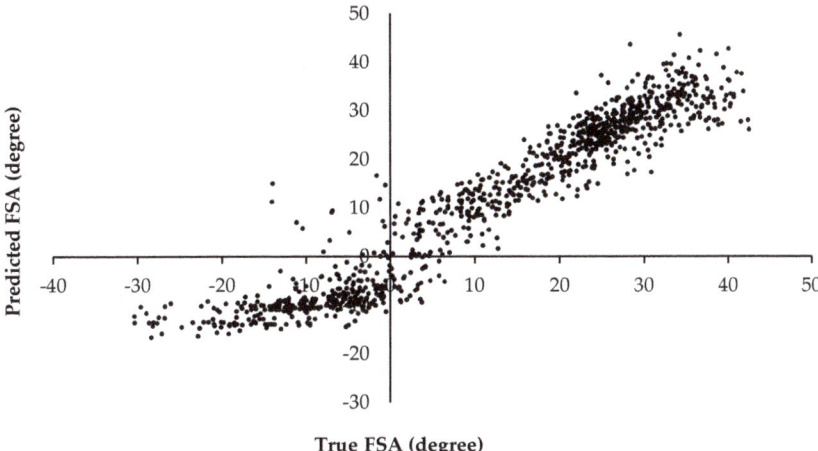

Figure 4. The relationship between the true foot strike angle (FSA) and that predicted by the multiple regression is shown for the distribution of the foot falls included in the study. The strike patterns can be discerned from the following scale: fore foot: FSA < −1.6°; mid foot: −1.6° ≤ FSA ≤ 8.0°; rear foot: FSA > 8.0°.

Importantly, the midfoot and more extreme RF strikes are not as well predicted by the MR than by the $FRST_{PRED}$ (Figure 3). However, both models exhibit higher numbers of residuals outside of the Bland–Altman limits of agreement at the extremes of FF foot strike pattern. Additional proportional bias may be evidenced in the extreme FF range of the MR. However, because these extreme foot strike patterns were considered "exaggerated" to the participants (as was their instruction), the bias present there may not influence the practical application of such models. Further, the stratification seen in the $TREE_{PRED}$ Bland–Altman makes it apparent that it's use for continuous FSA prediction is limited to the number of outcomes (i.e., maximum tree depth) included in the model (Figure 3). Ultimately, the $TREE_{PRED}$ appears to be better suited for discrete classification problems, whereas the $FRST_{PRED}$ is arguably the most appropriate model for prediction problems that include a large range of FSAs or number of MF strikes.

4.2. FSP Classification

Although the overall classification accuracy of the MR was greater than 90%, the MF strike was only properly classified with 38% recall (Table 4). Conversely, $TREE_{CLASS}$ and $FRST_{CLASS}$ classified the MF strike with approximately 73% and 75% recall (Table 4). This is similar to the findings of Delgado-Gonzalo and colleagues [53], who found that the MF condition was classified with the least recall and precision using accelerometer-based inputs. Importantly, the MF strike pattern in the current study may have been classified with the least accuracy because it had the least number of samples in the training set (MF = 197, RF = 1495, FF = 650). Supporting this theory, the RF pattern classified with the highest recall in the MR and $TREE_{CLASS}$ methods (98–99%) and was the greatest sample contributor in the training set. Further, the most important variable for the $FRST_{CLASS}$ was RFD_Aft (Figure 2), which is consistent with the first splitting node variable of $TREE_{CLASS}$. The models may be best suited to distinguish between RF and FF strikes primarily due to the lack of independent variable or sensor differentiation regarding the middle region of the foot. Thus, a three-part sensor insole that highlights the central region of the foot (thus allowing a variable such as the mid-region rate of force development) may be better suited for MF classifications. However, Lieberman and colleagues [9] found that habitually shod runners primarily perform RF strike patterns, therefore the current models should serve recreational runners well.

For populations of shod runners who have consciously altered or retrained their running foot strike pattern (i.e., those investigated by Cheung and Davis [11]), the higher accuracy of the $FRST_{CLASS}$ may provide further confidence in the MF classifications. However, the future use of simple methods like the MR or $TREE_{CLASS}$ methods should not be discounted because equal class sizes in the training set may improve the recall of MF classifications and overall model accuracy.

4.3. Application

The results of the current study support that a two sensor (fore and aft) pressure insoles can be used to predict and classify foot strike with sufficient accuracy. Compared to previous works with the aim of estimating FSA using IMU sensors [15], the current results boast lower bias when compared to a reference 3D motion capture camera system ($FRST_{PRED}$ of current study = −0.11° vs. IMU = 3.9°) and only slightly worse precision ($FRST_{PRED}$ of current study = 14.30° vs. IMU = 10.6°). This raises the potential of an insole sensor to provide the holistic pairing of kinetic and kinematic information regarding performance and injury indicators during running. An ankle joint torque MR prediction model has already been developed with adequate accuracy ($R^2_{ADJUSTED}$ = 0.831, RMSE = 6.91 Nm) using the independent input of 99-sensor pressure insoles [54]. Further, vertical GRF from pressure insoles have been used to predict the 3D GRF components using MR and Artificial Neural Networks, supporting that power and injury related variables can be considered a possibility via simple wearable sensors [55]. From an application standpoint, although many independent variables are used in the models of the current study, they all are derived from a single system. The use of a single system thus reduces the necessity of the synchronization and additional processing power of a supplementary system. A larger range of running conditions could be studied in the future, which may allow for the reduction of independent variables and further encourage the potential to transition toward "real time" foot strike pattern and angle detection.

The current study thus lays the framework for FSA and FSP detection in insoles with larger numbers of sensors (like those used by Billing et al. and Fong et al. [54,55]). This framework may be useful in the push to define and detect running power accurately. The calculation of power during running is a controversial topic due to the complexity of the human biomechanical system, and many of the current commercial systems do not have proven validity in calculating the metric [56]. Therefore, a kinetic approach may exceed current IMU-based calculation methods (i.e., Stryd^{TM} foot pods) due to the immense information a multi-sensor pressure insole can provide.

5. Conclusions

The current study supports the feasibility of two-sensor pressure insoles to detect FSA and FSP, and therefore aids in the research and coaching of running movements, as well as consumer-based shoe prescription. Simple machine learning techniques can be used to predict and classify runners' foot strike patterns with accuracies greater than 90%. However, foot falls that are a true MF strike are incorrectly classified more often than RF or FF strikes by these methods. A greater accuracy can be accomplished with the application of a more complex machine learning technique like a FRST. The current study was limited in its collection of MF steps, therefore more MF steps or using over- or under-sampling techniques may improve the classification of the MF pattern in the future. Further, the machine learning techniques should be applied to running with higher ecological validity that encompasses variable metabolic intensities (i.e., speeds), and limited changes of direction.

Author Contributions: Conceptualization, J.F., J.K., H.S., and S.R.M.; Data Curation, J.F. and S.R.M.; Formal Analysis, C.K. and S.R.M.; Funding Acquisition, T.S. and H.S.; Investigation, J.F.; Methodology, J.F., C.K., and S.R.M.; Project Administration, H.S.; Resources, T.S. and H.S.; Software, C.K. and S.R.M.; Supervision, J.K. and H.S.; Validation, C.K. and S.R.M., Visualization, S.R.M.; Writing—Original Draft, S.R.M.; Writing—Review & Editing, C.K., J.K., J.F., T.S., and H.S. All authors have read and agreed to the published version of the manuscript.

Funding: No funding was received for this work from the National Institutes of Health, the Welcome Trust, the Howard Hughes Medical Institute, or other funding agencies to PubMed Central. Funding was provided based on the Salzburg "Trans-4-Tech" project "Sport Sense" and by the Austrian Ministry for Transport, Innovation and Technology, the Federal Ministry for Digital and Economic Affairs, and the federal state of Salzburg under the research program COMET—Competence Centers for Excellent Technologies—in the project Digital Motion in Sports, Fitness and Well-being (DiMo).

Acknowledgments: The authors would like to thank Martin Seiser and Cory Snyder for their support during data collection, as well as Aaron Martinez for his critical feedback.

Conflicts of Interest: The authors declare no conflict of interest.

References

1. Moore, I.S. Is There an Economical Running Technique? A Review of Modifiable Biomechanical Factors Affecting Running Economy. *Sports Med.* **2016**, *46*, 793–807. [CrossRef] [PubMed]
2. Paradisis, G.P.; Cooke, C. Kinematic and postural characteristics of sprint running on sloping surfaces. *J. Sports Sci.* **2001**, *19*, 149–159. [CrossRef] [PubMed]
3. Nigg, B.M.; Baltich, J.; Hoerzer, S.; Enders, H. Running shoes and running injuries: Mythbusting and a proposal for two new paradigms: 'preferred movement path' and 'comfort filter'. *Br. J. Sports Med.* **2015**, *49*, 1290–1294. [CrossRef] [PubMed]
4. Sinclair, J.; Shore, H.; Dillon, S. The effect of minimalist, maximalist and energy return footwear of equal mass on running economy and substrate utilisation. *Comp. Exerc. Physiol.* **2016**, *12*, 49–54. [CrossRef]
5. Lindorfer, J.; Kröll, J.; Schwameder, H. Does enhanced footwear comfort affect oxygen consumption and running biomechanics? *Eur. J. Sport Sci.* **2019**, *20*, 468–476. [CrossRef]
6. Mohr, M.; Meyer, C.; Nigg, S.; Nigg, B. The relationship between footwear comfort and variability of running kinematics. *Footwear Sci.* **2017**, *9*, S45–S47. [CrossRef]
7. Malisoux, L.; Chambon, N.; Delattre, N.; Gueguen, N.; Urhausen, A.; Theisen, D. Injury risk in runners using standard or motion control shoes: A randomised controlled trial with participant and assessor blinding. *Br. J. Sports Med.* **2016**, *50*, 481–487. [CrossRef]
8. Zrenner, M.; Ullrich, M.; Zobel, P.; Jensen, U.; Laser, F.; Groh, B.H.; Duemler, B.; Eskofier, B.M. Kinematic Parameter Evaluation for the Purpose of a Wearable Running Shoe Recommendation. In Proceedings of the 2018 IEEE 15th International Conference on Wearable and Implantable Body Sensor Networks (BSN), Las Vegas, NV, USA, 4–7 March 2018; pp. 106–109.
9. Lieberman, D.E.; Venkadesan, M.; Werbel, W.A.; Daoud, A.I.; D'Andrea, S.; Davis, I.S.; Mang'Eni, R.O.; Pitsiladis, Y. Foot strike patterns and collision forces in habitually barefoot versus shod runners. *Nat. Cell Biol.* **2010**, *463*, 531–535. [CrossRef]
10. Hamill, J.; Gruber, A.H.; Derrick, T.R. Lower extremity joint stiffness characteristics during running with different footfall patterns. *Eur. J. Sport Sci.* **2012**, *14*, 130–136. [CrossRef]
11. Cheung, R.; Davis, I.S. Landing Pattern Modification to Improve Patellofemoral Pain in Runners: A Case Series. *J. Orthop. Sports Phys. Ther.* **2011**, *41*, 914–919. [CrossRef]
12. Maiwald, C.; Sterzing, T.; Mayer, T.; Milani, T. Detecting foot-to-ground contact from kinematic data in running. *Footwear Sci.* **2009**, *1*, 111–118. [CrossRef]
13. Seiberl, W.; Jensen, E.; Merker, J.; Leitel, M.; Schwirtz, A. Accuracy and precision of loadsol® insole force-sensors for the quantification of ground reaction force-based biomechanical running parameters. *Eur. J. Sport Sci.* **2018**, *18*, 1100–1109. [CrossRef] [PubMed]
14. Altman, A.R.; Davis, I.S. A kinematic method for footstrike pattern detection in barefoot and shod runners. *Gait Posture* **2012**, *35*, 298–300. [CrossRef] [PubMed]
15. Falbriard, M.; Meyer, F.; Mariani, B.; Millet, G.P.; Aminian, K. Contact Time and Foot Strike Angles Estimation Using Foot Worn Inertial Sensors in Running. *ISBS Proc. Arch.* **2017**, *35*, 213. Available online: https://commons.nmu.edu/isbs/vol35/iss1/213 (accessed on 4 March 2020).
16. Shiang, T.-Y.; Hsieh, T.-Y.; Lee, Y.-S.; Wu, C.-C.; Yu, M.-C.; Mei, C.-H.; Tai, I.-H. Determine the Foot Strike Pattern Using Inertial Sensors. *J. Sens.* **2016**, *2016*. [CrossRef]

17. Iosa, M.; Picerno, P.; Paolucci, S.; Morone, G. Wearable Inertial Sensors for Human Movement Analysis. *Expert Rev. Med. Devices* **2016**, *13*, 641–659. [CrossRef]
18. Aubry, R.L.; Power, G.A.; Burr, J.F. An Assessment of Running Power as a Training Metric for Elite and Recreational Runners. *J. Strength Cond. Res.* **2018**, *32*, 2258–2264. [CrossRef]
19. García-Pinillos, F.; Latorre-Román, P.Á.; Roche-Seruendo, L.E.; García-Ramos, A. Prediction of power output at different running velocities through the two-point method with the Stryd™ power meter. *Gait Posture* **2019**, *68*, 238–243. [CrossRef]
20. García-Pinillos, F.; Roche-Seruendo, L.E.; Marcén-Cinca, N.; Marco-Contreras, L.A.; Latorre-Román, P.A. Absolute Reliability and Concurrent Validity of the Stryd System for the Assessment of Running Stride Kinematics at Different Velocities. *J. Strength Cond. Res.* **2018**. [CrossRef]
21. Arampatzis, A.; Knicker, A.; Metzler, V.; Brüggemann, G.-P. Mechanical power in running: A comparison of different approaches. *J. Biomech.* **2000**, *33*, 457–463. [CrossRef]
22. Ancillao, A.; Tedesco, S.; Barton, J.; O'Flynn, B. Indirect Measurement of Ground Reaction Forces and Moments by Means of Wearable Inertial Sensors: A Systematic Review. *Sensors* **2018**, *18*, 2564. [CrossRef] [PubMed]
23. Cheung, R.; Zhang, J.H.; Chan, Z.Y.; An, W.W.; Au, I.P.H.; MacPhail, A.; Davis, I.S. Shoe-mounted accelerometers should be used with caution in gait retraining. *Scand. J. Med. Sci. Sports* **2019**, *29*, 835–842. [CrossRef]
24. Ngueleu, A.M.; Blanchette, A.K.; Bouyer, L.J.; Maltais, D.B.; McFadyen, B.J.; Moffet, H.; Batcho, C.S. Design and Accuray of an Instrumented Insole Using Pressure Sensors for Step Count. *Sensors* **2019**, *19*, 984. [CrossRef] [PubMed]
25. Roth, N.; Martindale, C.F.; Eskofier, B.M.; Gaßner, H.; Kohl, Z.; Klucken, J. Synchronized Sensor Insoles for Clinical Gait Analysis in Home-Monitoring Applications. *Curr. Dir. Biomed. Eng.* **2018**, *4*, 433–437. [CrossRef]
26. Cheung, R.T.; Ivan, P.H.A.; Au, I.P.H.; Zhang, J.H.; Chan, Z.Y.S.; Man, A.; Lau, F.O.Y.; Lam, M.K.Y.; Lau, K.K.; Leung, C.Y.; et al. Measurement agreement between a newly developed sensing insole and traditional laboratory-based method for footstrike pattern detection in runners. *PLoS ONE* **2017**, *12*, e0175724. [CrossRef]
27. Fritz, J.; Brunauer, R.; Snyder, C.; Kröll, J.; Stöggl, T.; Schwameder, H. Foot strike angle calculation during running based on in-shoe pressure measurements. *Footwear Sci.* **2019**, *11*, S147–S149. [CrossRef]
28. Bruening, D.A.; Cooney, K.M.; Buczek, F.L. Analysis of a kinetic multi-segment foot model. Part I: Model repeatability and kinematic validity. *Gait Posture* **2012**, *35*, 529–534. [CrossRef]
29. Panero, E.; Gastaldi, L.; Rapp, W. Two-Segments Foot Model for Biomechanical Motion Analysis. In *Advances in Mechanism and Machine Science*; Springer Science and Business Media LLC: Berlin, Germany, 2017; Volume 49, pp. 988–995.
30. Burns, G.T.; Zendler, J.D.; Zernicke, R.F. Validation of a wireless shoe insole for ground reaction force measurement. *J. Sports Sci.* **2019**, *37*, 1129–1138. [CrossRef]
31. Renner, K.E.; Williams, D.B.; Queen, R.M. The Reliability and Validity of the Loadsol®under Various Walking and Running Conditions. *Sensors* **2019**, *19*, 265. [CrossRef]
32. Alpaydin, E. *Introduction to Machine Learning*, 3rd ed.; Massachusetts Institute of Technology: Cambridge, MA, USA, 2014; Available online: http://dl.matlabyar.com/siavash/ML/Book/Ethem%20Alpaydin-Introduction%20to%20Machine%20Learning-The%20MIT%20Press%20(2014).pdf (accessed on 12 March 2020).
33. Fahrmeir, L.; Kneib, T.; Lang, S. *Regression: Modelle, Methoden und Anwendungen*; Springer: Berlin, Germany, 2009.
34. Hothorn, T.; Hornik, K.; Zeileis, A. Unbiased Recursive Partitioning: A Conditional Inference Framework. *J. Comput. Graph. Stat.* **2006**, *15*, 651–674. [CrossRef]
35. Breiman, L. Random Forests. *Mach. Learn.* **2001**, *45*, 5–32. [CrossRef]
36. Fernandez-Delgado, M.; Cernadas, E.; Barro, S.; Amorim, D. Do we Need Hundreds of Classifiers to Solve Real World Classification Problems? *J. Mach. Learn. Res.* **2014**, *15*, 3133–3181.
37. Moore, S.R.; Fritz, J.; Kröll, J.; Stöggl, T.; Schwameder, H. Consistency and validity of acute foot-strike pattern alterations during laboratory-based running. *ISBS Proc. Arch.* **2020**, *38*, 848.
38. Selbie, W.S.; Hamill, J.; Kepple, T. Chapter 7: Three Dimensional Kinetics. In *Research Methods in Biomechanics*, 2nd ed.; Robertson, G., Caldwell, G., Hamill, J., Whittlesey, S., Eds.; Human Kinetics: Champaign, IL, USA, 2004; pp. 151–176.
39. C-Motion, Inc. Visual3D Wiki Documentation. 2017. Available online: https://c-motion.com/v3dwiki/index.php?title=Main_Page (accessed on 24 January 2020).

40. Neto, E.C.; Pratap, A.; Perumal, T.M.; Tummalacherla, M.; Snyder, P.; Bot, B.M.; Trister, A.D.; Friend, S.H.; Mangravite, L.; Omberg, L. Detecting the impact of subject characteristics on machine learning-based diagnostic applications. *NPJ Digit. Med.* **2019**, *2*, 1–6. [CrossRef]
41. Little, M.A.; Varoquaux, G.; Saeb, S.; Lonini, L.; Jayaraman, A.; Mohr, D.C.; Kording, K.P. Using and understanding cross-validation strategies. Perspectives on Saeb et al. *GigaScience* **2017**, *6*. [CrossRef] [PubMed]
42. Saeb, S.; Lonini, L.; Jayaraman, A.; Mohr, D.C.; Kording, K.P. The need to approximate the use-case in clinical machine learning. *GigaScience* **2017**, *6*. [CrossRef]
43. Field, A. *Discovering Statistics Using IBM SPSS Statistics*, 3rd ed.; Sage Publications: London, UK, 2013.
44. R Core Development Team. *R: A Language and Environment for Statistical Computing*; R Foundation for Statistical Computing: Vienna, Austria, 2018; Available online: https://www.r-project.org/ (accessed on 29 July 2020).
45. Hothorn, T.; Zeileis, A. Partykit: A modular toolkit for recursive partytioning in R. *J. Mach. Learn. Res.* **2015**, *16*, 3905–3909.
46. Liaw, A.; Wiener, M. Classification and Regression by randomForest. *R News* **2002**, *2*, 18–22.
47. Probst, P.; Boulesteix, A.-L. To tune or not to tune the number of trees in random forest? *J. Mach. Learn. Res.* **2017**, *18*, 6673–6690.
48. Kuhn, M. Caret: Classification and Regression Training. Available online: https://CRAN.R-project.org/package=caret (accessed on 9 June 2020).
49. Calle, M.L.; Urrea, V. Letter to the Editor: Stability of Random Forest importance measures. *Brief. Bioinform.* **2011**, *12*, 86–89. [CrossRef]
50. Galdi, P.; Tagliaferri, R. Data Mining: Accuracy and Error Measures for Classification and Prediction. In *Encyclopedia of Bioinformatics and Computational Biology*; Elsevier BV: Amsterdam, The Netherlands, 2019; pp. 431–436.
51. Bland, J.M.; Altman, D.G. Statistical methods for assessing agreement between two methods of clinical measurement. *Int. J. Nurs. Stud.* **2010**, *47*, 931–936. [CrossRef]
52. Mason, C.H.; Perreault, W.D. Collinearity, Power, and Interpretation of Multiple Regression Analysis. *J. Mark. Res.* **1991**, *28*, 268. [CrossRef]
53. Delgado-Gonzalo, R.; Hubbard, J.; Renevey, P.; Lemkaddem, A.; Vellinga, Q.; Ashby, D.; Willardson, J.; Bertschi, M. Real-Time Gait Analysis with Accelerometer-Based Smart Shoes. In Proceedings of the 2017 39th Annual International Conference of the IEEE Engineering in Medicine and Biology Society (EMBC), Jeju Island, Korea, 11–15 July 2017; pp. 148–148c.
54. Fong, D.T.-P.; Chan, Y.-Y.; Hong, Y.; Yung, P.S.-H.; Fung, K.-Y.; Chan, K.-M. A three-pressure-sensor (3PS) system for monitoring ankle supination torque during sport motions. *J. Biomech.* **2008**, *41*, 2562–2566. [CrossRef] [PubMed]
55. Billing, D.C.; Nagarajah, C.R.; Hayes, J.P.; Baker, J. Predicting ground reaction forces in running using micro-sensors and neural networks. *Sports Eng.* **2006**, *9*, 15–27. [CrossRef]
56. Cerezuela-Espejo, V.; Hernández-Belmonte, A.; Courel-Ibáñez, J.; Conesa-Ros, E.; Mora-Rodriguez, R.; Pallarés, J.G. Are we ready to measure running power? Repeatability and concurrent validity of five commercial technologies. *Eur. J. Sport Sci.* **2020**, 1–10. [CrossRef] [PubMed]

Publisher's Note: MDPI stays neutral with regard to jurisdictional claims in published maps and institutional affiliations.

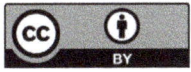

© 2020 by the authors. Licensee MDPI, Basel, Switzerland. This article is an open access article distributed under the terms and conditions of the Creative Commons Attribution (CC BY) license (http://creativecommons.org/licenses/by/4.0/).

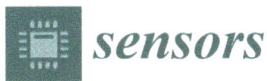
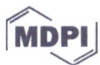

Article

Wearable Sensors Detect Differences between the Sexes in Lower Limb Electromyographic Activity and Pelvis 3D Kinematics during Running

Iván Nacher Moltó [1,*], Juan Pardo Albiach [2], Juan José Amer-Cuenca [1], Eva Segura-Ortí [1], Willig Gabriel [3] and Javier Martínez-Gramage [1]

[1] Department of Physiotherapy, Universidad Cardenal Herrera-CEU, CEU Universities, 46113 Valencia, Spain; juanjoamer@uchceu.es (J.J.A.-C.); esegura@uchceu.es (E.S.-O.); jmg@uchceu.es (J.M.-G.)
[2] Embedded Systems and Artificial Intelligence Group, Universidad Cardenal Herrera-CEU, CEU Universities, 46113 Alfara del Patriarca, Spain; juaparal@uchceu.es
[3] Laboratorio de Investigaciones Biomecánicas, Cátedra de Anatomía Funcional y Biomecánica, Universidad de Buenos Aires, Buenos Aires 1107, Argentina; gwillig@fmed.uba.ar
* Correspondence: ivan.nacher.molto@gmail.com; Tel.: +34-605-450-061

Received: 13 October 2020; Accepted: 10 November 2020; Published: 12 November 2020

Abstract: Each year, 50% of runners suffer from injuries. Consequently, more studies are being published about running biomechanics; these studies identify factors that can help prevent injuries. Scientific evidence suggests that recreational runners should use personalized biomechanical training plans, not only to improve their performance, but also to prevent injuries caused by the inability of amateur athletes to tolerate increased loads, and/or because of poor form. This study provides an overview of the different normative patterns of lower limb muscle activation and articular ranges of the pelvis during running, at self-selected speeds, in men and women. Methods: 38 healthy runners aged 18 to 49 years were included in this work. We examined eight muscles by applying two wearable superficial electromyography sensors and an inertial sensor for three-dimensional (3D) pelvis kinematics. Results: the largest differences were obtained for gluteus maximus activation in the first double float phase ($p = 0.013$) and second stance phase ($p = 0.003$), as well as in the gluteus medius in the second stance phase ($p = 0.028$). In both cases, the activation distribution was more homogeneous in men and presented significantly lower values than those obtained for women. In addition, there was a significantly higher percentage of total vastus medialis activation in women throughout the running cycle with the median (25th–75th percentile) for women being 12.50% (9.25–14) and 10% (9–12) for men. Women also had a greater range of pelvis rotation during running at self-selected speeds ($p = 0.011$). Conclusions: understanding the differences between men and women, in terms of muscle activation and pelvic kinematic values, could be especially useful to allow health professionals detect athletes who may be at risk of injury.

Keywords: running; kinematics; surface electromyography; wearables

1. Introduction

Recreational running is becoming an increasingly popular pastime [1], with approximately 15% and 70% of amateur athletes currently engaging in this activity in the United Kingdom and the United States, respectively [2,3]. Various studies have shown that 50% of runners suffer an injury each year [4], although there are discrepancies in the literature, due to incidence values that vary from 18.2% to 92.4% [5] and reported prevalence ranging from 46% to 90% among amateur runners [6,7].

In recent years, an increasing number of studies have been published in relation to the biomechanics of running, including factors that could help prevent and treat injuries in runners [8–11]. Running is a popular recreational activity, but a lack of adequate training in correct running techniques may account for the reported increase in injuries among these athletes [12]. Thus, in this work, we aimed to provide an overview of the different normative patterns of lower limb muscle activation and pelvic joint ranges during running at self-selected speeds in men and women. We analyzed the biomechanics of running by measuring the activation of the main muscles involved in this activity, as well as the dynamic ranges of joint movement, especially in the pelvis [13].

The choice of a preferred speed could be affected by the level of performance and the intensity of the training habits [14]. It is reasonable to expect that amateur runners, with a higher level of performance, will train at higher intensities and, therefore, select a higher running speed for pleasure and metabolic cost [14,15].

Portable dynamic surface electromyography (sEMG) measurement devices, together with inertial sensor units (IMUs), are currently used for this type of analysis [16,17]. These systems provide information about muscle use intensity and activation time, and reflect the different contraction strategies, neuromuscular control systems, and three-dimensional (3D) pelvic kinematics used during running [18–20]. The use of wearable systems for these biomechanical measurements allow the data to be captured under more realistic conditions [21].

Given the intrinsic variability of these biomechanical values, the field still lacks a set of reliable reference values for use when assessing both the status and evolution of injured individuals. Some studies have determined these values based on the dynamic range of the pelvis and level of muscle activation by using sEMG for the main muscles involved in running [21–27]. One study noted increased hamstring and hip flexor tension in runners caused by excess anteroposterior pelvic movement or tilt [23], while in another, back pain was correlated with limited lower knee range [24].

Many studies, exploring the differences in muscle activation in the stance and swing phases of running, are now available in the literature [19,28–30]. However, none have systematically categorized the values for muscle function and pelvic kinematics during the different phases of running. Moreover, running mechanics also differ between the sexes, but the differences in the normative patterns of muscle activation, in different phases of running between male and female amateur runners, has not yet been determined [31].

Measuring and characterizing human movements during activity to evaluate athlete performance, improve technique, and prevent injuries is a crucial part of modern training programs [32]. Collecting these data will increase scientific knowledge of kinematic patterns and the degree of muscle activation in runners. Therefore, the purpose of this study was to establish the differences between the sexes in terms of lower limb sEMG activity and three-dimensional (3D) kinematics of the pelvis during running.

2. Materials and Methods

2.1. Participants

Healthy participants were recruited, who typically engaged in at least 90 min of continuous running training per week, and who had not suffered any injury in the prior year that could have changed their movement patterns. In addition, we excluded individuals who reported having suffered an orthopedic, neurological, or surgical injury in the prior year that could have affected their movement patterns. We explained the nature of the study to all of the participants and they signed their informed consent to participation prior to the start of the work. The entire study was carried out according to the principles of the Declaration of Helsinki, was approved by the ethics committee at CEU Cardenal Herrera University (reference number: CEI18/137), and was registered as a clinical trial (ClinicalTrials.gov registration №: NCT04221698).

2.2. Procedure

In this study, we measured the level of activation in the muscles of the dominant leg as well as the pelvic dynamic range of each participant. We used a treadmill (BH Fitness Columbia Pro

130 cm × 40 cm) to establish standardized conditions under which the kinematic variables of running would be more reproducible. We set the incline to 1° and allowed each participant to select the speed [31,32] at which they regularly trained. The participants used their own shoes and were allowed a 15-min warm-up period in order to adjust to the treadmill. According to protocols used in previous running biomechanics studies [28,33–35], the initial speed was progressively increased over 2 min and was then maintained for 3 min while the data were collected.

The dynamic range of the pelvis was assessed using an inertial sensor (BTS G-Sensor 2) with an ergonomic belt at the height of S1 to capture different kinematic and spatiotemporal variables. This IMU comprised a 16-axis triaxial accelerometer with multiple sensitivities (±2, ±4, ±6, ±8, and ±16 g) with a frequency of 4 Hz to 1000 Hz, a triaxial gyroscope with multiple sensitivities (±250, ±500, ±1000, ±2000 o/s), with a frequency oscillating between 4 Hz to 8000 Hz, and a triaxial 13-bit magnetometer (±1200 uT), with a frequency exceeding 100 Hz.

Muscle activation was simultaneously studied by sEMG in eight muscles: the gluteus maximus, gluteus medius, rectus femoris, vastus medialis, biceps femoris, semitendinosus, medial gastrocnemius, and soleus. The skin was prepared according to SENIAM guidelines [36], and then two 20 mm pre-gelled self-adhesive bipolar Ag/AgCl disposable surface electrodes (Infant Electrode, Lessa, Barcelona) were placed on each muscle with a 20 mm interelectrode distance between them. A 10 g wireless probe (41.5 × 24, 8 × 14 mm) was placed on each pair of electrodes to capture the sEMG signal and send the information by Wi-Fi to the capture system (BTS FREEMG 1000, BTS Bioengineering, Milan, Italy) via a signal receiver (Wireless IEEE802.15.4) connected to a computer via USB [37].

The running phases analyzed by sEMG were the percentage of the stride cycle and percentage of each subphase. The start of the stride cycle corresponded to the initial contact and start of the contact of the same foot. The running subphases were: the first stance, first double float, second stance, and second double float (Figure 1). Thus, for the right leg, the first stance occurred from the initial contact of the right foot to the take-off of the right toe. The first double float occurred from the initial float phase of the right foot to the contact of the contralateral foot. This was then followed by the second stance, from the time of initial contact of the left foot to take-off of the left toe, and the second double float from the initial float phase of the left foot until contact of the contralateral foot.

1st ST   1st SW   2nd ST   2nd SW

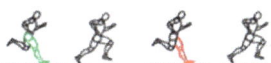

Figure 1. Figure of the running stride cycle sub-cycles: the first stance (1st St), first double float (1st Sw), second stance (2nd St), and second double float (2nd Sw).

2.3. Data Analysis

The EMG signal was recorded simultaneously using a FREEEMG 1000 and EMG Analyzer (BTS Bioengineering, Milan, Italy) that was set to a sampling rate of 1000 Hz per channel, and the signals were band-pass filtered from 20 Hz to 450 Hz. The EMG signals were subsequently full-wave rectified and low pass filtered using a bidirectional, 6th order Butterworth filter, with a cutoff frequency of 5 Hz. The root mean square (RMS) in several subphases was detected. The IMU sensor detected every event performed, initial contact, and toe-off of each foot. Moreover, at the same time, the sEMG signal was recorded, so that the system selected the right and left strides and the different subphases (first stance phase, first float phase, second stance phase, second float phase), as described in Figure 1.

2.4. Statistical Analysis

To describe the demographic data of the population sample, descriptive statistics were calculated separately by sex for the participant age, height, weight, and training sessions performed during the chosen week and for the running dynamics data. The data from the study variables were analyzed to check for extreme outlying values using Chauvenet's criterion, because these may have represented abnormalities in the measurements, musculature, or nerve conduction of the participants.

After testing compliance with the assumptions of normality (Shapiro–Wilk test) and homogeneity of variances (Levene's test), we decided to use non-parametric methods in our analyses. We used the Wilcoxon rank sum method (based on the Mann–Whitney U test) to compare the sex factor in the biomechanical patterns of pelvis use, muscular activation during the complete running cycle, and the mean activation between men and women at their self-selected speeds. G*Power software was used to calculate the sample size; to detect an effect size of 0.8 with a statistical power of 0.8, we calculated that we would require at least 21 participants in each group. We finally obtained data from 22 men and 16 women, and post-hoc calculations gave us a statistical power of 0.75. RStudio Desktop software (version 1.2.5 for macOS; RStudio Inc., Boston, MA, USA) was used for all of our statistical analyses.

3. Results

A total of 48 individuals initially participated in the study, of which eight were considered excluded values because of injury ($n = 7$) or Bluetooth receiver failure ($n = 1$). The demographics of these participants are described in Table 1.

Table 1. Participant characteristics *.

	Value	
	Female	Male
Participants, n	16	22
Age, years	27.07 ± 9.16	26.39 ± 6.61
Weight, Kg	58.31 ± 7.06	70.14 ± 8.3
Height, cm	166.3 ± 0.06	177.5 ± 0.07
Weekly number of training sessions	3.93 ± 1.03	4.87 ± 1.14

* Values represented as the mean and standard deviation (SD).

Once the data from the 40 participants included in the trial had been analyzed, 2 participants were excluded because they were considered outliers, leaving a final sample of 38 individuals. Regarding the self-selected speed, the mean for women was 9.22 (±1.59) km/h, and for men it was 10.61 (±1.56) km/h, with this difference being statistically significant. Table 2 shows the mean value and the p-value of the difference between the speed and distance between the sexes, calculated using Mann–Whitney U tests.

Table 2. Statistics and significance between sex and the speed and distance variables *.

	Female (avg)	Female SD	Male (avg)	Male SD	Wilcoxon p-Value
Speed (km/h)	9.22	1.59	10.61	1.56	0.009 *
Distance (Km)	0.79	0.13	0.9	0.14	0.02 *

* Significant differences at $p < 0.05$. Speed expressed in kilometers/hour and distance measured in kilometers.

3.1. Kinematics of the Pelvis

Significant differences in the range of pelvic rotation (Figure 2) were observed between the sexes, with female runners presenting a greater range of rotation during running at their self-selected speed, but no significant differences were observed in the tilt or obliquity between the sexes (Table 3).

Table 3. Differences between men and women in the kinematics of the pelvis during sprinting at a self-selected speed *.

Variable	Mean Men	Mean Women	p-Value
Rotation	12.53 (SD: 3.2)	17.04 (SD: 5.72)	0.011 *
Obliquity	7.57 (SD: 1.99)	7.82 (SD: 1.61)	0.391
Tilt	7.41 (SD: 1.68)	8.51 (SD: 2.11)	0.086

* Mean values with their standard deviations (SD) are shown. * Statistically significant differences at $p < 0.05$.

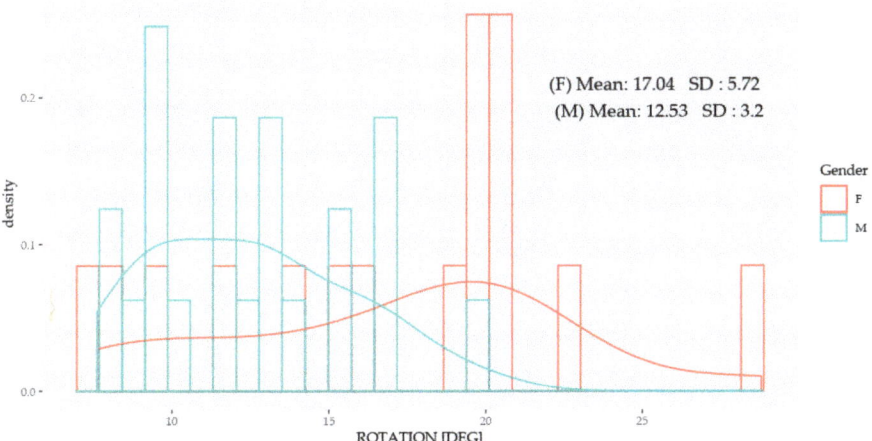

Figure 2. Variation of the rotation between women (F) and men (M), with each bar representing one participant. The lines summarize the distribution of the mean.

3.2. Mean Running Cycle Muscle Activation

Table 4 shows the statistics for each of the recorded muscles compared by sex for the percentage factor of total muscle activation during each running cycle. The vastus medialis showed a significantly higher percentage of activation in women throughout the running cycle (Figure 3) with a significantly different distribution between the sexes; there was greater muscle activation dispersion in women, indicating increased variability, while the vastus medialis activation homogeneity was reduced in men.

Table 4. Statistics and significance of the percentage of total muscle activation during the running cycle *.

Muscle	% Activation Women	% Activation Men
Gluteus maximus	12 (11.25–15.50)	12 (11–13)
Gluteus medius	12 (11–13)	11.50 (10.75–13)
Femoral rectus	12 (11–14)	13.50 (12–15.25)
Vastus medial	12.50 (9.25–14) *	10 (9–12) *
Semitendinosus	14 (13–15.75)	13 (11.75–16)
Femoral biceps	14.50 (13.25–17.30)	15.00 (13–15)
Medial gastrocnemius	10.50 (9–12)	11.00 (10–12)
Soleus	10.00 (10–11.75)	12 (11–13.70)

* Percentage value of the median (25th–75th percentile). * Significant differences at $p < 0.05$.

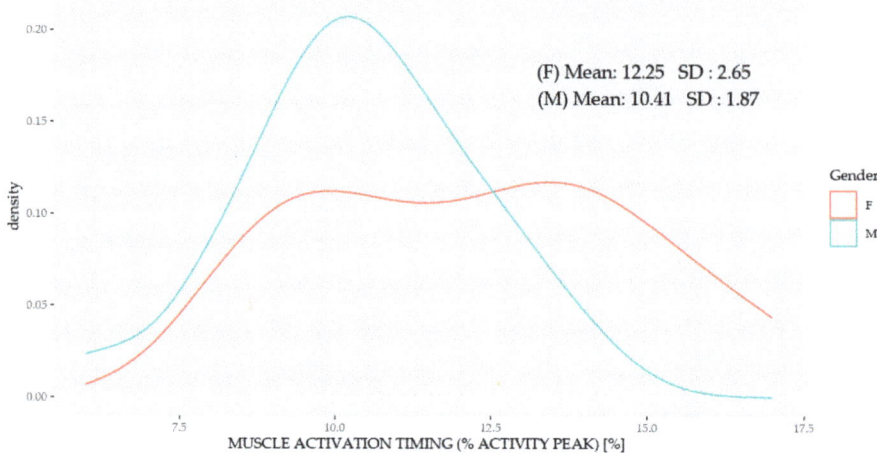

Figure 3. Percentage of the total activation of the vastus medialis during the running cycle distributed between women (F) and men (M). The distribution of the mean and *SD* were more homogeneous in men.

3.3. Muscle Activation for Each of the Phases

There were significant differences in the muscle activation measurements for each of the phases in each of the main muscles (Table 5). Figure 4 shows the difference in the gluteus maximus muscle activation between women and men running at their self-selected speeds. The distribution of the muscle activation in men was more homogeneous and presented significantly lower values than for women. Figure 5 shows the difference in gluteus medius muscle activation between women and men during the second stance, showing lower homogeneity in women and greater activation than in men.

Table 5. The *p*-values of the mean in the muscles with significant differences between the sexes in different phases.

Muscle	1st Stance	1st Double Float	2nd Stance	2nd Double Float
Gluteus maximus	$p = 0.114$	$p = 0.013$ *	$p = 0.003$ *	$p = 0.647$
Gluteus medius	$p = 0.198$	$p = 0.057$	$p = 0.028$ *	$p = 0.584$

* Significant differences at $p < 0.05$.

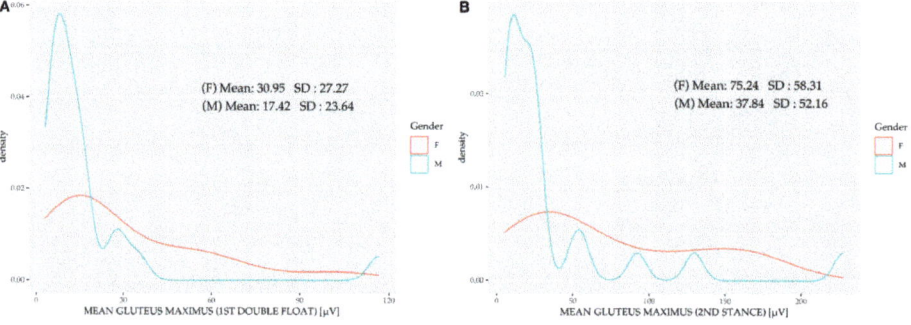

Figure 4. Variation by sex in the gluteus maximus in the first double float (**A**) and second stance (**B**).

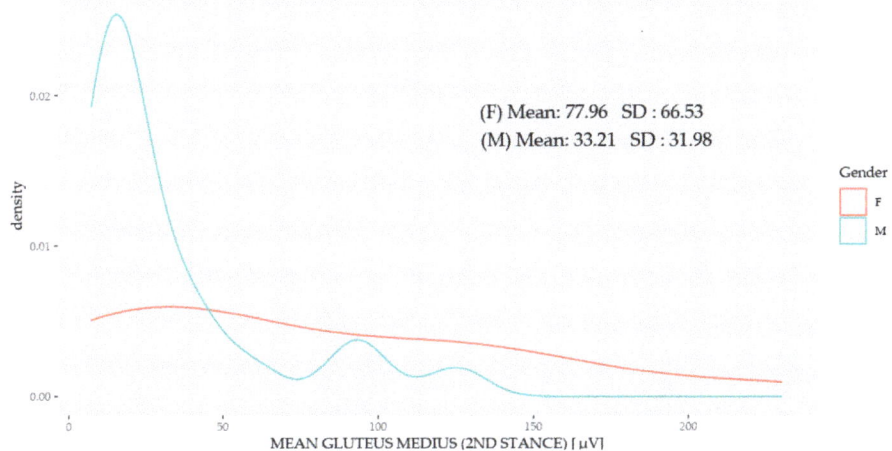

Figure 5. Variation between the sexes in the mean gluteus medius activation during the second stance.

4. Discussion

The main objective of this study was to establish whether there were differences between the sexes in muscular activation or in the 3D kinematics of the pelvis during the entire running cycle and in each of the running phases. We started with the hypothesis that the sex factor could determine the level of muscle activation throughout the running cycle and its component phases. Our results show that there were differences between the sexes, in terms of the total percentage of muscle activation during the entire running cycle in the vastus medialis. In addition, there were differences in the use of this muscle and the gluteus maximus between the sexes in the individual running phases. Moreover, there were sex differences in the rotation of the pelvis. The differences between the sexes in terms of the speed and distance traveled were similar to those previously described in the literature [21].

Similar to the cohorts used in other studies [19,38–40], the participants in this work were recruited through random sampling, following established inclusion criteria, from among a population of amateur runners of different ages. We allowed the participants to self-select the speed at which they ran because, in addition to the effects of the age and body mass and body composition factors [17], running speed is directly related to cardiovascular factors, such as individual aerobic threshold and performance [16], and with biomechanical factors, such as stability, flight time, and leg contact time [41]. In this same sense, work by Zamprano et al. [14] and Lussiana et al. [41] indicated that the speed chosen by each participant is related to their energy saving strategy. Thus, imposing a set speed upon runners, rather than allowing them to select the speed at which they are comfortable running, caused lower limb biomechanical changes and produced alterations in the muscle activation pattern and pelvis dynamics. These data are reinforced by those published by Kong et al. [42], which concluded that self-selected velocities would eliminate abnormal kinematic patterns.

In this work, we placed the inertial sensor at the S1 level as a reference to quantify the kinematics of the pelvis. However, we are unable to compare our data with other methodologies, because no previously published work contrasted the kinematic data of the pelvis during running at self-selected speeds, except for the work by Perpiñá et al. [24], who also placed the sensor at level S1. There were no significant differences between the sexes for the tilt range or pelvic obliquity kinematic values obtained. These values coincided with the expected normal values and were not novel. However, we did find that the mean lower pelvic rotation range for women (17.04° ± 5.72°) was significantly higher than the values found for men (12.53° ± 3.2°). Furthermore, the rotational ranges in men were lower than the reference values of 16°–18° provided in studies that dynamically measured the pelvis during running, perhaps because of differences in the speed used [28,43].

When the toes take off during the propulsion phase in running, the pelvis presents its maximum anterior tilt level, slight ipsilateral obliquity to support, and slight external rotation [27,42]. This limits hip flexion and makes rotation the most advantageous mechanism to lengthen the stride. This increased pelvic rotation in women seems to be related to a genetic predisposition towards greater flexibility [44] and a lower capacity for elastic energy storage [45]. All of this is associated with a decrease in the peak vertical forces used by female runners [46]; thus, requiring rotational compensation at every speed. Therefore, women must increase their dynamic range of rotation to increase their hip extension without altering the other kinematic variables and muscle activation factors. This would lead to greater stability and running economy in women due to structural differences in the female pelvis and hips compared to males [22].

We also found different muscle activation responses in the different running phases according to the muscles studied. The gluteus medius is activated in women because they have increased pelvis–hip joint movement and the main function of this muscle is to stabilize these joints. Thus, when the ground reaction force is absorbed in the first part of the first or second stance, the gluteus medius performs more eccentric work in women than in men [39]. In contrast, this muscle causes hip abduction in the first and second take-off phases [47,48]. Therefore, women require increased gluteus medius activation to meet the biomechanical requirements of running, particularly in the second stance. This can lead to the appearance of injuries, either because of a lack of activation or because of fatigue, which are both of primary clinical importance because these factors strongly correlate with the appearance of injuries [49–53].

The gluteus maximus is activated when the foot first contacts the ground and stops hip and trunk flexion in this phase [51]. This muscle also performs trunk extension and strengthens the knee when it is fully extended by acting through the iliotibial tract [54]. Gluteus maximus activity increases during the flight and swing phases because, together with the hamstrings and psoas, it behaves as a hip and knee accelerator during this phase [55]. In agreement with the data from this current study, several other authors also believe that contraction of this muscle at the midpoint of the oscillation phase (between the first double float and second stance) is involved in leg deceleration [56] and may also be related to passive extension of the knee.

We obtained a mean gluteus maximus activation of less than 30.95 µV for men in the first double float phase in this study, which may correspond to a gluteus maximus activation deficit. In contrast, activation of this muscle in female runners in the second stance was below 75.24 µV. Furthermore, the hamstring muscles in this study showed increased activity to control hip flexion when the trunk was flexed, which was causally related to pelvis stabilization [57–59]. Maximal medial and lateral hamstring activity during running occurs through eccentric contraction in the middle of the swing phase in order to decelerate the leg just before maximal hip flexion, and immediately after the start of the knee extension [60,61].

The increase in vastus medialis muscle activity we observed in women compared to men (as a percentage of the overall running cycle), as well as during the swing in the first double float and second stance phases, may be because women tend to be less stiff than men. This would reduce their energy storage capacity in the transverse and frontal planes of the trunk and hip muscles [45], thus, decreasing the stability of passive structures and increasing their range of motion, in turn leading to greater stabilization at the muscular level [62–64].

Another function attributed to the vastus medialis is stabilization of the patella within the trochlear groove [63–65], thus, generating a medializing force vector upon the patella, which would cause its rotation when in extension [66–68]. The quadriceps are also active during the swing phase of running, in preparation to receive the weight load [69]. Interestingly, women seem to have increased quadriceps activation when performing sports activities [70], which can substantially contribute to physiologically significant [71–73] changes in muscle strength between the sexes [71].

Our data also agreed with previous work showing that vastus medialis activation for hip muscle recruitment differs in women when in positions that are neutral or with a slight medial hip rotation [74,75]. Indeed, Montgomery et al. concluded that contraction of this muscle is required in the swing phase to provide knee extension, thus, stabilizing the patella before the heel strike [73]. In addition, compared to men, we found structural and anatomical differences in the lower limbs of women during running. This reduced normative pattern of vastus medialis activation in women may help them cope with external forces. This is important because it would generate a neuromuscular imbalance between the vastus of the quadriceps, thus, producing a greater risk of injuries, such as patellofemoral pain in female runners [72,76].

To the best of our knowledge, this is the first time normative patterns for the running kinematics of the major muscles and range of motion of the pelvis have been specifically established for each sex. Our results support the stabilizing role the gluteus medius has on the pelvis and knee, as well as the role of the vastus medialis in balancing the patella and controlling the knee valgus during running. The co-contraction of these muscles, together with that of the gluteus maximus and hamstrings, produces adequate motor control. These data could prove useful in clinical settings to prevent the injuries most frequently found in female amateur runners.

One of the limitations of this work may be its sample size (although it was similar to the cohort sizes used in other studies) because it could limit statistical interpretation with the aim of establishing normative data. Furthermore, we did not consider the influence of age, which could have affected the choice of our participants' running speeds, as well as their running economies [40]. Finally, this study was novel, so the lack of publications about normative muscle activation levels and normative pelvic kinematic patterns limited our ability to compare these data with other work; this makes it harder to understand the true causes of the differences we found between the sexes. Future studies should analyze the differences between healthy individuals and those with certain running injuries in order to analyze their possible origins. This could allow personalized training and prevention plans to be established, and could increase the recovery speed in individuals who already have an injury.

5. Conclusions

In conclusion, these differences between the sexes, in terms of muscle activation and pelvic kinematic values, could be especially useful for detecting athletes who may be at risk, allowing healthcare professionals to intervene before possible injuries appear. Here, we found a normative pattern of increased pelvic rotation as well as an increase in gluteus maximus, gluteus medius, and vastus medialis muscle activation in female runners. Further studies will be required to examine whether these differences in pelvic kinematics and muscle activation are related to the injuries commonly experienced by female and male recreational runners.

Author Contributions: Conceptualization, I.N.M. and J.M.-G.; methodology, I.N.M. and J.M.-G.; software, J.P.A.; validation, W.G., J.J.A.-C., and E.S.-O.; formal analysis, J.J.A.-C.; investigation, I.N.M. and J.M.-G.; resources, W.G.; data curation, E.S.-O.; writing—original draft preparation, I.N.M.; writing—review and editing, I.N.M.; visualization, J.P.A.; supervision, I.N.M. and J.M.-G.; project administration, J.M.-G. All authors have read and agreed to the published version of the manuscript.

Funding: This research received no external funding.

Acknowledgments: We appreciate the voluntary participation of all the runners and their invaluable kindness.

Conflicts of Interest: The authors declare no conflict of interest.

References

1. Vidal, A.B.; Monezi, L.A.; Sarro, K.; De Barros, R.M.L. Analysis of required coefficient of friction in running and walking. *Sports Biomech.* **2019**, 1–13. [CrossRef]
2. Bramah, C.; Preece, S.J.; Gill, N.; Herrington, L. Is There a Pathological Gait Associated With Common Soft Tissue Running Injuries? *Am. J. Sports Med.* **2018**, *46*, 3023–3031. [CrossRef]
3. Abadía, S.; Medina, F.X.; Sánchez, R.; Bantulà, J.; Fornons, D.; Bastida, N.; Augé, A.; Corderas, F.; Vega, S.; Pujadas, X. Entre el boom atlético y la cooperación social. Las carreras solidarias y el ejemplo de la Trailwalker España 2013. *Península Inval.* **2014**, *9*, 105–123. [CrossRef]

4. Fields, K.B. Running Injuries—Changing Trends and Demographics. *Curr. Sports Med. Rep.* **2011**, *10*, 299–303. [CrossRef] [PubMed]
5. Saragiotto, B.T.; Di Pierro, C.; Lopes, A.D. Risk factors and injury prevention in elite athletes: A descriptive study of the opinions of physical therapists, doctors and trainers. *Braz. J. Phys. Ther.* **2014**, *18*, 137–143. [CrossRef] [PubMed]
6. Salas Sanchez, J.; Latorre Roman, P.A.; Soto Hermoso, V.M. Body Composition and Strength of the Veteran Athlete: Effect of Aging. *Apunt. Med. Sport* **2013**, *48*, 137–142.
7. Boling, M.; Padua, D.; Marshall, S.; Guskiewicz, K.; Pyne, S.; Beutler, A. Gender differences in the incidence and prevalence of patellofemoral pain syndrome. *Scand. J. Med. Sci. Sports* **2010**, *20*, 725–730. [CrossRef]
8. Preece, S.J.; Bramah, C.; Mason, D. The biomechanical characteristics of high-performance endurance running. *Eur. J. Sport Sci.* **2019**, *19*, 784–792. [CrossRef]
9. Williams, D.S.B.; Welch, L.M. Male and female runners demonstrate different sagittal plane mechanics as a function of static hamstring flexibility. *Rev. Bras. Fisioter.* **2015**, *19*, 421–428. [CrossRef]
10. Barnes, K.R.; Hopkins, W.G.; McGuigan, M.R.; Northuis, M.E.; Kilding, A.E. Effects of Resistance Training on Running Economy and Cross-country Performance. *Med. Sci. Sports Exerc.* **2013**, *45*, 2322–2331. [CrossRef]
11. Taunton, J.E.; Ryan, M.B.; Clement, D.B.; McKenzie, D.C.; Lloyd-Smith, D.R.; Zumbo, B.D. A prospective study of running injuries: The Vancouver Sun Run "In Training" clinics. *Br. J. Sports Med.* **2003**, *37*, 239–244. [CrossRef] [PubMed]
12. Taunton, J.E.; Ryan, M.B.; Clement, D.B.; McKenzie, D.C.; Lloyd-Smith, D.R.; Zumbo, B.D. A retrospective case-control analysis of 2002 running injuries. *Br. J. Sports Med.* **2002**, *36*, 95–101. [CrossRef] [PubMed]
13. Dorn, T.W.; Schache, A.G.; Pandy, M.G. Muscular strategy shift in human running: Dependence of running speed on hip and ankle muscle performance. *J. Exp. Biol.* **2012**, *215*, 1944–1956. [CrossRef] [PubMed]
14. Zamparo, P.; Perini, R.; Peano, C.; Di Prampero, P.E. The Self Selected Speed of Running in Recreational Long Distance Runners. *Int. J. Sports Med.* **2001**, *22*, 598–604. [CrossRef]
15. Ekkekakis, P.; Hall, E.; Petruzzello, S. Affective Responses to a Graded Treadmill Test: Is the Ventilatory Threshold the Turning Point Toward Negativity? *J. Sport Exerc. Psychol.* **2002**, *24*, 52–53.
16. Liu, S.-H.; Lin, C.-B.; Chen, Y.; Chen, W.; Huang, T.-S.; Hsu, C.-Y. An EMG Patch for the Real-Time Monitoring of Muscle-Fatigue Conditions during Exercise. *Sensors* **2019**, *19*, 3108. [CrossRef]
17. Yoong, N.K.M.; Perring, J.; Mobbs, R.J. Commercial Postural Devices: A Review. *Sensors* **2019**, *19*, 5128. [CrossRef]
18. Stirling, L.M.; Von Tscharner, V.; Kugler, P.; Nigg, B.M. Classification of muscle activity based on effort level during constant pace running. *J. Electromyogr. Kinesiol.* **2011**, *21*, 566–571. [CrossRef]
19. Von Tscharner, V.; Eskofier, B.; Federolf, P. Removal of the electrocardiogram signal from surface EMG recordings using non-linearly scaled wavelets. *J. Electromyogr. Kinesiol.* **2011**, *21*, 683–688. [CrossRef]
20. Farina, D.; Merletti, R.; Enoka, R.M.; Cope, K.A.; Watson, M.T.; Foster, W.M.; Sehnert, S.S.; Risby, T.H. The extraction of neural strategies from the surface EMG. *J. Appl. Physiol.* **2004**, *96*, 1486–1495. [CrossRef]
21. Schubert, A.G.; Kempf, J.; Heiderscheit, B.C. Influence of Stride Frequency and Length on Running Mechanics: A Systematic Review. *Sports Health* **2014**, *6*, 210–217. [CrossRef] [PubMed]
22. Howard, R.M.; Conway, R.; Harrison, A.J. Muscle activity in sprinting: A review. *Sports Biomech.* **2018**, *17*, 1–17. [CrossRef] [PubMed]
23. León Sánchez, J.M. Determinación De Los Datos Normativos De La Actividad Muscular Del Miembro Inferior Y De Los Parámetros Espacio-Temporales Durante La Carrera. Ph.D. Thesis, Universidad CEU Cardenal Herrera, Moncada, Spain, 2017.
24. Perpiñá, S.M. Fiabilidad Del Sistema Inercial Durante El Análisis Biomecánico De La carrera a Pie En Triatletas: Establecimiento Del Patrón Cinemático Normativo. Ph.D. Thesis, Universidad CEU Cardenal Herrera, Moncada, Spain, 2017.
25. Heise, G.D.; Shinohara, M.; Binks, L. Biarticular Leg Muscles and Links to Running Economy. *Int. J. Sports Med.* **2008**, *29*, 688–691. [CrossRef] [PubMed]
26. Bergamini, E.; Picerno, P.; Pillet, H.; Natta, F.; Thoreux, P.; Camomilla, V. Estimation of temporal parameters during sprint running using a trunk-mounted inertial measurement unit. *J. Biomech.* **2012**, *45*, 1123–1126. [CrossRef]
27. Gazendam, M.G.J.; Hof, A.L. Averaged EMG profiles in jogging and running at different speeds. *Gait Posture* **2007**, *25*, 604–614. [CrossRef]

28. Cappellini, G.; Ivanenko, Y.P.; Poppele, R.E.; Lacquaniti, F. Motor Patterns in Human Walking and Running. *J. Neurophysiol.* **2006**, *95*, 3426–3437. [CrossRef]
29. Wall-Scheffler, C.M.; Myers, M.J. The Biomechanical and Energetic Advantages of a Mediolaterally Wide Pelvis in Women. *Anat. Rec.* **2017**, *300*, 764–775. [CrossRef]
30. Schache, A.G.; Blanch, P.; Rath, D.; Wrigley, T.; Bennell, K. Differences between the sexes in the three-dimensional angular rotations of the lumbo-pelvic-hip complex during treadmill running. *J. Sports Sci.* **2003**, *21*, 105–118. [CrossRef]
31. Ferber, R.; Davis, I.M.; Iii, D.S.W. Gender differences in lower extremity mechanics during running. *Clin. Biomech.* **2003**, *18*, 350–357. [CrossRef]
32. Taborri, J.; Keogh, J.; Kos, A.; Santuz, A.; Umek, A.; Urbanczyk, C.; Van Der Kruk, E.; Rossi, S. Sport Biomechanics Applications Using Inertial, Force, and EMG Sensors: A Literature Overview. *Appl. Bionics Biomech.* **2020**, *2020*, 1–18. [CrossRef]
33. Queen, R.M.; Gross, M.T.; Liu, H.-Y. Repeatability of lower extremity kinetics and kinematics for standardized and self-selected running speeds. *Gait Posture* **2006**, *23*, 282–287. [CrossRef] [PubMed]
34. Lavcanska, V.; Taylor, N.F.; Schache, A.G. Familiarization to treadmill running in young unimpaired adults. *Hum. Mov. Sci.* **2005**, *24*, 544–557. [CrossRef] [PubMed]
35. McNair, P.J.; Marshall, R.N. Kinematic and kinetic parameters associated with running in different shoes. *Br. J. Sports Med.* **1994**, *28*, 256–260. [CrossRef] [PubMed]
36. Hermens, H.J.; Freriks, B.; Disselhorst-Klug, C.; Rau, G. Development of recommendations for SEMG sensors and sensor placement procedures. *J Electromyogr. Kinesiol.* **2000**, *10*, 361–374. [CrossRef]
37. BTS. 2020. Available online: Https://www.Btsbioengineering.Com/ (accessed on 12 November 2020).
38. Stegeman, D.F.; Blok, J.H.; Hermens, H.J.; Roeleveld, K. Surface EMG models: Properties and applications. *J. Electromyogr. Kinesiol.* **2000**, *10*, 313–326. [CrossRef]
39. Stegeman, D.F.; Linsenn, W.F. Muscle fiber action potential changues and surface EMG: A simulation study. *J. Electromyogr. Kinesiol.* **1992**, *2*, 130–140. [CrossRef]
40. Õunpuu, S. The Biomechanics of Walking and Running. *Clin. Sports Med.* **1994**, *13*, 843–863. [CrossRef]
41. Lussiana, T.; Gindre, C. Feel your stride and find your preferred running speed. *Biol. Open* **2016**, *5*, 45–48. [CrossRef]
42. Kong, P.W.; Candelaria, N.G.; Tomaka, J. Perception of self-selected running speed is influenced by the treadmill but not footwear. *Sports Biomech.* **2009**, *8*, 52–59. [CrossRef]
43. Novacheck, T.F. Running injuries: A biomechanical approach. *J. Bone Jt. Surg. Am.* **1998**, *80A*, 1220–1233. [CrossRef]
44. Lewis, C.L.; Laudicina, N.M.; Khuu, A.; Loverro, K.L. The Human Pelvis: Variation in Structure and Function During Gait. *Anat. Rec.* **2017**, *300*, 633–642. [CrossRef] [PubMed]
45. Aura, O.; Komi, P.V. Mechanical Efficiency of Pure Positive and Pure Negative Work with Special Reference to the Work Intensity. *Int. J. Sports Med.* **1986**, *7*, 44–49. [CrossRef]
46. Anderson, P.T. Biomechanics and Running Economy. *Sports Med.* **1996**, *22*, 76–89. [CrossRef]
47. Novacheck, T.F. The biomechanics of running. *Gait Posture* **1998**, *7*, 77–95. [CrossRef]
48. Vaughan, C.L. Biomechanics of running gait. *Crit. Rev. Biomed. Eng.* **1984**, *12*, 1–48.
49. Bramah, C.; Preece, S.J.; Gill, N.; Herrington, L. A 10% Increase in Step Rate Improves Running Kinematics and Clinical Outcomes in Runners With Patellofemoral Pain at 4 Weeks and 3 Months. *Am. J. Sports Med.* **2019**, *47*, 3406–3413. [CrossRef]
50. Neal, M.; Fleming, N.; Eberman, L.; Games, K.; Vaughan, J. Effect of Body-Weight-Support Running on Lower-Limb Biomechanics. *J. Orthop. Sports Phys. Ther.* **2016**, *46*, 784–793. [CrossRef]
51. Bazuelo-Ruiz, B.; Durá, J.-V.; Palomares, N.; Medina, E.; Llana-Belloch, S. Effect of fatigue and gender on kinematics and ground reaction forces variables in recreational runners. *PeerJ* **2018**, *6*, e4489. [CrossRef]
52. Lessi, G.C.; Dos Santos, A.F.; Batista, L.F.; De Oliveira, G.C.; Serrão, F.V. Effects of fatigue on lower limb, pelvis and trunk kinematics and muscle activation: Gender differences. *J. Electromyogr. Kinesiol.* **2017**, *32*, 9–14. [CrossRef]
53. Willson, J.D.; Loss, J.R.; Willy, R.W.; Meardon, S.A. Sex differences in running mechanics and patellofemoral joint kinetics following an exhaustive run. *J. Biomech.* **2015**, *48*, 4155–4159. [CrossRef]

54. Clemente, C.J.; Dick, T.J.M.; Wheatley, R.; Gaschk, J.; Nasir, A.F.A.A.; Cameron, S.F.; Wilson, R.S. Moving in complex environments: A biomechanical analysis of locomotion on inclined and narrow substrates. *J. Exp. Biol.* **2019**, *222*, jeb189654. [CrossRef] [PubMed]
55. Orchard, J.W. Hamstrings are most Susceptible to Injury during the Early Stance Phase of Sprinting. *Br. J. Sports Med.* **2012**, *46*, 88–89. [CrossRef] [PubMed]
56. Lieberman, D.E.; Venkadesan, M.; Werbel, W.A.; Daoud, A.I.; D'Andrea, S.; Davis, I.S.; Mang'Eni, R.O.; Pitsiladis, Y. Foot strike patterns and collision forces in habitually barefoot versus shod runners. *Nature* **2010**, *463*, 531–535. [CrossRef]
57. Higashihara, A.; Nagano, Y.; Ono, T.; Fukubayashi, T. Differences in activation properties of the hamstring muscles during overground sprinting. *Gait Posture* **2015**, *42*, 360–364. [CrossRef]
58. Gantchev, G.N.; Draganova, N. Muscular synergies during different conditions of postural activity. *Acta Physiol. Pharmacol. Bulg.* **1986**, *12*, 58–65.
59. Okada, M. An electromyographic estimation of the relative muscular load in different human postures. *J. Hum. Ergol.* **1973**, *1*, 75–93.
60. Evangelidis, P.E.; Pain, M.T.G.; Folland, J. Angle-specific hamstring-to-quadriceps ratio: A comparison of football players and recreationally active males. *J. Sports Sci.* **2015**, *33*, 309–319. [CrossRef]
61. Chumanov, E.S.; Wille, C.M.; Michalski, M.P.; Heiderscheit, B. Changes in muscle activation patterns when running step rate is increased. *Gait Posture* **2012**, *36*, 231–235. [CrossRef]
62. Yu, B.; Li, L. Research in prevention and rehabilitation of hamstring muscle strain injury. *J. Sport Health Sci.* **2017**, *6*, 253–254. [CrossRef]
63. Gleim, G.W.; Stachenfeld, N.S.; Nicholas, J.A. The influence of flexibility on the economy of walking and jogging. *J. Orthop. Res.* **1990**, *8*, 814–823. [CrossRef]
64. Asmussen, E.; Bonde-Petersen, F. Apparent Efficiency and Storage of Elastic Energy in Human Muscles during Exercise. *Acta Physiol. Scand.* **1974**, *92*, 537–545. [CrossRef] [PubMed]
65. Panagiotopoulos, E.; Strzelczyk, P.; Herrmann, M.; Scuderi, G. Cadaveric study on static medial patellar stabilizers: The dynamizing role of the vastus medialis obliquus on medial patellofemoral ligament. *Knee Surg. Sports Traumatol. Arthrosc.* **2006**, *14*, 7–12. [CrossRef] [PubMed]
66. Mellor, R.; Hodges, P.W. Effect of knee joint angle on motor unit synchronization. *J. Orthop. Res.* **2006**, *24*, 1420–1426. [CrossRef] [PubMed]
67. Lin, C.-F.; Liu, H.; Garrett, W.E.; Yu, B. Effects of a Knee Extension Constraint Brace on Selected Lower Extremity Motion Patterns during a Stop-Jump Task. *J. Appl. Biomech.* **2008**, *24*, 158–165. [CrossRef] [PubMed]
68. Bennett, H.J.; Shen, G.; Cates, H.E.; Zhang, S. Effects of toe-in and toe-in with wider step width on level walking knee biomechanics in varus, valgus, and neutral knee alignments. *Knee* **2017**, *24*, 1326–1334. [CrossRef] [PubMed]
69. Sharma, S.K.; Yadav, S.L.; Singh, U.; Wadhwa, S. Muscle Activation Profiles and Co-Activation of Quadriceps and Hamstring Muscles around Knee Joint in Indian Primary Osteoarthritis Knee Patients. *J. Clin. Diagn. Res.* **2017**, *11*, RC09–RC14. [CrossRef]
70. McLean, S.G.; Neal, R.J.; Myers, P.T.; Walters, M.R. Knee joint kinematics during the sidestep cutting maneuver: Potential for injury in women. *Med. Sci. Sports Exerc.* **1999**, *31*, 959–968. [CrossRef]
71. Oya, Y.; Nakamura, M.; Tabata, E.; Morizono, R.; Mori, S.; Kimuro, Y.; Horikawa, E. Fall risk assessment and knee extensor muscle activity in elderly people. *Nippon. Ronen Igakkai Zasshi. Jpn. J. Geriatr.* **2008**, *45*, 308–314. [CrossRef]
72. Tenan, M.S.; Hackney, A.C.; Griffin, L. Entrainment of vastus medialis complex activity differs between genders. *Muscle Nerve* **2016**, *53*, 633–640. [CrossRef]
73. Tucker, R.; Noakes, T.D. The physiological regulation of pacing strategy during exercise: A critical review. *Br. J. Sports Med.* **2009**, *43*, e1. [CrossRef]
74. Peng, Y.-L.; Tenan, M.S.; Griffin, L. Hip position and sex differences in motor unit firing patterns of the vastus medialis and vastus medialis oblique in healthy individuals. *J. Appl. Physiol.* **2018**, *124*, 1438–1446. [CrossRef] [PubMed]
75. Montgomery, W.H.; Pink, M.; Perry, J. Electromyographic Analysis of Hip and Knee Musculature during Running. *Am. J. Sports Med.* **1994**, *22*, 272–278. [CrossRef] [PubMed]

76. Foss, K.D.B.; Myer, G.D.; Hewett, T.E. Epidemiology of Basketball, Soccer, and Volleyball Injuries in Middle-School Female Athletes. *Phys. Sportsmed.* **2014**, *42*, 146–153. [CrossRef] [PubMed]

Publisher's Note: MDPI stays neutral with regard to jurisdictional claims in published maps and institutional affiliations.

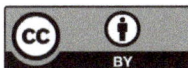
© 2020 by the authors. Licensee MDPI, Basel, Switzerland. This article is an open access article distributed under the terms and conditions of the Creative Commons Attribution (CC BY) license (http://creativecommons.org/licenses/by/4.0/).

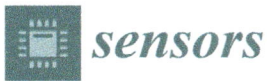 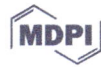

Article

A Random Forest Machine Learning Framework to Reduce Running Injuries in Young Triathletes

Javier Martínez-Gramage [1,*], Juan Pardo Albiach [2], Iván Nacher Moltó [1], Juan José Amer-Cuenca [1], Vanessa Huesa Moreno [3] and Eva Segura-Ortí [1]

[1] Department of Physiotherapy, Universidad Cardenal Herrera-CEU, CEU Universities, 46115 Valencia, Spain; ivan.nacher.molto@gmail.com (I.N.M.); juanjo@uchceu.es (J.J.A.-C.); esegura@uchceu.es (E.S.-O.)
[2] Embedded Systems and Artificial Intelligence Group, Universidad Cardenal Herrera-CEU, CEU Universities, 46115 Valencia, Spain; juaparal@uchceu.es
[3] Triathlon Technification Program, Federación Triatlón Comunidad Valencian, 46940 Manises, Spain; vanessa.huesa@triatlocv.org
* Correspondence: jmg@uchceu.es; Tel.: +34-617024366

Received: 6 October 2020; Accepted: 6 November 2020; Published: 9 November 2020

Abstract: Background: The running segment of a triathlon produces 70% of the lower limb injuries. Previous research has shown a clear association between kinematic patterns and specific injuries during running. Methods: After completing a seven-month gait retraining program, a questionnaire was used to assess 19 triathletes for the incidence of injuries. They were also biomechanically analyzed at the beginning and end of the program while running at a speed of 90% of their maximum aerobic speed (MAS) using surface sensor dynamic electromyography and kinematic analysis. We used classification tree (random forest) techniques from the field of artificial intelligence to identify linear and non-linear relationships between different biomechanical patterns and injuries to identify which styles best prevent injuries. Results: Fewer injuries occurred after completing the program, with athletes showing less pelvic fall and greater activation in gluteus medius during the first phase of the float phase, with increased trunk extension, knee flexion, and decreased ankle dorsiflexion during the initial contact with the ground. Conclusions: The triathletes who had suffered the most injuries ran with increased pelvic drop and less activation in gluteus medius during the first phase of the float phase. Contralateral pelvic drop seems to be an important variable in the incidence of injuries in young triathletes.

Keywords: running; kinematics; gait retraining

1. Introduction

Triathlon is a growing sport with broad participation spanning three disciplines (swimming, cycling, and running) in the same event. This has led to an increase in the incidence of injuries, varying from 37% to 91% in the adult population [1]. In Spain, participation in triathlon has increased by more than 200% among young athletes of school age in recent years (Spanish Triathlon Federation). In the United States, the increase in the participation of children and adolescents in sports, as well as more intense training and specialization at an early age, has contributed to musculoskeletal injuries normally observed in the adult population becoming more common among younger athletes, especially those caused by excessive and repeated use [2]. The risk of musculoskeletal injury in young athletes is related to growth and development which, together with factors such as the rapid increase in the intensity, duration, and volume of physical activity, poor condition, or insufficient sport-specific training, leads to injuries in articular cartilage or other muscle-tendon structures as the result of the exertion of repetitive and excessive stress on the tissues coupled with their lack of adaptation [2–4].

Most triathlon injuries are related to the running segment (58–72%) [5,6] and the incidence of such injuries is similar to that of athletics runners [7]. The anatomical area of injury corresponds to the lower extremities [5,7,8], especially the knee [6]. The most frequent types of injuries in running are patellofemoral pain (PFP), iliotibial band syndrome (ITBS), medial tibial stress syndrome (MTSS), Achilles tendinopathy (AT), plantar fasciitis, stress fractures, and muscle strains [9]. The factors related to the development of running-related injuries are multifactorial and diverse; however, it is widely accepted that kinematic alterations during running may also be related [9].

Gait retraining is a clinical intervention based on real-time feedback from wearables which aims to reduce the risk of injury and improve performance and motivation [10]. Current evidence indicates that this technique, alongside traditional therapeutic interventions, should be considered for use in the treatment of injured runners and to address potentially harmful running mechanics in the healthy population [11]. Various authors have shown a decrease in pain in runners with PFP [12–15] and a 62% reduction in the incidence of injuries in adult athletes [16] as a result of the use of these techniques. Furthermore, Bramah et al. [12] showed an improvement in peak contralateral pelvic drop, hip adduction, and knee flexion after a session of gait retraining, increasing cadence by 10%. Chumanov et al. [17] showed an increase in gluteus medius and gluteus maximus muscle activation associated with an increase in cadence during the final phase of oscillation. To date, there is no evidence on the effect of gait retraining in young triathletes in order to prevent injuries during running.

The objective of this study was to examine the kinematics of the pelvis and activation of the gluteus medius muscle in the float phase to assess their effect on the neuromuscular stability of the pelvis and the incidence of injuries during running in young triathletes over a seven-month observation period after having completed a gait retraining program.

2. Materials and Methods

2.1. Participants

The participants belonged to the Triathlon Technification Plan in High Performance of the Valencian Community in Spain. The study was approved by the Ethics Committee for Biomedical research at the CEU-Cardenal Herrera University, (reference №: CEI18/137) and is registered as a clinical trial (ClinicalTrials.gov registration №: NCT04221698).

Inclusion/exclusion criteria:

19 triathletes (10 males, 9 females) were enrolled in this study (Table 1). Using G*Power software, we calculated that we would need at least 17 subjects in order to detect a large effect size of 0.8, having a power of 0.87 and a critical alpha of 0.05. This calculation was based on the use of t-tests for two dependent means, to detect differences before and after the gait retraining, as we evaluated the same individuals at two different moments."

Table 1. Participant characteristics [a].

	Healthy ($n = 10$)	Injured ($n = 9$)
Age	14.8 ± 1.9	14.4 ± 1.7
Weight, kg	52.7 ± 7.9	56.1 ± 10.9
Height, cm	167.1 ± 8.1	169.1 ± 9.6
Body mass index, kg/m^2	18.8 ± 1.6	19.4 ± 1.8
Years in competition	7.2 ± 1.7	6.8 ± 1.8
Training hours per week	19.2 ± 5.7	17.9 ± 5.1

[a] Values are presented as the mean ± SD.

Participants were included if they reported running a minimum of 2 days per week for the 3 months prior with no reported injuries and with their worst pain rated a minimum of 3 out 10 on a numerical rating scale (NRS) for pain (0 = no pain; 10 = worst possible pain) [12]. Participants were excluded if they reported any previous musculoskeletal surgery, neurological impairment, structural deformity in the knee, pain suffered by trauma or sports activities, having stopped running, or having received additional treatment outside of this study.

2.2. Data Collection

The data were collected via a self-report questionnaire, similar to previous research in triathletes performed to document the incidence of overuse injuries during the 2018 season and in the post-gait-retraining protocol season (during 2019) [18]. Prior to testing, all the participants performed a 5-min warm-up on a treadmill (HP Cosmos Quasar, Nussdorf-Traunstein, Germany) at their preferred speed [12]. Kinematic and dynamic surface electromyography (sEMG) data were collected over 5 min at 90% of the maximum aerobic power speed (as obtained from the Wasserman protocol) to determine the VO2max [19].

Kinematic data were collected from all participants while running on a treadmill. For the 3D pelvis kinematics, the inertial measurement unit (IMU) was placed in S1 with a belt and raw data was recorded by GSensor and GSTUDIO software version 2.8.16.1. (BTS Bioengineering, Garbagnate, Italy). The validity of the IMU system has previously been shown for the measurement of 3D joint kinematics [20,21]. The 3D pelvis kinematics recorded were the difference in pelvic obliquity for the left and right leg, the tilt, and the rotation. A range of kinematic parameters at both initial contact and midstance were selected for analysis in the sagittal plane from a 2-dimensional video [22]. All the videos were recorded (120 frames per second) with the same camera mounted to a portable tripod and Apple iPad Air tablet computer (Apple Inc, Cupertino, CA). The kinematics angles were measured by using the Hudl Technique video analysis application. Parameters at initial contact included foot-strike pattern, tibial inclination, knee flexion, and forward trunk angles. Peak and midstance angles included dorsiflexion, knee flexion, and forward trunk lean angles. Parameters were selected based on previous research to identify running injury patterns [9,22].

sEMG was simultaneously recorded with the kinematics by placing sEMG electrodes on the gluteus medius [23,24]. The SEMG sensors used in this study were pre-gelled self-adhesive bipolar Ag/AgCl disposable surface electrodes of 20 mm (Infant Electrode, Lessa, Barcelona), with 2 cm interelectrode distance. SEMG electrodes were longitudinally placed on the muscle belly of the dominant leg according to SENIAM recommendations [23]. The EMG signal was recorded simultaneously using a FREEEMG 1000 and EMG Analyzer (BTS Bioengineering, Milan, Italy) that was set to a sampling rate of 1000 Hz per channel, and the signals were band-pass filtered from 20 Hz to 450 Hz. The EMG signals were subsequently full-wave rectified and low pass filtered using a bidirectional, 6th order Butterworth filter with a cutoff frequency of 5 Hz. The root mean square (RMS) in several sub-phases was detected. The IMU sensor detected every event performed; initial contact and toe-off of each foot. Moreover, at the same time, the sEMG signal was recorded, so that the system selected the right and left strides and the different subphases; (first stance phase, first float phase, second stance phase, second float phase).

2.3. Retraining Protocol

All participants included completed the 7 months gait retraining program. After baseline assessment, a number of global kinematic contributors to common running injuries were identified and were used for the real-time feedback during the retraining protocol; these were, cadence [12,25], greater peak contralateral pelvic drop (CPD), and trunk forward lean, as well as an extended knee and dorsiflexed ankle at initial contact [9]. Participants were asked to run at a self-selected speed with a 10% increase in their original step rate [11,12,16,25,26]. A modified gait retraining protocol according to Chan et al. [16] was used. In brief, the triathletes participated in four sessions of gait modification over four weeks with one session per week. During the training, the athletes were asked to run at a self-selected speed on a treadmill. Visual biofeedback in the form of a sagittal plane video of the triathlete was displayed on the monitor in front of them (Figure 1).

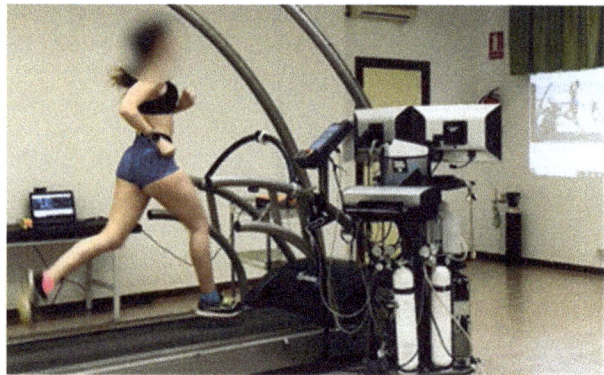

Figure 1. Visual real-time biofeedback during the retraining protocol.

Participants were instructed by the physiotherapist to modify kinematic variables such as the position of their trunk, contact of the foot with the ground, and knee flexion at initial contact. During the first 5 min, participants were instructed to match their footstep to an audible metronome set to the new step rate which increased their original step rate by 10% [12]. The training time was gradually increased from 15 min to 30 min over the four sessions, and visual/audible feedback was progressively reduced in the last 2 sessions (Table 2). Triathletes were then instructed to maintain their new running pattern during their daily running practice only with their watch cadence as feedback.

Table 2. Gait retraining protocol [a].

	VSP	A.M	WCd	Time Session
Session 1 (min)	10'	5'	—	15'
Session 2 (min)	15'	5'	—	20'
Session 3 (min)	10'	—	15'	25'
Session 4 (min)	—	—	30'	30'

[a] Training time and biofeedback time arrangement. VSP, video sagittal plane; AM, audible metronome; WCd, watch cadence.

2.4. Statistical Analysis

With the aim of discovering which variables were more strongly related with the risk of injury among triathletes, we applied machine learning techniques from the artificial intelligence field. Specifically, an ensemble learning method for classification, known as random forests (RF; Breiman, L., 2001) was used to extract the variables that best discriminated between participants who were injured or not in the first period of the study, i.e., before the gait retraining phase. A total of 71 variables were collected from these participants in an excel sheet, although not all these characteristics were selected for the purpose of this present study. Thus, we initially conducted a feature selection protocol to retain only 47 characteristics in order to construct the final dataset as input for the machine learning algorithms. Such variables were selected according to the literature [9,22], to collect data on kinematics, sEMG and running dynamics.

Hence, once the participant data were acquired from the overall observational system, i.e., from the sensors, accelerometers, and video recordings, a raw data set was constructed. After we cleaned this dataset, we converted it into a classification problem for use with machine learning classification techniques. Thus, the problem was added to a supervised learning area' in which the algorithm tried to learn patterns from data previously labeled for a classification. In our case, a new feature named "injured" was used to classify the triathletes who were injured before the retraining (during 2018) and was our dependent variable.

Once most of the important variables were obtained, we also statistically analyzed them through paired t-tests (with an alpha of 0.05) to compare differences in the pre- and post-test measurements, i.e., before and after the retraining phase. To select the appropriate test, first the normality of the data was checked through the Shapiro–Wilk test ($p \geq 0.05$). In case normality was not met an equivalent non-parametric alternative to paired t-test is used, in that case the paired samples Wilcoxon test was employed.

3. Results

A total of 19 volunteer triathletes initially participated in the study. All of them successfully completed the program and there were no losses to follow-up.

3.1. Random Forest Analysis

RF is a well-known algorithm belonging to the family of tree-based methods which yields significant improvements in classification accuracy from large problem sets. It is based on an ensemble of trees which vote for the most popular class [27]. Moreover, trees can capture complex interaction structures with relative bias from among the data and is more competitive than some linear methods [28,29] To develop the model used in this work we used the caret package that integrates the "RandomForest" library [30]. The discriminating ability of the model was assessed by calculating the receiver operating characteristic (ROC) curve to compare different models internally. Additionally, to minimize model overfitting, we used a K-fold cross-validation resampling technique to estimate the efficacy of the model [30], the K value was defined at 10. After testing 15 models, the final AUC-ROC was 0.8 (95% CI 0.6–0.9) and the "mtry" parameter (which defines the number of variables randomly sampled as candidates at each split) was 9. The sensitivity was 0.6 (95% CI 0.3–0.8), the specificity was 0.8 (95% CI 0.5–0.9), the NPV (negative predicted value) was 0.7 (95% CI 0.4-0.9) and the MCC (Matthews correlation coefficient) obtained was 0.4. About the values resulted from the confusion matrix, TP (true positives) were 5 and FP (false positives) were 2, nevertheless the TN (true negatives) were 8 and FN (false negatives) 4.

3.2. Variable Importance

RF is considered a black-box model because gaining insights on a RF prediction rule is difficult because of the large number of trees generated. Notwithstanding, there is a common approach to extract interpretable information about the contribution of different variables [31] which requires computing so-called variable importance measures to rank the variables (i.e., the features) with respect to their relevance in prediction [32].

Figure 2 shows the variable importance calculation obtained from the RF in this study. The features that appeared were the characteristics that were best able to discriminate the classification of an individual as injured during 2018 or not, i.e., they were the most important global kinematic contributors. Thus, these variables were the objective of this current study. As shown, the pelvic kinematics, knee flexion, ankle dorsiflexion at initial contact, and gluteus medius sEMG were the most important variables in this work.

Once the variables that potentially has the strongest influence on distinguishing injured from non-injured triathletes were identified, we calculated the differences in these variables before and after the retraining program. Table 3 shows which features had the strongest influence on the probability of the triathletes being injured.

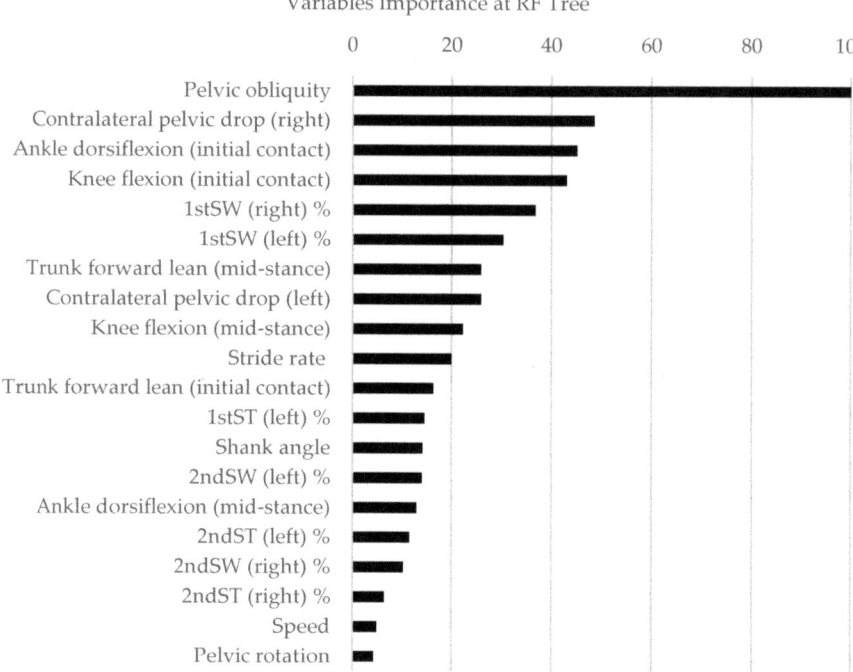

Figure 2. Importance of the variables, scaled according to the "varImp" method in the caret R library for the complete data set.

Table 3. Analysed variables [a].

	PRE	POST	*p* Value
Stride rate, steps/min	174.4 ± 8.3	181.4 ± 7.7	0.00 [b]
Speed, km/h	15.9 ± 1.7	16.5 ± 2.3	0.2
Run cycle, sec	0.69 ± 0.0	0.66 ± 0.0	0.00 [b]
Pelvic obliquity, deg	3 ± 2.1	1 ± 1.8	0.01 [b]
Pelvic tilt, deg	9.4 ± 1.2	9.9 ± 2.3	0.41
Pelvic rotation, deg	21 ± 5.7	19.7 ± 5.2	0,13
Trunk forward lean, deg (initial contact)	7.2 ± 5.3	3.6 ± 2.2	0.00 [b]
Knee flexion, deg (initial contact)	18.8 ± 6.5	22.1 ± 3.1	0.03 [b]
Ankle dorsiflexion, deg (initial contact)	6.8 ± 13.3	0.7 ± 6.6	0.03 [b]
Shank angle, deg (initial contact)	10.6 ± 3.9	5.4 ± 3	0.00 [b]
Knee flexion, deg (mid-stance)	44.4 ± 5.3	36.8 ± 9.6	0.00 [b]
Ankle dorsiflexion, deg (mid-stance)	19.1 ± 7.9	16.6 ± 4	0.28
Trunk forward lean, deg (mid-stance)	11.1 ± 3.8	9.7 ± 2.9	0.24
Contralateral pelvic drop (left), deg	6.7 ± 2.3	2.5 ± 1.6	0.00 [b]
Contralateral pelvic drop (right), deg	5.2 ± 2.4	4.1 ± 1.5	0.04 [b]
1stST (right), %	52.2 ± 15.7	56.1 ± 26.6	0.6
1stSW (right), %	57.9 ± 13.4	72.6 ± 23.6	0.01 [b]
2ndST (right), %	69.7 ± 14.3	96.6 ± 102.7	0.65
2ndSW (right), %	63.4 ± 26.8	61.5 ± 18	0.68
1stST (left), %	66.2 ± 57.4	46.9 ± 24.6	0.06
1stSW (left), %	61.8 ± 14.2	69.4 ± 13.4	0.01 [b]
2ndST (left), %	80.7 ± 42	67 ± 23.8	0.46
2ndSW (left), %	58.7 ± 11.9	78.6 ± 40.8	0.08

[a] Values are presented as the mean ± SD using paired t-tests. 1stST, first stance phase; 1stSW, first float phase; 2ndST, second stance phase; 2ndSW, second float phase. [b] Statistical significance was set at $p \leq 0.05$.

Figure 3 shows the difference between the values obtained before and after retraining, as well as their density curves. After retraining, the difference in pelvic obliquity in the right and left limb (A), ankle dorsiflexion in the initial contact (B), contralateral pelvic drop (C, D), and gluteus medius activation during the first phase of flight (E, F) had reduced in almost all of the participants.

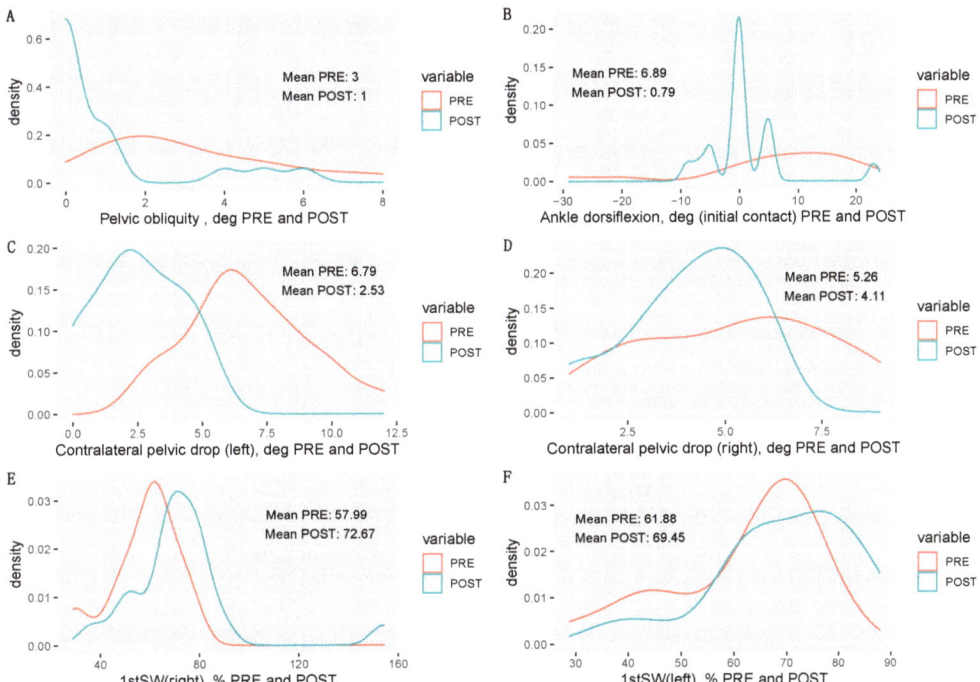

Figure 3. Density plots showing the differences between pre- and post-values obtained before and after the retraining phase. Higher density values on the ordinate axis point out which are the most probable values on the abscissa axis. The difference in pelvic obliquity in the right and left limb (**A**), ankle dorsiflexion in the initial contact (**B**), contralateral pelvic drop (**C,D**), and gluteus medius activation during the first phase of flight (**E,F**).

Figure 4 shows, in more detail, the differences in pelvic obliquity between participants who were injured during the 2018 season and those who were not injured after retraining. Athletes who were not injured had an average pelvic obliquity of around 2 degrees, while those who were injured had a pelvic obliquity twice that value at 4.22 degrees (A), before retraining (B), after retraining both groups had corrected their pelvic obliquity levels with their mean values homogenizing and coming much closer to zero, thus indicating that they had obtained near symmetry.

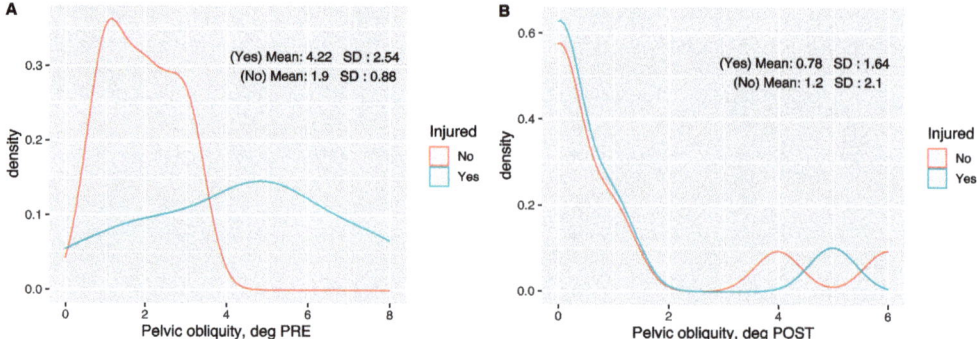

Figure 4. Density plots comparing the differences between injured and non-injured triathletes in terms of the degree of pelvic obliquity between the (**A**) pre-retraining; (**B**) and post-retraining phase values. Higher density values on the ordinate axis point out which are the most probable values on the abscissa axis.

Figure 5 shows, the differences in gluteus medius (right) sEMG before and after retraining protocol. Note the increase in activation during the 1st SW.

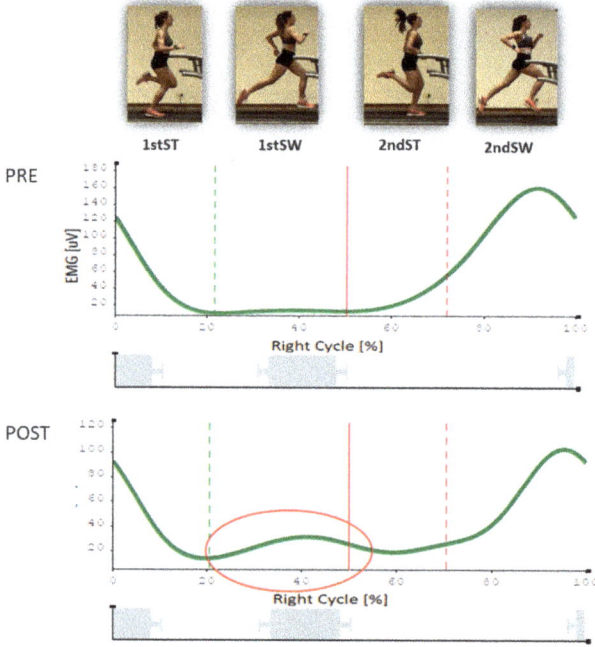

Figure 5. Gluteus medius (right) sEMG plot pre and post.

Figure 6 shows, the differences in pelvic kinematics before and after retraining protocol. Note the reduction in contralateral pelvic drop.

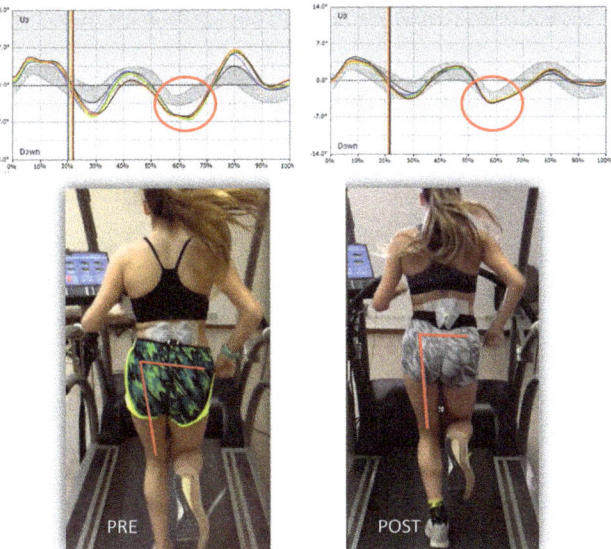

Figure 6. Pelvis kinematics before and after retraining protocol.

4. Discussion

This study identified a number of biomechanical variables that allowed the risk of suffering an injury while running to be detected (Figure 2). To the best of our knowledge, the evidence presented in this work is the first to demonstrate the effect of a gait retraining program in young triathletes in the prevention of injuries. In particular, the triathletes who suffered injuries in the 2018 season had an increased difference in their pelvic obliquity, contralateral fall of the pelvis in the mid-stance phase, increased ankle dorsiflexion during initial contact, and decreased gluteus medius sEMG readings in the first phase of float (Figure 3). We found that differences in pelvic obliquity and contralateral pelvic drop were the most important predictive variables of injury when classifying triathletes as injured or non-injured. These kinematic patterns coincide with the results obtained in previous studies [9,12], except that our study was carried out in a young population for which no similar data is yet available.

Various authors [12,33] have hypothesized that the delay in gluteus medius activation during the stance phase of running could alter neuromuscular control in the hip and pelvis, thus facilitating the loss of stability in the frontal plane. In this study, a significant increase in gluteus medius activation was achieved during the first phase of float. This increase occurred prior to the strike of the contralateral foot, facilitating neuromuscular control in the frontal plane, improving both the difference in the range of obliqueness in each limb and in the fall of the contralateral pelvis. In agreement with other studies that also obtained positive results [12,25,26], this increase in muscle activation seemed to be the result of the increased cadence established during the gait retraining program (by 10% compared to their cadence from the initial assessment), but did not seem to be related to an increase in pelvis stability, making this work the first to show this effect. Bonacci et al. demonstrated that movement patterns in triathletes during the transition from cycling to running are altered at the neuromuscular level [34]. Even in veterans and highly trained triathletes, there is altered muscle recruitment after cycling, which can lead to tibial stress fractures from overuse which may be associated with increased bone load caused by impaired neuromuscular control [35].

Various authors have pointed out that the knee is the most common location for acute and overuse problems in triathletes, followed by the lower leg, lumbar area, and shoulder [5]. Overuse was the reported cause in 41% of the injuries, two-thirds of which occurred during running [36]. Many triathletes continue to train, albeit on a modified routine, after an injury and so further injurious exposures may occur [7]. Defective movement patterns have previously been associated with injuries and pain, although there is no homogeneity between the running pattern and its location. Studies have shown that strengthening exercises alone do not alter these patterns and so a different approach to treatment targeting the motor level is necessary to effect these changes [26]. Therefore, movement retraining, while still adhering to basic principles of motor control, should be part of the intervention skill set [15]. Our study echoes these results but, unlike the studies published to date, focused on young triathletes. Thus, the concepts discussed above could help explain the decrease in the number of injuries produced after the gait retraining program.

Although, one of the most commonly used statistical learning models for discriminant analysis is logistic regression, we were concerned that this technique would only capture linearities in data. However, because RF is a non-parametric machine learning technique, it has additional, powerful capabilities for this type of analysis. This is why this technique is preferred in many medical applications, both for its excellent prediction performance but also its ability to identify important variables [37]. Thus, we decided to implement tree techniques such as RF in this current work. These techniques are simple and powerful machine learning models, that can generate a set of highly interpretable conditions that are straightforward to implement [31].

Limitations of the Study and Future Activities

One of the limitations of the study is the lack of a control group. However, all the included triathletes fulfilled homogeneous inclusion criteria running a minimum of two days per week for the three months prior with no reported injuries and with their worst pain rated a minimum of 3 out 10 on a numerical rating scale (NRS) for pain (0 = no pain; 10 = worst possible pain). A second limitation of this work is the sample size, since this only allows us to obtain clues about what we are investigating although encourages us to continue working in this line as the results seem very promising. However, we must also take into account that obtaining data on high-performance athletes is quite difficult since it is a very small population and therefore the sample can never be too large. Nevertheless, it is also true that the sample, despite being small, is quite homogeneous. This allows us to think that the conclusions of the research could be generalized to other athletes, who will have very similar characteristics to the sample we are working on. On the contrary, is difficult to profit all the potential of the present artificial intelligence techniques that bring a new framework to study the data, such models need from large datasets. The future directions of this work should be addressed towards the application of these results in the field of training of young triathletes to reduce running injuries. Future research should determine biomechanical running patterns that indicate a lower incidence of injury in young athletes.

5. Conclusions

This study identified a number of scaled and related variables based on their importance in preventing injuries during running. In particular, we found an increase in the obliquity of the pelvis, fall of the contralateral pelvis, the extension of the knee, dorsiflexion of the ankle in the initial contact, and less activation of the gluteus medium during the first phase of float in triathletes who suffered injuries. After the gait retraining program, the number of injuries was reduced by improving the neuromuscular stability of the pelvis of these athletes, thus providing an easy way to assess and readjust their running style in clinical practice.

Author Contributions: Conceptualization, J.M.-G. and V.H.M.; methodology, J.M.-G. and I.N.M.; machine learning models, J.P.A.; validation, J.P.A. and E.S.-O.; formal analysis, I.N.M.; research, J.M.-G. and I.N.M.; resources, V.H.M.; data curation, J.J.A.-C.; writing—original draft preparation, J.M.-G.; writing—review and editing, J.M.-G., I.N.M., and J.P.A.; visualization, J.J.A.-C.; supervision, E.S.-O.; project administration, E.S.-O. All authors have read and agreed to the published version of the manuscript.

Funding: This research received no external funding.

Acknowledgments: We appreciate the voluntary participation of young athletes from Triathlon Technification Plan in High Performance of the Valencian Community in Spain.

Conflicts of Interest: The authors declare no conflict of interest.

References

1. McHardy, A.; Pollard, H.; Fernandez, M. Triathlon Injuries: A Review of the Literature and Discussion of Potential Injury Mechanisms. *Clin. Chiropr.* **2006**, *3*, 129–138.
2. Patel, D.R.; Yamasaki, A.; Brown, K. Epidemiology of Sports-Related Musculoskeletal Injuries in Young Athletes in the United States. *Transl. Pediatr.* **2017**, *6*, 160–166. [CrossRef] [PubMed]
3. Brenner, J.S.; American Academy of Pediatrics Council on Sports Medicine and Fitness. Overuse Injuries, Overtraining, and Burnout in Child and Adolescent Athletes. *Pediatrics* **2007**, *119*, 1242–1245. [CrossRef] [PubMed]
4. Patel, D.R.; Baker, R.J. Musculoskeletal Injuries in Sports. *Prim. Care: Clin. Off. Pr.* **2006**, *33*, 545–579. [CrossRef] [PubMed]
5. Vleck, V.E.; Garbutt, G. Injury and Training Characteristics of Male Elite, Development Squad, and Club Triathletes. *Int. J. Sports Med.* **1998**, *19*, 38–42. [CrossRef] [PubMed]
6. Clements, K.; Yates, B.; Curran, M. The Prevalence of Chronic Knee Injury in Triathletes. *Br. J. Sports Med.* **1999**, *33*, 214–216. [CrossRef] [PubMed]
7. Cipriani, D.J.; Swartz, J.D.; Hodgson, C.M. Triathlon and the Multisport Athlete. *J. Orthop. Sports Phys. Ther.* **1998**, *27*, 42–50. [CrossRef]
8. Burns, J.; Keenan, A.M.; Redmond, A.C. Factors Associated with Triathlon-Related Overuse Injuries. *J. Orthop. Sports Phys. Ther.* **2003**, *33*, 177–184. [CrossRef] [PubMed]
9. Bramah, C.; Preece, S.J.; Gill, N.; Herrington, L. Is there a Pathological Gait Associated with Common Soft Tissue Running Injuries? *Am. J. Sports Med.* **2018**, *46*, 3023–3031. [CrossRef]
10. Van Hooren, B.; Goudsmit, J.; Restrepo, J.; Vos, S. Real-Time Feedback by Wearables in Running: Current Approaches, Challenges and Suggestions for Improvements. *J. Sports Sci.* **2019**, *38*, 214–230. [CrossRef]
11. Agresta, C.; Brown, A. Gait Retraining for Injured and Healthy Runners using Augmented Feedback: A Systematic Literature Review. *J. Orthop. Sports Phys. Ther.* **2015**, *45*, 576–584. [CrossRef]
12. Bramah, C.; Preece, S.J.; Gill, N.; Herrington, L. A 10% Increase in Step Rate Improves Running Kinematics and Clinical Outcomes in Runners with Patellofemoral Pain at 4 Weeks and 3 Months. *Am. J. Sports Med.* **2019**, *47*, 3406–3413. [CrossRef]
13. Noehren, B.; Scholz, J.; Davis, I. The Effect of Real-Time Gait Retraining on Hip Kinematics, Pain and Function in Subjects with Patellofemoral Pain Syndrome. *Br. J. Sports Med.* **2011**, *45*, 691–696. [CrossRef]
14. Willy, R.W.; Scholz, J.P.; Davis, I.S. Mirror Gait Retraining for the Treatment of Patellofemoral Pain in Female Runners. *Clin. Biomech.* **2012**, *27*, 1045–1051. [CrossRef] [PubMed]
15. Davis, I.S.; Tenforde, A.S.; Neal, B.S.; Roper, J.L.; Willy, R.W. Gait Retraining as an Intervention for Patellofemoral Pain. *Curr. Rev. Musculoskelet. Med.* **2020**, *13*, 103–114. [CrossRef]
16. Chan, Z.Y.S.; Zhang, J.H.; Au, I.P.H.; An, W.W.; Shum, G.L.K.; Ng, G.Y.F.; Cheung, R.T.H. Gait Retraining for the Reduction of Injury Occurrence in Novice Distance Runners: 1-Year Follow-Up of a Randomized Controlled Trial. *Am. J. Sports Med.* **2018**, *46*, 388–395. [CrossRef]
17. Chumanov, E.S.; Wille, C.M.; Michalski, M.P.; Heiderscheit, B.C. Changes in Muscle Activation Patterns when Running Step Rate is Increased. *Gait Posture* **2012**, *36*, 231–235. [CrossRef] [PubMed]
18. Manninen, J.S.; Kallinen, M. Low Back Pain and Other Overuse Injuries in a Group of Japanese Triathletes. *Br. J. Sports Med.* **1996**, *30*, 134–139. [CrossRef]
19. Beltz, N.M.; Gibson, A.L.; Janot, J.M.; Kravitz, L.; Mermier, C.M.; Dalleck, L.C. Graded Exercise Testing Protocols for the Determination of VO2max: Historical Perspectives, Progress, and Future Considerations. *J. Sports Med.* **2016**, *2016*. [CrossRef]
20. Al-Amri, M.; Nicholas, K.; Button, K.; Sparkes, V.; Sheeran, L.; Davies, J.L. Inertial Measurement Units for Clinical Movement Analysis: Reliability and Concurrent Validity. *Sensors* **2018**, *18*, 719. [CrossRef]
21. Teufl, W.; Miezal, M.; Taetz, B.; FrÃ¶hlich, M.; Bleser, G. Validity of Inertial Sensor Based 3D Joint Kinematics of Static and Dynamic Sport and Physiotherapy Specific Movements. *PLoS ONE* **2019**, *14*. [CrossRef]

22. Pipkin, A.; Kotecki, K.; Hetzel, S.; Heiderscheit, B. Reliability of a Qualitative Video Analysis for Running. *J. Orthop. Sports Phys. Ther.* **2016**, *46*, 556–561. [CrossRef] [PubMed]
23. SENIAM. European Recommendations for Surface Electromyography, Results of the SENIAM Project. *Mt. Res. Dev.* **1999**, *8*, 13–54.
24. Hermens, H.J.; Freriks, B.; Disselhorst-Klug, C.; Rau, G. Development of Recommendations for SEMG Sensors and Sensor Placement Procedures. *J. Electromyogr. Kinesiol.* **2000**, *10*, 361–374. [CrossRef]
25. Hafer, J.F.; Brown, A.M.; deMille, P.; Hillstrom, H.J.; Garber, C.E. The Effect of a Cadence Retraining Protocol on Running Biomechanics and Efficiency: A Pilot Study. *J. Sports Sci.* **2015**, *33*, 724–731. [CrossRef]
26. Adams, D.; Pozzi, F.; Willy, R.W.; Carrol, A.; Zeni, J. Altering Cadence Or Vertical Oscillation during Running: Effects on Running Related Injury Factors. *Int. J. Sports Phys. Ther.* **2018**, *13*, 633–642. [CrossRef] [PubMed]
27. Breiman, L. Random Forests. *Mach. Learn.* **2001**, *45*, 5–32. [CrossRef]
28. Hastie, T.; Friedman, J.; Tibshirani, R. *The Elements of Statistical Learning*; Springer Series in Statistics: New York, NY, USA, 2001; p. 189.
29. Couronne, R.; Probst, P.; Boulesteix, A.L. Random Forest Versus Logistic Regression: A Large-Scale Benchmark Experiment. *BMC Bioinformatics* **2018**, *19*, 270. [CrossRef]
30. Kuhn, M.; Johnson, K. *Applied Predictive Modeling*; Springer: New York, NY, USA, 2013; Volume 26, p. 386.
31. Climent, M.T.; Pardo, J.; Munoz-Almaraz, F.J.; Guerrero, M.D.; Moreno, L. Decision Tree for Early Detection of Cognitive Impairment by Community Pharmacists. *Front. Pharmacol.* **2018**, *9*, 1232. [CrossRef]
32. Greenwell, B.M.; Boehmke, B.C.; McCarthy, A.J. A Simple and Effective Model-Based Variable Importance Measure. *arXiv* **2018**, arXiv:arXiv:1805.04755.
33. Willson, J.D.; Kernozek, T.W.; Arndt, R.L.; Reznichek, D.A.; Scott Straker, J. Gluteal Muscle Activation during Running in Females with and without Patellofemoral Pain Syndrome. *Clin. Biomech.* **2011**, *26*, 735–740. [CrossRef] [PubMed]
34. Bonacci, J.; Saunders, P.U.; Alexander, M.; Blanch, P.; Vicenzino, B. Neuromuscular Control and Running Economy is Preserved in Elite International Triathletes After Cycling. *Sports Biomech.* **2011**, *10*, 59–71. [CrossRef]
35. Chapman, A.R.; Vicenzino, B.; Blanch, P.; Hodges, P.W. Is Running Less Skilled in Triathletes than Runners Matched for Running Training History? *Med. Sci. Sports Exerc.* **2008**, *40*, 557–565. [CrossRef] [PubMed]
36. Korkia, P.K.; Tunstall-Pedoe, D.S.; Maffulli, N. An epidemiological investigation of training and injury patterns in British triathletes. *Br. J. Sports Med.* **1994**, *28*, 191–196. [CrossRef] [PubMed]
37. Saarela, M.; Ryynanen, O.P.; Ayramo, S. Predicting Hospital Associated Disability from Imbalanced Data using Supervised Learning. *Artif. Intell. Med.* **2019**, *95*, 88–95. [CrossRef]

Publisher's Note: MDPI stays neutral with regard to jurisdictional claims in published maps and institutional affiliations.

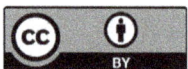

© 2020 by the authors. Licensee MDPI, Basel, Switzerland. This article is an open access article distributed under the terms and conditions of the Creative Commons Attribution (CC BY) license (http://creativecommons.org/licenses/by/4.0/).

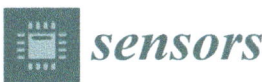

Systematic Review

Is This the Real Life, or Is This Just Laboratory? A Scoping Review of IMU-Based Running Gait Analysis

Lauren C. Benson [1,2,*], Anu M. Räisänen [1,3], Christian A. Clermont [1,4] and Reed Ferber [1,5,6]

1. Faculty of Kinesiology, University of Calgary, Calgary, AB T2N 1N4, Canada; araisanen@westernu.edu (A.M.R.); christian.clermont@ucalgary.ca (C.A.C.); rferber@ucalgary.ca (R.F.)
2. Tonal Strength Institute, Tonal, San Francisco, CA 94107, USA
3. Department of Physical Therapy Education, College of Health Sciences—Northwest, Western University of Health Sciences, Lebanon, OR 97355, USA
4. Sport Product Testing, Canadian Sport Institute Calgary, Calgary, AB T3B 6B7, Canada
5. Cumming School of Medicine, Faculty of Nursing, University of Calgary, Calgary, AB T2N 1N4, Canada
6. Running Injury Clinic, Calgary, AB T2N 1N4, Canada
* Correspondence: lauren.benson@ucalgary.ca

Abstract: Inertial measurement units (IMUs) can be used to monitor running biomechanics in real-world settings, but IMUs are often used within a laboratory. The purpose of this scoping review was to describe how IMUs are used to record running biomechanics in both laboratory and real-world conditions. We included peer-reviewed journal articles that used IMUs to assess gait quality during running. We extracted data on running conditions (indoor/outdoor, surface, speed, and distance), device type and location, metrics, participants, and purpose and study design. A total of 231 studies were included. Most (72%) studies were conducted indoors; and in 67% of all studies, the analyzed distance was only one step or stride or <200 m. The most common device type and location combination was a triaxial accelerometer on the shank (18% of device and location combinations). The most common analyzed metric was vertical/axial magnitude, which was reported in 64% of all studies. Most studies (56%) included recreational runners. For the past 20 years, studies using IMUs to record running biomechanics have mainly been conducted indoors, on a treadmill, at prescribed speeds, and over small distances. We suggest that future studies should move out of the lab to less controlled and more real-world environments.

Keywords: biomechanics; wearable devices; injury; running conditions

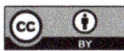

1. Introduction

Wearable technology has been adopted among sports science researchers and practitioners to capture movement in the conditions in which sports take place [1]. Inertial measurement units (IMUs) are a type of wearable technology that can be used to measure running biomechanics [2]. The use of IMUs for real-world monitoring of running biomechanics may provide insights that are different from observations in controlled conditions [3–5]. Historically, the space and computational costs of onboard data storage and processing have created challenges for long-term monitoring of running biomechanics [2]. However, as device capabilities and approaches to big data have improved, the large amounts of data produced by IMUs have changed from a liability to an opportunity for real-world running biomechanical analyses.

While several editorials and commentaries have indicated the capability of IMUs to study running biomechanical gait patterns out of the laboratory and recommend that investigators do so [2–4,6,7], these suggestions were not based on systematic evidence. Therefore, we do not know how many studies are using IMUs to record running biomechanics and in which settings. In 2018, a systematic review identified only 14 studies that used wearables for running gait analysis for distances greater than 200 m [8]. As the use of wearables is a trending topic in the field of running biomechanics, we expect the number of studies that analyze running gait using IMUs in real-world settings to dramatically increase.

Thus, the purpose of this review is to systematically identify the scope of how IMUs are used to record running biomechanics in all settings. Our primary focus is on the conditions (i.e., location, surface, speed, and distance) in which IMUs capture running quality. Our secondary objectives were to identify the devices and sensors used, the calculated metrics and analyses from the IMU signals, the characteristics of the participants in the studies, and the study details such as the purpose and study design. By identifying the scope of IMU-based running biomechanical studies, we aim to mark the progress made and the steps that remain for analyzing running gait in real-world settings.

2. Materials and Methods

2.1. Registration

The review protocol was registered through the Open Science Framework on 24 August 2020 (https://osf.io/gsmvj/?view_only=cc97d0034c5341bca4ac181878770ec7, accessed on 16 February 2022).

2.2. Eligibility Criteria

This review was designed to capture all journal articles that used IMUs to assess gait quality during running, published in English since 2001. Exclusion criteria were: not original research article (e.g., review papers, conference proceedings, and dissertations); the study did not involve human subjects; the study did not involve running; running quality was analyzed as part of another athletic task (e.g., change of direction and playing a team sport); only spatiotemporal variables were analyzed (e.g., speed, cadence, and step length); there was no use of IMUs; the sole purpose of the study was the use of IMUs for any purpose other than gait analysis; the study primarily focused on development of new technology or methods rather than gait analysis; and running was only with the use of robotic orthoses, exoskeletons, or virtual reality environments.

2.3. Search Strategy

The search was executed in the scientific databases CINAHL, Embase, HealthSTAR, MEDLINE, PsycINFO, PubMed, SPORTDiscus and Web of Science. Databases were searched for articles related to IMUs and running using the following terms and logic: (Wearable Electronic Devices/OR Accelerometry/OR wearable* OR inertial sensor* OR inertial measurement unit* OR imu OR imus OR gyroscope* OR magnetometer* OR acceleromet*) AND (Running/OR running OR jogging), where/indicates a MESH term and * indicates the search term can have any ending. The final search was conducted on 24 April 2021.

2.4. Study Selection

One author (LCB) searched each database, combined the resulting records from each database, and performed initial screening for duplicates, format, and language. The records that passed initial screening were uploaded to an online review management platform (Covidence, Melbourne, Australia). Two authors (LCB and AMR) screened the title and abstract of all records for eligibility, with one author (CAC) serving as the tiebreaker. One author (LCB) obtained and uploaded the full text of the records that passed the title and abstract screening. The full-text review was conducted by two authors (LCB and AMR), and the reason for exclusion was indicated for articles deemed ineligible. In the case where multiple exclusion criteria were relevant, the criterion highest in the list above was chosen. One author (CAC) served as the tiebreaker for conflicts on whether an article should be included or excluded as well as conflicts on the selected reason for exclusion.

2.5. Data Extraction

Each included study was assigned to an author (LCB, AMR, and CAC) who extracted data related to the study, participants, conditions, device(s), and analysis.

2.5.1. Conditions
Location

Categorized as: indoor, outdoor, or indoor and outdoor.

Running Surface

Categorized as: track, pavement or sidewalk, grass (includes real or artificial), trail (includes gravel), treadmill, floor or platform, or not controlled.

Speed

Categorized as: exact (minimum speed of 1.67 m/s except for incremental runs that started with walking but ended with running; recorded in units of m/s), relative—calculated (based on a race time or a specific test [e.g., VO2max and heart rate]), relative—subjective (self-selected or based on participant interpretation [e.g., maximal, slow, and moderate]), and not controlled (races or training runs).

Full Distance or Duration

For each surface, the complete distance or duration was calculated by multiplying the distance or duration by the number of trials and number of days and reported using units from the study. Exceptions for using the reported units for the full distance or duration include more than 180 s (converted to minutes) and more than 5000 m (converted to km).

Analyzed Distance

For each surface, the amount of IMU data analyzed was categorized as: single step or stride per trial for one or more trials, consecutive steps for less than 200 m per trial for one or more trials, consecutive steps over 200 m to 1000 m per trial for one or more trials, consecutive steps over more than 1000 m for one trial, consecutive steps over more than 1000 m for multiple trials. A trial was a repeated run on the same or different course, or a repeated or different segment run on the same or different days. If not provided, the analyzed distance was calculated from the reported speed. If only the number of steps or insufficient information was reported for determining the analyzed distance, equivalences between 200 m, 60 s, and 150 steps/min were used—200 m in 60 s corresponds with a speed of 3.33 m/s, which is a common intermediate running speed [9,10], and 150 steps/min is on the low end of preferred running cadence [11–14], representing a low threshold of number of steps that equates to 200 m.

2.5.2. Device(s)
Brand and Model

As reported.

Device Location(s)

Categorized as: foot (any portion of foot or shoe), shank (includes tibia/shin, calf, ankle), thigh, lower back (includes pelvis, lumbar spine), upper back (includes thoracic, cervical spine), chest, arm (includes wrist), head. If multiple devices were placed on the same location (e.g., both feet), the location was only recorded once.

Sensors

The number of axes were recorded for each type of sensor: Accelerometer, gyroscope, magnetometer.

2.5.3. Analysis
Statistical Approach

Categorized as: descriptive, inferential, or machine learning. Descriptive was only used when it was the only type of analysis performed. Machine learning was included only when it was used as part of the statistical approach and not to generate metrics (e.g., estimated ground reaction forces from accelerations using an artificial neural network).

Metrics

Categorized as: vertical/axial magnitude (e.g., peak and RMS), anterior–posterior magnitude (e.g., peak and RMS), medial–lateral magnitude (e.g., peak, RMS), resultant magnitude (e.g., peak and RMS), axis ratio (e.g., axis RMS/resultant RMS), variability—any axis (e.g., SD and CV), loading rate, power, PlayerLoad, shock attenuation—time domain, shock attenuation—frequency domain, frequency content, spectral power or spectral energy, stiffness, joint angles or ROM, joint angular velocity, segment rotation, segment rotation velocity, COM displacement (e.g., bounce, oscillation, and trajectory), COM change in velocity (e.g., braking), symmetry or regularity (based on autocorrelation of signal), stability (e.g., Lyapunov exponent), or entropy. Due to the large number of studies investigating shock absorption using an accelerometer placed on the tibia, when the axis for tibial acceleration magnitude was not specified, it was assumed to be vertical. For other situations where the axis of acceleration magnitude was not reported, it was assumed to be the resultant.

2.5.4. Participants
Sex

Females, males, or females and males.

Type

Non-runner (includes sedentary, adults, recreational team sport athletes), recreational runner (described as a runner; includes runners with defined weekly mileage, well-trained runners), and competitive runner (competes at a high level; includes elite, member of a collegiate or higher sports team).

Injury Status

Injured or uninjured.

Age

The central tendency and variability of age were recorded across all participant types. If the study only reported age for each participant group, the overall mean age was calculated.

2.5.5. Study Details
Country

Based on ethics approval, or if not reported, the first author's first affiliation.

Study Design

Randomized controlled trial, quasi-experimental, case study, case series, case control, prospective cohort, retrospective cohort, or cross-sectional.

Purpose

Equipment intervention, training intervention, validity or reliability of metric(s), compare metrics, compare groups, identify changes due to fatigue, identify changes between sessions, identify changes between conditions, associate with injury or associate with performance. Some studies had multiple purposes.

2.6. Quality Assessment

A formal quality assessment was not part of this scoping review. However, we evaluated the amount of information reported (adequate or lacking) and the relevance to running and IMUs (appropriate or not appropriate) for each set of data extracted (study, participants, conditions, device(s), and analysis) of each study.

3. Results

3.1. Study Selection

A total of 16,023 records were identified across all databases (Figure 1) and 7336 records were excluded during title and abstract screening. Of the 402 full-text articles that were assessed, 171 were excluded and 231 studies met all eligibility criteria and were included.

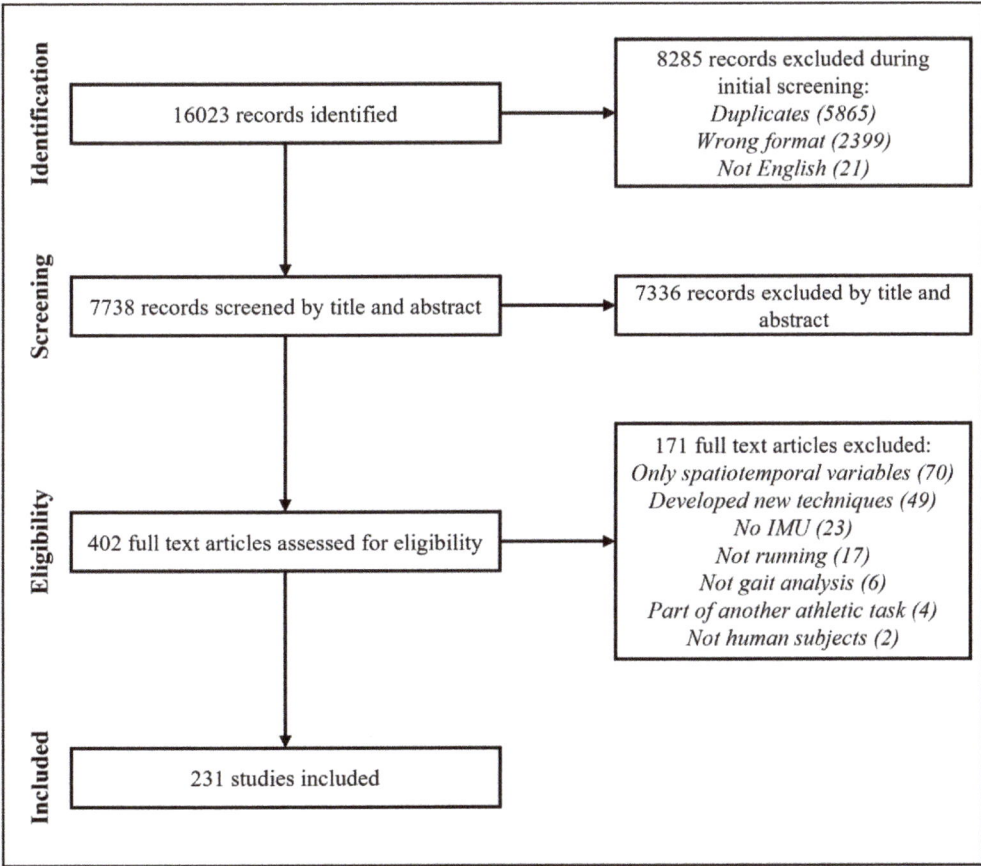

Figure 1. Flowchart of the study selection process.

3.2. Data Extraction

The complete data extracted for each included study are reported as an appendix. The conditions, devices, analysis, participants, and study details are summarized here with key details provided in Tables 1–6.

Table 1. Study characteristics where the analyzed distance is one step/stride.

Ref.	Author	Year	Location	Surface	Speed	Distance/Duration	Type	Number (Sex)	Overall Age	Metric(s)
[15]	Aubol, et al.	2020	Indoor	Floor	3.0 m/s	30 m	Rec.	19 (10 F, 9 M)	Mean: 31; SD: 6	VT, Res.
[16]	Blackah, et al.	2013	Indoor	Treadmill	3.83 m/s	2 min	Rec.	9 (0 F, 9 M)	Mean: 19; SD: 1	VT, Shock-time, Shock-frequency
[17]	Boyer and Nigg	2006	Indoor	Floor	3 m/s	320 m	Non	5 (0 F, 5 M)	Mean: 24.6; SD: 2.5	VT, Shock-frequency
[18]	Chadefaux, et al.	2019	Indoor	Floor	3.1 m/s	175 m	Rec.	10 (0 F, 10 M)	Mean: 21; SD: 3	VT, AP, ML, Res., Freq.
[19]	Clansey, et al.	2012	Indoor	Floor	4.5 m/s	270 m	Rec.	21 (0 F, 21 M)	Mean: 36.2; SD: 12.5	VT, Loading Rate
[20]	Crowell and Davis	2011	Indoor	Floor	3.7 m/s	230 m	Rec.	10 (6 F, 4 M)	Mean: 26; SD: 7	VT, Loading Rate
[21]	Edwards, et al.	2019	Indoor	Floor	3.3, 5.0, and 6.7 m/s	≥450 m	Comp.	10 (0 F, 10 M)	Mean: 21; SD: 2	VT
[22]	Gil-Rey, et al.	2021	Indoor	Track	incremental from 1.69 m/s	≥40 min	Non	82 (82 F, 0 M)	Mean: 59.1; SD: 5.4	VT, AP, ML
[23]	Hagen, et al.	2009	Indoor	Floor	3.3 m/s	NR	Rec.	20 (0 F, 20 M)	Mean: 32; SD: 10	VT
[24]	Havens, et al.	2018	Indoor	Floor	self-selected	90 m	Non	14 (7 F, 7 M)	Mean: 29; SD: 12	VT
[25]	Higgins, et al.	2021	Indoor	Floor	self-selected	368 m	Non	30 (15 F, 15 M)	Mean: 23.0; SD: 4.5	VT, Res.
[26]	Lam, et al.	2018	Indoor	Floor	3.0 and 6.0 m/s	230 m	Comp.	18 (0 F, 18 M)	Mean: 25.0; SD: 2.3	VT
[27]	Laughton, et al.	2003	Indoor	Floor	3.7 m/s	≥57 m	Rec.	15 (NS)	Mean: 22.46; SD: 4	VT
[28]	Mavor, et al.	2020	Indoor	Floor	self-selected	30 m	Non	18 (9 F, 9 M)	Mean: 23.7; SD: 3.44	Joint ROM VT, Res.,
[29]	Meinert, et al.	2016	Indoor	Floor	2.9 m/s	30 m	Rec.	20 (0 F, 20 M)	Mean: 22.7; SD: 2.9	Shock-frequency, Spectral Energy
[30]	Mercer, et al.	2005	Indoor	Treadmill	2.9 m/s comfortable, faster, slower	10 s	Non	6 (NS)	Mean: 26; SD: 4.0	VT, Shock-time
[31]	Milner, et al.	2020	Indoor	Floor	3.0 m/s	≥30 m	Rec.	19 (10 F, 9 M)	Mean: 31; SD: 6	VT, AP, ML, Res., Seg. Rot.
[32]	Milner, et al.	2006	Indoor	Floor	3.7 m/s	115 m	Rec.	40 (40 F, 0 M)	Mean: 26; SD: 9	VT
[33]	Nedergaard, et al.	2018	Indoor	Floor	2, 3, 4, and 5 m/s	≥64 m	Non	20 (0 F, 20 M)	Mean: 22; SD: 4	Res.
[34]	Ogon, et al.	2001	Indoor	Floor	slow	144 m	Non	12 (5 F, 7 M)	Mean: 32.9; SD: 7.9	VT
[35]	Rowlands, et al.	2012	Indoor	Floor	self-selected	320 m	Non	10 (5 F, 5 M)	Mean: 29.4; SD: 7.3	VT, Res., Loading Rate
[36]	Sayer, et al.	2020	Indoor	Floor	2.8–3.2 m/s	NR	Non	64 (64 F, 0 M)	Mean: 13.7; SD: 2.3	VT, AP
[37]	Sinclair and Dillon	2016	Indoor	Floor	4 m/s	110 m	Rec.	12 (0 F, 12 M)	Mean: 23.59; SD: 2	VT, Loading Rate
[38]	Sinclair and Sant	2017	Indoor	Floor	4 m/s	NR	Non	13 (0 F, 13 M)	Mean: 27.81; SD: 7.02	VT, Loading Rate
[39]	Sinclair, et al.	2016	Indoor	Floor	4 m/s	NR	Rec.	12 (0 F, 12 M)	Mean: 23.11; SD: 5.01	VT, Loading Rate

Table 1. Cont.

Ref.	Author	Year	Location	Surface	Speed	Distance/Duration	Type	Number (Sex)	Overall Age	Metric(s)
[40]	Sinclair, et al.	2015	Indoor	Floor	4 m/s	110 m	Rec.	12 (12 F; 0 M)	Mean: 21.45; SD: 2.98	VT, Loading Rate
[41]	Sinclair, et al.	2017	Indoor	Grass	4 m/s	NR	Comp.	12 (0 F; 12 M)	Mean: 22.47; SD: 1.13	VT
[42]	Thompson, et al.	2016	Indoor	Floor	self-selected	450 m	Rec.	10 (5 F; 5 M)	Mean: 26; SD: 7.3	Res.
[43]	Trama, et al.	2019	Indoor	Track	2.22, 2.92, 3.61, and 4.31 m/s	≥60 m	Rec.	20 (0 F; 20 M)	Mean: 23.9; SD: 2.1	VT, Shock-frequency, Freq., Spectral Energy
[44]	Van den Berghe, et al.	2019	Indoor	Floor	2.55, 3.20, and 5.10 m/s	768 m	Rec.	13 (NS)	NR	VT, Res.
[45]	Wundersitz, et al.	2013	Indoor	Floor	maximal	50 m	Non	17 (5 F; 12 M)	Mean: 21; SD: 2	VT, Res.

Note: NR = not reported; Pavement = pavement or sidewalk; Floor = floor or platform; Rec. = recreational; Comp. = competitive; Non = non-runners; Disp. = displacement; Δv = change in velocity; Sym. = symmetry or regularity; Res. = resultant magnitude; VT = vertical/axial magnitude; AP = anterior-posterior magnitude; ML = medial-lateral magnitude; Seg. Rot. = segment rotation; Joint = joint angles or range of motion; Joint ω = joint angular velocity; Freq. = frequency content. = shock attenuation—frequency domain; Joint ROM = joint angles or range of motion; Shock—time = shock attenuation—time domain; Shock—frequency

Table 2. Study characteristics where the analyzed distance is <200 m.

Ref.	Author	Year	Location	Surface	Speed	Distance/Duration	Type	Number (Sex)	Overall Age	Metric(s)
[46]	Adams, et al.	2016	Indoor	Treadmill	comfortable	2 min	Rec.	20 (8 F; 12 M)	Mean: 30.0; SD: 7.0	COM Disp.
[47]	Adams, et al.	2018	Indoor	Treadmill	comfortable	90 s	Rec.	20 (NS)	NR	COM Disp.
[48]	Argunsah Bayram, et al.	2021	Indoor	Treadmill	preferred	15 min	Non	24 (10 F; 14 M)	Mean: 22.2; SD: 0.9	Joint ROM, COM Disp., Sym. or Reg.
[49]	Armitage, et al.	2021	Indoor	Floor	sprint	21 m	Non	16 (0 F; 16 M)	Mean: 17; SD: 1	Res.
			Indoor	Treadmill	3.0 m/s	1 min				
[50]	Backes, et al.	2020	Indoor	Treadmill	2.78 and 3.33 m/s	2 min	Rec.	39 (6 F; 33 M)	Mean: 41.8; SD: 9.8	COM Disp.
[51]	Bailey and Harle	2015	Indoor	Treadmill	2.3, 2.7, 3.0, and 3.4 m/s	6 min	Rec.	3 (1 F; 2 M)	NR	Res., Seg. Rot.
			Outdoor	Grass	steady state	100 m				
			Outdoor	Pavement	steady state	100 m				
			Outdoor	Track	steady state	100 m				
			Outdoor	Trail	steady state	100 m				

Table 2. Cont.

Ref.	Author	Year	Location	Surface	Speed	Distance/Duration	Type	Number (Sex)	Overall Age	Metric(s)
[52]	Barnes, et al.	2021	Outdoor	Grass	2.1, 2.9, and 4.4 m/s	140 m	Comp.	29 (0 F, 29 M)	Mean: 25.2; SD: 3.5	PlayerLoad
[53]	Bastiaansen, et al.	2020	NR	NR	maximal sprint	90 m	Non	5 (0 F, 5 M)	Mean: 22.5; SD: 2.1	Joint ROM, Joint ω
[54]	Benson, et al.	2018	Indoor	Treadmill	preferred	2 min	Rec.	44 (18 F, 26 M)	Mean: 13.9; SD: 12.3	VT, AP, ML, Res.
[55]	Bergamini, et al.	2012	Outdoor	Track	sprint	180 m	Comp. Rec.	5 (2 F, 3 M) 6 (2 F, 4 M)	NR	Res., Joint ω
[56]	Boey, et al.	2017	NR NR NR	Pavement Track Trail	3.06 m/s 3.06 m/s 3.06 m/s	90 m 90 m 90 m	Rec. Non	23 (11 F, 12 M) 12 (6 F, 6 M)	Mean: 23.3; SD: 3.0	VT
[57]	Boyer and Nigg	2007	Indoor	Track	4.8 m/s	NR	Non	13 (NS)	NR	VT, Freq.
[58]	Boyer and Nigg	2004	Indoor	Floor	2.0, 3.0, 4.0, and 5.5 m/s	960 m	Non	10 (0 F, 10 M)	Mean: 25; SE: 4.2	VT, Freq.
[59]	Brayne, et al.	2018	Indoor	Treadmill	2.5, 3.5, and 4.5 m/s	120 s	Rec.	13 (0 F, 13 M)	Mean: 30; SD: 7	VT
[60]	Buchheit, et al.	2015	Indoor	Treadmill	2.78, 4.72, and 6.67 m/s	450 s	Non	1 (0 F, 1 M)	Exact: 36; NA	Stiffness
[61]	Butler, et al.	2003	Indoor	Floor	3.4 m/s	375 m	Rec.	15 (NS)	NR; Range: 18–45	VT
[62]	Camelio, et al.	2020	Indoor	Treadmill	preferred	36 min	Rec.	17 (9 F, 8 M)	Mean: 27; SD: 7	VT
[63]	Carrier, et al.	2020	Indoor	Treadmill	self-selected	6 min	Rec.	17 (8 F, 9 M)	Mean: 28.1; SD: 7.38	COM Disp.
[64]	Castillo and Lieberman	2018	Indoor	Treadmill	3.0 m/s	2 min	Non	27 (13 F, 14 M)	NR; Range: 18–45	Shock-frequency, Spectral Energy, Joint ROM, Joint ω
[65]	Chen, et al.	2021	Indoor	Treadmill	2.5 m/s	3 min	Non	24 (0 F, 24 M)	NR	Spectral Energy
[66]	Cheung, et al.	2018	Indoor	Treadmill	typical	12 min	Rec.	16 (5 F, 11 M)	Mean: 28.3; SD: 6.2	VT, Loading Rate
[67]	Cheung, et al.	2019	Indoor	Treadmill	2.78 m/s	10 min	Rec.	14 (7 F, 7 M)	Mean: 26.4; SD: 11.2	VT, Loading Rate
[68]	Ching, et al.	2018	Indoor	Treadmill	self-selected	20 min	Rec.	16 (9 F, 7 M)	Mean: 25.1; SD: 7.9	VT, Loading Rate
[69]	Chu and Caldwell	2004	Indoor	Treadmill	4.17 m/s	≥75 s	Rec.	10 (0 F, 10 M)	Mean: 26; SD: 6	VT, Shock-frequency, Spectral Energy
[70]	Clark, et al.	2010	Indoor	Treadmill	2.78 m/s	12 min	Non	36 (36 F, 0 M)	Mean: 30.3; SD: 5.8	VT, AP, ML
[71]	Creaby and Franttenovich Smith	2016	Indoor	Treadmill	3 m/s	50 min	Rec.	22 (0 F, 22 M)	Mean: 25.4; SD: 6.2	VT
[72]	Crowell, et al.	2010	Indoor	Treadmill	self-selected	25 min	Rec.	5 (5 F, 0 M)	Mean: 26; SD: 2	VT, Loading Rate
[73]	Day, et al.	2021	Indoor	Treadmill	3.8, 4.1, 4.9, and 5.4 m/s	NR	Comp.	30 (21 F, 9 M)	NR	VT, Spectral Energy
[74]	De la Fuente, et al.	2019	Indoor	Treadmill	typical	10 min	Rec.	20 (0 F, 20 M)	Mean: 30.5; SD: 9.3	VT, Res, Freq.

Table 2. *Cont.*

Ref.	Author	Year	Location	Surface	Speed	Distance/Duration	Type	Number (Sex)	Overall Age	Metric(s)
[75]	Deflandre, et al.	2018	Indoor	Treadmill	2.22 and 4.44 m/s	6 min	Rec.	20 (0 F, 20 M)	Mean: 26; SD: 9.5	Stiffness, Joint ROM, COM Disp., Sym. or Reg.
[76]	DeJong and Hertel	2020	Outdoor	Grass	2.22, 2.78, and 3.33 m/s	720 m	Non	10 (0 F, 10 M)	Mean: 20; SD: 2	Joint ROM
[77]	Derrick, et al.	2002	Indoor	Treadmill	2.68 and 3.6 m/s	180 s	Comp.	20 (12 F, 8 M)	Mean: 25.8; SD: 7.0	VT, Shock-time, Shock-frequency, Spectral Energy, Joint ω, Seg. Rot.
[78]	Dufek, et al.	2009	Indoor	Treadmill	3.2 km pace	run to exhaustion	Rec.	10 (NS)	Mean: 24.9; SD: 4	VT, Shock-time
[79]	Eggers, et al.	2018	Indoor	Track	preferred, 10% slower	102 s	Rec.	14 (7 F, 7 M)	Mean: 24.9; SD: 4	VT, Stiffness, COM Disp.
[80]	Encarnación-Martínez, et al.	2020	Indoor	Treadmill	3.33 m/s	400 m	Non	17 (7 F, 10 M)	NR; Range: 18–40	VT, Shock-frequency, Spectral Energy
[81]	Encarnación-Martínez, et al.	2018	Outdoor	Grass	3.33 and 4.00 m/s	480 m	Non	12 (0 F, 12 M)	Mean: 24.3; SD: 3.7	VT, Shock-time
[82]	Encarnación-Martínez, et al.	2021	Indoor	Treadmill	2.78 m/s	10 min	Non	30 (10 F, 20 M)	Mean: 26.3; SD: 7.0	VT
[83]	Friesenbichler, et al.	2011	Outdoor	NR	10 km pace	run to exhaustion	Rec.	10 (7 F, 3 M)	Mean: 31.7; SD: 7.3	VT, AP, ML, Freq., Spectral Energy
[84]	Fu, et al.	2015	Indoor/Outdoor/Outdoor/Outdoor	Treadmill/Grass/Pavement/Track	3.33 m/s / 3.33 m/s / 3.33 m/s / 3.33 m/s	6 min / 90 m / 90 m / 90 m	Rec.	13 (0 F, 13 M)	Mean: 23.7; SD: 1.2	VT
[85]	Gantz and Derrick	2018	Indoor	Treadmill	self-selected	≥6 min	Rec.	16 (7 F, 9 M)	Mean: 22.9; SD: 3.3	VT, Shock-frequency, Spectral Energy
[86]	Garcia, et al.	2021	Outdoor	Pavement	self-selected	200 m	Rec.	15 (12 F, 3 M)	Mean: 27.7; SD: 9.1	VT, AP, ML, Res., Shock-time
[87]	García-Pérez, et al.	2014	Indoor	Treadmill	4 m/s	800 m	Rec.	20 (9 F, 11 M)	Mean: 34; SD: 8	VT, Loading Rate, Shock-time

Table 2. Cont.

Ref.	Author	Year	Location	Surface	Speed	Distance/Duration	Type	Number (Sex)	Overall Age	Metric(s)
[88]	Giandolini, et al.	2014	Outdoor Indoor	Track Treadmill	4 m/s 3.89 and 4.44 m/s	800 m 8 min	Rec.	48 (18 F, 30 M)	Mean: 38.4; SD: 6.7	VT
[89]	Giandolini, et al.	2013	Outdoor	Trail Treadmill	2.78 and 3.33 m/s	6 min 60 min	Non	30 (8 F, 22 M)	Mean: 18.3; SD: 4.5	VT
[90]	Glassbrook, et al.	2020	Indoor	Treadmill	60%–100% of maximal	435 s	Non	16 (6 F, 10 M)	Mean: 24.5; SD: 4.5	Res.
[91]	Gullstrand, et al.	2009	Indoor	Treadmill	2.78, 3.33, 3.89, 4.44, 5.00, 5.56, and 6.11 m/s	≥210 s	Rec.	13 (0 F, 13 M)	Mean: 22.7; NR	COM Disp.
[92]	Hardin and Hamill	2002	Indoor	Treadmill	3.4 m/s	30 min	Rec.	24 (0 F, 24 M)	NR	VT
[93]	Iosa, et al.	2014	Indoor	Floor	self-selected	10 m	Non	25 (NS)	Mean: 15.3; SD: 3.9	VT, AP, ML, Stability
[94]	Iosa, et al.	2013	Indoor	Floor	self-selected	10 m	Non	40 (16 F, 24 M)	Mean: 5.5; SD: 2.5	VT, AP, ML, Res, Freq.
[95]	Johnson, et al.	2020	Indoor	Treadmill	90% marathon pace	30 s	Rec.	192 (87 F, 105 M)	Mean: 44.9; SD: 10.8	VT, Res.
[96]	Johnson, et al.	2021	Outdoor	Pavement	not controlled	42.2 km	Rec.	18 (8 F, 10 M)	Mean: 33; SD: 11	AP, ML
[97]	Johnson, et al.	2020	Indoor	Treadmill	self-selected	16 s	Rec.	18 (8 F, 10 M)	Mean: 33; SD: 11	VT, Res, Loading Rate
[98]	Kawabata, et al.	2013	Indoor	Treadmill	self-selected	32 s	Non	13 (0 F, 13 M)	Mean: 23.3; SD: 0.6	VT, AP, ML
[99]	Kenneally-Dabrowski, et al.	2018	Outdoor Indoor	Track	slow, preferred, fast slow, preferred, fast	18 min 4800 m 120 m	Comp.	13 (0 F, 13 M)	Mean: 23.8; SD: 2.4	VT
[100]	Khassetarash, et al.	2015	Indoor	Treadmill	maximal sprint 4 m/s	run to exhaustion (10 km max)	Comp.	8 (0 F, 8 M)	Mean: 26; SD: 3.6	Shock-frequency
[101]	Kobsar, et al.	2014	Indoor	Treadmill	self-selected	135 s	Rec.	42 (42 F, 0 M)	Mean: 33; SD: 6	VT, AP, ML, Res., Freq., Axis Ratio, Sym. or Reg.
[102]	Koldenhoven and Hertel	2018	Indoor	Treadmill	comfortable	1.5 miles	Rec.	12 (6 F, 6 M)	Mean: 23.1; SD: 5.5	Seg. Rot., Seg. Rot. Velocity
[103]	Le Bris, et al.	2006	NR	Track	maximal aerobic	run to exhaustion	Comp.	6 (0 F, 6 M)	Mean: 21.6; SD: 4	Res., Freq., Spectral Energy, Sym. or Reg.

Table 2. Cont.

Ref.	Author	Year	Location	Surface	Speed	Distance/Duration	Type	Number (Sex)	Overall Age	Metric(s)
[104]	Leduc, et al.	2020	Outdoor	NR	5.00 m/s	240 m	Comp.	17 (0 F, 17 M)	Mean: 21.0; SD: 1.3	VT, AP, ML, Res., PlayerLoad
[105]	Lee, et al.	2010	Indoor	Treadmill	self-selected, 0.28 m/s above and below	15 min	Comp.	10 (4 F, 6 M)	Mean: 30; SD: 8	VT
[106]	Lee, et al.	2015	Indoor	Treadmill	2.0 and 3.5 m/s	30 s	Non	15 (0 F, 15 M)	Mean: 26.9; SD: 3.1	VT, AP, ML, Res., Seg. Rot. Velocity
[107]	Lin, et al.	2014	Indoor	Treadmill	1.67, 2.22, 2.50, and 3.33 m/s	4 min	Comp.	10 (0 F, 10 M)	Mean: 50.30; SD: 9.40	VT, AP, ML
			Outdoor	Not Controlled	not controlled	12 hours				
[108]	Lindsay, et al.	2016	Indoor	Treadmill	2.22, 2.78, and 3.33 m/s	8.5 min	Non	15 (4 F, 11 M)	Mean: 23.7; SD: 4.7	VT, AP, ML, Res.
[109]	Lindsay, et al.	2014	Indoor	Treadmill	2.22, 2.78, and 3.33 m/s	180 s	Non	18 (0 F, 18 M)	Mean: 24.0; SD: 4.2	VT, AP, ML, Res.
[110]	Lucas-Cuevas, et al.	2017	Indoor	Treadmill	2.22, 2.78, and 3.33 m/s	6 min	Rec.	30 (0 F, 30 M)	Mean: 27.3; SD: 6.4	VT, Shock-time, Shock-frequency, Freq., Spectral Energy
[111]	Lucas-Cuevas, et al.	2016	Indoor	Treadmill	60% maximal aerobic	3 min	Rec.	22 (NS)	Mean: 28.4; SD: 5.8	VT, Loading Rate, Shock-time
[112]	Lucas-Cuevas, et al.	2017	Indoor	Treadmill	3.33 m/s	16 min	Rec.	38 (18 F, 20 M)	Mean: 29.8; SD: 5.3	VT, Loading Rate, Shock-time
[113]	Macadam, et al.	2019	Indoor	Track	maximal sprint	160 m	Comp.	1 (0 F, 1 M)	Exact: 32; NA	Seg. Rot., Seg. Rot. Velocity
[114]	Macadam, et al.	2020	NR	NR	sprint	200 m	Comp.	15 (0 F, 15 M)	Mean: 21.0; SD: 2.5	Seg. Rot., Seg. Rot. Velocity
[115]	Macadam, et al.	2020	Indoor	Treadmill	maximal sprint	80 s	Non	14 (NS)	Mean: 24.9; SD: 4.2	Seg. Rot., Seg. Rot. Velocity
[116]	Macdermid, et al.	2017	Indoor	Treadmill	2.61 m/s	9 min	Rec.	8 (NS)	Mean: 25; SD: 12	Res., Loading Rate
[117]	Mangubat, et al.	2018	Indoor	Treadmill	preferred	90 s	Rec.	13 (5 F, 8 M)	Mean: 27.1; SD: 5.1	VT
[118]	Masci, et al.	2013	Indoor	Floor	maximal	15 m	Non	54 (NS)	Mean: 5; SD: 3	VT, AP, ML, Res., Stiffness
[119]	McGregor, et al.	2009	Indoor	Treadmill	incremental from 0.56 m/s	run to exhaustion	Comp.	7 (0 F, 7 M)	Mean: 21.4; SD: 1.7; Range: 19–24	VT, AP, ML, Res., Entropy

Table 2. Cont.

Ref.	Author	Year	Location	Surface	Speed	Distance/Duration	Type	Number (Sex)	Overall Age	Metric(s)
[120]	Mercer and Chona	2015	Indoor	Treadmill	100%, 110%, 120%, and 130% of preferred	16 min	Non	10 (6 F, 4 M)	Mean: 21.4; SD: 2.0	VT
[121]	Mercer, et al.	2002	Indoor	Treadmill	50%, 60%, 70%, 80%, 90%, and 100% of maximal	120 s	Non	8 (0 F, 8 M)	Mean: 25; SD: 4.6	VT, Shock-frequency
[122]	Mercer, et al.	2003	Indoor	Treadmill	3.8 m/s	140 s	Rec.	10 (0 F, 10 M)	Mean: 24; SD: 5.8	Shock-frequency, Spectral Energy
[123]	Mercer, et al.	2010	Indoor	Floor	preferred preferred, 0.5 m/s faster and slower	200 m	Non	18 (7 F, 11 M)	Mean: 10.3; SD: 1	VT, Shock-time
			Indoor	Treadmill		6 min				
[124]	Mercer, et al.	2003	Indoor	Treadmill	3.1 and 3.8 m/s	40 s	Non	10 (0 F, 10 M)	Mean: 24; SD: 6	VT, Shock-frequency, Spectral Energy
[125]	Meyer, et al.	2015	Indoor	Floor	1.67 and 2.78 m/s	140 m	Non	13 (3 F, 10 M)	Mean: 10.1; SD: 3.0; Range: 5-16	VT
[126]	Meyer, et al.	2018	Indoor	Track	3.5 m/s	900 m	Non	36 (18 F, 18 M)	Mean: 25.4; SD: 3.5	VT, AP, ML, Variability-any axis
			Indoor	Treadmill	3.0 m/s	1 min				
			Outdoor	Grass	3.0 m/s	1 min				
			Outdoor	Pavement	3.0 m/s	1 min				
[127]	Mitschke, et al.	2017	Indoor	Track	2.5 and 3.5 m/s	450 m	Rec.	24 (NS)	Mean: 24.7; SD: 4.1	Seg. Rot. Velocity
[128]	Mitschke, et al.	2017	Indoor	Track	3.5 m/s	450 m	Rec.	21 (0 F, 21 M)	Mean: 28.9; SD: 10.8	VT, Seg. Rot., Seg. Rot. Velocity
[129]	Mitschke, et al.	2018	Indoor	Track	self-selected	225 m	Rec.	21 (0 F, 21 M)	Mean: 24.4; SD: 4.2	VT, Seg. Rot.
[130]	Montgomery, et al.	2016	Indoor	Floor	natural jog, natural run	40 m	Non	15 (NS)	Mean: 24.2; SD: 3.8	VT, Loading Rate
			Indoor	Treadmill	natural jog, natural run	1 min				
[131]	Moran, et al.	2017	Indoor	Treadmill	75% of maximum HR	37 min	Rec.	15 (6 F, 9 M)	Mean: 20.4; SD: 2.4	VT
[132]	Morrow, et al.	2014	Indoor	Floor	slow, normal, fast	≥504 m	Non	11 (8 F, 3 M)	Mean: 33.4; SD: 10.5	VT, AP, ML
[133]	Neugebauer, et al.	2012	Indoor	Floor	consistent	540 m	Non	35 (20 F, 15 M)	Mean: 11.6; SD: 0.7	Res.
[134]	Nüesch, et al.	2017	Indoor	Treadmill	self-selected	6 min	Rec.	20 (12 F, 8 M)	Mean: 27.4; SD: 8.3	Joint ROM
[135]	O'Connor and Hamill	2002	Indoor	Treadmill	3.8 m/s	4 min	Non	12 (0 F, 12 M)	Mean: 27.6; SD: 5.3	VT

Table 2. Cont.

Ref.	Author	Year	Location	Surface	Speed	Distance/Duration	Type	Number (Sex)	Overall Age	Metric(s)
[136]	Provot, et al.	2017	Indoor	Treadmill	2.22, 2.78, 3.33, 3.89, 4.44, and 5.00 m/s	7 min	Non	1 (0 F, 1 M)	Exact: 33; NA	Res., Spectral Energy
[137]	Provot, et al.	2019	Indoor	Treadmill	2.22, 2.50, 2.78, 3.06, 3.33, 3.61, 3.89, 4.44, and 5.00 m/s	9 min	Rec.	18 (8 F, 10 M)	Mean: 31.4; SD: 8.9	Res., Freq., Spectral Energy, Stiffness
[138]	Rabuffetti, et al.	2019	Indoor	Treadmill	1.8 and 2.2 m/s	140 s	Non	25 (11 F, 14 M)	Mean: 26.5; SD: 4.5; Range: 20–40	Sym. or Reg.
[139]	Raper, et al.	2018	Indoor	Track	slow, medium, fast	50 m	Comp.	10 (6 F, 4 M)	Mean: 26.90; SD: 4.03	VT
[140]	Reenalda, et al.	2019	Outdoor	Track	10 km pace	20 min	Rec.	10 (0 F, 10 M)	Mean: 31; SD: 5	VT, Shock-time, Joint ROM
[141]	Schütte, et al.	2015	Indoor	Treadmill	3.2 km pace	run to exhaustion	Rec.	20 (8 F, 12 M)	Mean: 21.05; SD: 2.14	VT, AP, ML, Axis Ratio, Sym. or Reg., Entropy
[142]	Schütte, et al.	2016	Outdoor	Pavement	self-selected	180 m	Rec.	28 (14 F, 14 M)	Mean: 22.62; SD: 3.07	VT, AP, Freq., Axis Ratio, Sym. or Reg., Entropy
			Outdoor	Track	self-selected	180 m				
			Outdoor	Trail	self-selected	180 m				
[143]	Schütte, et al.	2018	Indoor	Treadmill	incremental from 2.22 or 2.50 m/s	run to exhaustion	Rec.	30 (14 F, 16 M)	Mean: 21.75; SD: 1.40	VT, AP, ML, Axis Ratio, Sym. or Reg., Entropy
[144]	Setuain, et al.	2017	Indoor	Floor	maximal sprint	60 m	Comp.	1 (0 F, 1 M)	Exact: 19, NA	VT, AP, Res., COM Disp., COM Δv
[145]	Setuain, et al.	2018	Indoor	Floor	maximal sprint	80 m	Rec.	16 (8 F, 8 M)	Mean: 28.8; SD: 5.35	AP, Res., COM Δv, Power
[146]	Sheerin, et al.	2018	Indoor	Treadmill	2.7, 3.0, 3.3, and 3.7 m/s	8 min	Rec.	14 (0 F, 14 M)	Mean: 33.6; SD: 11.6	Res.
[147]	Sheerin, et al.	2018	Indoor	Treadmill	2.7, 3.0, 3.3, and 3.7 m/s	8 min	Rec.	85 (20 F, 65 M)	Mean: 39.51; SD: 8.92	Res.
[148]	Shiang, et al.	2016	Indoor	Treadmill	1.94, 2.78, and 3.61 m/s	6 min	Non	6 (0 F, 6 M)	Mean: 25.4; SD: 1.7	Seg. Rot.
[149]	Simoni, et al.	2020	Indoor	Treadmill	self-selected	1 min	Rec.	87 (28 F, 59 M)	Mean: 41; SD: 10	VT, AP, ML

Table 2. Cont.

Ref.	Author	Year	Location	Surface	Speed	Distance/Duration	Type	Number (Sex)	Overall Age	Metric(s)
[150]	Stickford, et al.	2015	Indoor	Treadmill	3.88, 4.47, and 5.00 m/s	12 min	Comp.	16 (0 F, 16 M)	Mean: 22.4; SD: 3	Stiffness, COM Disp.
[151]	TenBroek, et al.	2014	Indoor	Treadmill	3 m/s	90 min	Rec.	10 (0 F, 10 M)	NR; Range: 18-55	VT, Shock-frequency
[152]	Tenforde, et al.	2020	Indoor	Treadmill	self-selected	3 min	Rec.	169 (74 F, 95 M)	Mean: 38.7; SD: 13.1	VT, Res.
[153]	Thomas and Derrick	2003	Indoor	Treadmill	preferred	10 min	Comp.	12 (6 F, 6 M)	Mean: 20.9; SD: 2.3	VT, Shock-time, Spectral Energy, Joint ROM, Joint ω
[154]	Tirosh, et al.	2019	Indoor	Treadmill	20% above walking	27 min	Non	37 (NS)	Mean: 9.2; SD: 1.3	VT
[155]	Tirosh, et al.	2017	Indoor	Treadmill	20% above walking	2 min	Non	24 (NS)	Mean: 8.5; SD: 0.9	VT
[156]	Tirosh, et al.	2020	Indoor	Treadmill	20% above walking	2 min	Non	32 (15 F, 17 M)	Mean: 9.26; SD: 1.18	VT, Shock-time
[157]	van Werkhoven, et al.	2019	Indoor	Treadmill	comfortable	3 min	Non	12 (NS)	NR; Range: 18-45	Joint ROM, Joint ω, Seg. Rot.
[158]	Walsh	2021	Indoor	Treadmill	100% and 120% of preferred	12 min	Non	18 (9 F, 9 M)	Mean: 29; SD: 6.5	Stability, Entropy
[159]	Waite, et al.	2021	Outdoor Outdoor	Grass Pavement	80% of 1 mile pace 80% of 1 mile pace	180 m 360 m	Rec.	13 (5 F, 8 M)	Mean: 20.07; SD: 0.95	VT
[160]	Winter, et al.	2016	Indoor	Floor	self-selected	8.2 km	Rec.	10 (4 F, 6 M)	Mean: 27.5; SD: 9.5	VT, AP, ML
[161]	Wixted, et al.	2010	Outdoor	Track	race effort	1500 m	Comp.	2 (NS)	NR	VT, AP, ML
[162]	Wood and Kipp	2014	Indoor	Treadmill	comfortable fast jog	25 min	Rec.	9 (6 F, 3 M)	Mean: 20; SD: 1.5	VT, AP, Res.
[163]	Wundersitz, et al.	2015	Indoor	Treadmill	3.3, 5.0, and 5.9 m/s	90 s	Non	39 (11 F, 28 M)	Mean: 24.2; SD: 2.5	Res.
[164]	Zhang, et al.	2019	Indoor	Treadmill	90%, 100%, and 110% of preferred	9 min	Rec.	13 (3 F, 10 M)	Mean: 41.1; SD: 6.9	VT
[165]	Zhang, et al.	2016	Indoor	Treadmill	preferred, 15% faster and slower	18 min	Non	10 (2 F, 8 M)	Mean: 23.6; SD: 3.8	VT

Note: NR = not reported; Pavement = pavement or sidewalk; Floor = floor or platform; Rec. = recreational; Comp. = competitive; Non = non-runners; Disp. = displacement; Δv = change in velocity; Sym. or Reg. = symmetry or regularity; Res. = resultant magnitude; VT = vertical/axial magnitude; AP = anterior-posterior magnitude; ML = medial-lateral magnitude; Seg. Rot. = segment rotation; Shock–time = shock attenuation—time domain; Shock–frequency = shock attenuation—frequency domain; Joint ROM = joint angles or range of motion; Joint ω = joint angular velocity; Freq. = frequency content.

Table 3. Study characteristics where the analyzed distance is 200–1000 m.

Ref.	Author	Year	Location	Surface	Speed	Distance/Duration	Type	Number (Sex)	Overall Age	Metric(s)
[166]	Aubry, et al.	2018	Indoor Outdoor	Treadmill Track	3.06–5.00 m/s 3.06–5.00 m/s	6 min 12 min	Comp. Rec.	11 (0 F, 11 M) 13 (0 F, 13 M)	Mean: 33.4; SD: 6.6	COM Disp., Power
[167]	Austin, et al.	2018	Indoor	Treadmill	85–89% VO2max	8 min	Comp.	17 (8 F, 9 M)	Mean: 20.6; SD: 2.3	Power
[168]	Barrett, et al.	2014	Indoor	Treadmill	incremental from 1.94 m/s	2 runs to exhaustion	Comp.	44 (NS)	Mean: 22; SD: 3	PlayerLoad
[5]	Benson, et al.	2020	Indoor Outdoor	Treadmill Pavement	preferred preferred	5 min 600 m run to exhaustion	Rec.	69 (31 F, 38 M)	Mean: 33.7; SD: 11.5	VT, AP, ML, Res., Sym. or Reg.
[169]	De Brabandere, et al.	2018	Indoor	Treadmill	incremental from 2.5 m/s to 4.58 m/s	60 min	Rec.	28 (16 F, 12 M)	Mean: 21.8; SD: 1.3	VT, AP, ML
[170]	Cher, et al.	2017	Indoor	Treadmill	slow, medium, fast	60 min	Non	12 (4 F, 8 M)	Mean: 29.4; SD: 6.8	VT, AP, ML, Res.
[171]	Clansey, et al.	2016	Indoor	Treadmill	95% of onset of blood lactate accumulation	40 min	Rec.	13 (0 F, 13 M)	Mean: 35.1; SD: 10.2	VT, Shock-frequency
[172]	Clermont, et al.	2019	Indoor	Treadmill	preferred	5 min	Rec.	41 (16 F, 25 M)	Mean: 32.5; SD: 12.7	VT, AP, ML, Res., Sym. or Reg.
[173]	Clermont, et al.	2020	Indoor	Track	self-selected	21 min	Rec.	17 (10 F, 7 M)	Mean: 39.8; SD: 9.6	VT, AP, ML, Res., Sym. or Reg.
[174]	Deriaz, et al.	2010	Outdoor Indoor	Track Treadmill	not controlled comfortable	6 km 15 min	Rec. Non	65 (0 F, 65 M) 16 (0 F, 16 M)	Mean: 36.0; SD: 6.8	VT
[175]	Enders, et al.	2014	Indoor	Treadmill	3.5 m/s	20 min	Rec.	12 (0 F, 12 M)	Mean: 25.56; SD: 2.88	VT, Shock-frequency, Freq., Spectral Energy
[176]	Garcia-Byrne, et al.	2020	Indoor	Floor	2.22 m/s	400 m	Comp.	36 (0 F, 36 M)	Mean: 25; SD: 3	PlayerLoad
[177]	Giandolini, et al.	2016	Outdoor	Pavement	self-selected	6.5 km	Rec.	23 (0 F, 23 M)	Mean: 39; SD: 11	VT, ML, Res., Shock-time, Shock-frequency
[178]	Giandolini, et al.	2017	Outdoor Outdoor Outdoor	Trail Pavement Trail	self-selected self-selected self-selected	6.5 km 6.5 km 6.5 km	Rec.	23 (0 F, 23 M)	Mean: 39; SD: 11	VT
[179]	Horvais, et al.	2019	Indoor	Treadmill	3.9 m/s	14 min	Rec.	10 (0 F, 10 M)	Mean: 27.3; SD: 5.4	VT, AP, Res., Spectral Energy
[180]	Hughes, et al.	2019	Indoor	Treadmill	3.89 and 5.00 m/s	9 min	Comp.	16 (NS)	Mean: 17.36; SD: 1.25	VT
[181]	Koska, et al.	2018	Indoor	Treadmill	2.78, 3.33, and 4.17 m/s	9 min	Rec.	51 (15 F, 36 M)	Mean: 33.9; SD: 8.2	Seg. Rot., Seg. Rot. Velocity

Table 3. Cont.

Ref.	Author	Year	Location	Surface	Speed	Distance/Duration	Type	Number (Sex)	Overall Age	Metric(s)
[182]	Melo, et al.	2020	Indoor	Treadmill	10 km pace typical	20 km	Rec.	13 (5 F, 8 M)	Mean: 36; SD: 4	COM Disp.
[183]	Moltó, et al.	2020	Indoor	Treadmill	3.06 m/s	3 min	Rec.	38 (16 F, 22 M)	Mean: 26.7; SD: 7.7	Seg. Rot.
[184]	Morio, et al.	2016	Indoor	Treadmill	incremental to reach [La]b concentration of 4 mmol/L	12 min	Rec.	8 (0 F, 8 M)	Mean: 26; SD: 2	VT, AP, ML
[185]	Murray, et al.	2017	Indoor	Treadmill		run to exhaustion	Comp.	6 (0 F, 6 M)	Mean: 15.6; SD: 1.2	VT, AP, ML, Entropy
[186]	Navalta, et al.	2019	Outdoor	Trail	self-selected	10 min	Non	20 (8 F, 12 M)	Mean: 22.2; SD: 5.8	Stiffness, COM Disp., Power
[187]	Olin and Gutierrez	2013	Indoor	Treadmill	comfortable	21 min	Rec.	18 (12 F, 6 M)	Mean: 31.2; SD: 7.9	VT
[188]	Perrotin, et al.	2021	Outdoor	Pavement	not controlled	1 km	Rec.	30 (3 F, 27 M)	Mean: 36.4; SD: 8	Stiffness, COM Disp., Power
[189]	Provot, et al.	2016	Indoor	Treadmill	3.33 m/s	40 min	Rec.	1 (0 F, 1 M)	Exact: 22; NA	Res., Freq., Spectral Energy, Stiffness
[190]	Reenalda, et al.	2016	Outdoor	Pavement	not controlled	42.2 km	Rec.	3 (0 F, 3 M)	Mean: 38.7; SD: 8.2; Range: 31–50	VT, Joint ROM, COM Disp.
[191]	Seeley, et al.	2020	Indoor	Treadmill	2.68, 3.13, and 3.58 m/s	12 min	Non	31 (14 F, 17 M)	Mean: 23; SD: 3	VT, AP, ML, Res.
[192]	Shih, et al.	2014	Indoor	Treadmill	70% of maximal	30 min	Rec.	15 (NS)	Mean: 24.5; SD: 1.7	Joint ROM, Joint ω
[193]	Tirosh, et al.	2019	Indoor	Floor	20% above walking	1 km	Non	10 (NS)	Mean: 10.7; SD: 1.27	VT
			Outdoor	Grass	3.33, 3.89, 4.44, and 5.00 m/s	12 min				
			Outdoor	Pavement	3.33, 3.89, 4.44, and 5.00 m/s	12 min				
			Outdoor	Track	3.33, 3.89, 4.44, and 5.00 m/s	12 min				
			Outdoor	Track	4.78 m/s	6 km				
[194]	Ueberschar, et al.	2019	Indoor	Treadmill	incremental from 1.67 m/s	run to exhaustion	Rec.	15 (0 F, 15 M)	Mean: 30; SD: 7	VT, Res.
[195]	Van den Berghe, et al.	2021	Indoor	Track	3.2 m/s	20 min	Rec.	10 (NS)	Mean: 33; SD: 9; Range: 24–49	VT
[196]	van der Bie and Krose	2015	Indoor	Treadmill	ventilatory threshold	run to exhaustion	Non	18 (14 F, 4 M)	Mean: 23; SD: 3	VT, AP, ML, Variability-any axis, Entropy

Table 3. Cont.

Ref.	Author	Year	Location	Surface	Speed	Distance/Duration	Type	Number (Sex)	Overall Age	Metric(s)
[9]	Watari, et al.	2016	Indoor	Treadmill	2.7, 3.0, 3.3, 3.6, and 3.9 m/s	5 min	Rec.	22 (8 F, 14 M)	Mean: 28.2; SD: 10.1	COM Disp.
[197]	Weich, et al.	2019	Indoor	Track	95% anaerobic threshold	5000 m	Rec. Non	25 (NS) 9 (NS)	Mean: 26.64; SD: 6.86	VT, AP, ML

Note: NR = not reported; Pavement = pavement or sidewalk; Floor = floor or platform; Rec. = recreational; Comp. = competitive; Non = non-runners; Disp. = displacement; Δv = change in velocity; Sym. or Reg. = symmetry or regularity; Res. = resultant magnitude; VT = vertical/axial magnitude; AP = anterior-posterior magnitude; ML = medial-lateral magnitude; Seg. Rot. = segment rotation; Shock—time attenuation—time domain; Shock—frequency = shock attenuation—frequency domain; Joint ROM = joint angles or range of motion; Joint ω = joint angular velocity; Freq. = frequency content.

Table 4. Study characteristics where the analyzed distance is >1000 m over a single run.

Ref.	Author	Year	Location	Surface	Speed	Distance/Duration	Type	Number (Sex)	Overall Age	Metric(s)
[198]	Bigelow, et al.	2013	Indoor	Track	self-selected	4 miles	Rec.	12 (NS)	Mean: 32.8; SD: 9.8	VT, ML
[199]	Brahms, et al.	2020	Indoor Indoor	Treadmill Track	self-selected 5 km pace	4 miles run to exhaustion	Comp. Rec.	16 (NS) 16 (NS)	Mean: 24; SD: 3.9	Res.
			Indoor	Treadmill	incremental from 2.5 m/s	run to exhaustion				
			Outdoor	Track	2.78 m/s	9 min				
			Outdoor	Track	incremental from 2.5 m/s	run to exhaustion				
[200]	Clermont, et al.	2019	Outdoor	Not Controlled	not controlled	42.2 km	Rec.	27 (15 F, 12 M)	Mean: 45.1; SD: 11.5	Joint ROM, Seg. Rot., COM Disp., COM Δv
[201]	DeJong and Hertel	2020	Outdoor	Pavement	not controlled	6–21.1 km	Comp.	5 (4 F, 1 M)	Mean: 30.2; SD: 3.3	VT, AP, Joint ω
			Outdoor	Trail	not controlled	5 km				
[202]	Giandolini, et al.	2015	Outdoor	Trail	not controlled	45 km	Comp.	1 (0 F, 1 M)	Exact: 26; NA	VT, AP, Res, Freq.

Table 4. Cont.

Ref.	Author	Year	Location	Surface	Speed	Distance/Duration	Type	Number (Sex)	Overall Age	Metric(s)
[203]	Gómez-Carmona, et al.	2020	Indoor	Treadmill	incremental from 2.22 m/s	run to exhaustion	Rec.	20 (0 F, 20 M)	Mean: 27.32; SD: 6.65	PlayerLoad
[204]	Hoenig, et al.	2019	Outdoor	Track	incremental from 2.22 m/s maximal	run to exhaustion	Rec.	30 (0 F, 30 M)	Mean: 27; SD: 6.0	Stability
[205]	Provot, et al.	2019	NR	Track	3.75 m/s	5000 m	Rec.	10 (5 F, 5 M)	Mean: 38.0; SD: 11.6	VT, AP, ML, Res., Freq, Spectral Energy, Stiffness
[206]	Rojas-Valverde, et al.	2019	Indoor	Treadmill	not controlled	run to exhaustion	Rec.	20 (0 F, 20 M)	Mean: 38.95; SD: 9.99	Res., Entropy, PlayerLoad
[207]	Rojas-Valverde, et al.	2020	Outdoor	Trail	not controlled	35.27 km	Rec.	18 (NS)	Mean: 38.78; SD: 10.38	Res.
[208]	Schütte, et al.	2018	Outdoor	Not Controlled	3.2 km pace	36 km	Rec.	16 (6 F, 10 M)	Mean: 20.23; SD: 0.78	VT, Shock-frequency, Spectral Energy, Axis Ratio, Sym. or Reg., Entropy
[209]	Ueberschar, et al.	2019	Outdoor	Track	3.17 m/s	3200 m	Rec. Non	14 (6 F, 8 M) 10 (NS)	Mean: 10.7; SD: 1.27	VT

Note: NR = not reported; Pavement = pavement or sidewalk; Floor = floor or platform; Rec. = recreational; Comp. = competitive; Non = non-runners; Disp. = displacement; Δv = change in velocity; Sym. or Reg. = symmetry or regularity; Res. = resultant magnitude; VT = vertical/axial magnitude; AP = anterior-posterior magnitude; ML = medial-lateral magnitude; Seg. Rot. = segment rotation; Shock—time = shock attenuation—time domain; Shock—frequency = shock attenuation—frequency domain; Joint ROM = joint angles or range of motion; Joint ω = joint angular velocity; Freq. = frequency content.

Table 5. Study characteristics where the analyzed distance is >1000 m over multiple runs.

Ref.	Author	Year	Location	Surface	Speed	Distance/Duration	Type	Number (Sex)	Overall Age	Metric(s)
[210]	Ahamed, et al.	2019	Outdoor	Not Controlled	not controlled	29 km	Rec.	11 (10 F, 1 M)	Mean: 44.1; SD: 9.1	Joint ROM, Seg. Rot., COM Disp., COM Δv
[211]	Ahamed, et al.	2018	Outdoor	Pavement	not controlled	≥24 km	Rec.	6 (5 F, 1 M)	Mean: 44.4; NR	Seg. Rot., COM Disp., COM Δv

Table 5. Cont.

Ref.	Author	Year	Location	Surface	Speed	Distance/Duration	Type	Number (Sex)	Overall Age	Metric(s)
[212]	Ahamed, et al.	2019	Outdoor	Not Controlled	not controlled	7 runs	Rec.	35 (25 F, 10 M)	Mean: 49.7; SD: 9.6	Joint ROM, Seg. Rot., COM Disp., COM Δv
[213]	Benson, et al.	2019	Outdoor	Not Controlled	not controlled	10 runs	Rec.	12 (9 F, 3 M)	Mean: 48.5; SD: 12.0	Joint ROM, Seg. Rot., COM Disp., COM Δv
[214]	Carton-Llorente, et al.	2021	Indoor	Treadmill	submaximal	120 min	Rec.	22 (0 F, 22 M)	Mean: 34; SD: 7.5	Power
[215]	Cerezuela-Espejo, et al.	2020	Indoor	Treadmill	2.78 m/s	24 min	Rec.	12 (0 F, 12 M)	Mean: 25.7; SD: 7.9	Power
[216]	Colapietro, et al.	2020	Outdoor	Track	slow, fast	3200 m	Rec.	18 (10 F, 8 M)	Mean: 22.7; SD: 4.7	VT, AP, Joint ROM, Joint ω
[217]	Gregory, et al.	2019	Outdoor	Track	hard	1600 m	Non	12 (6 F, 6 M)	Mean: 22.0; SD: 1.9	VT, AP, Joint ROM, Joint ω
[218]	Hollander, et al.	2021	Indoor	Treadmill	70% VO2max	105 min	Non	41 (20 F, 21 M)	Mean: 25.2; SD: 3.1	Stability
[219]	Hollis, et al.	2019	Outdoor	Grass	moderate, hard	3200 m	Rec.	15 (8 F, 7 M)	Mean: 20; SD: 3.1	VT, AP, Joint ROM, Joint ω
			Outdoor	Track	moderate, hard	3200 m				
[220]	Kiernan, et al.	2018	Outdoor	Not Controlled	not controlled	60 day training period	Comp.	9 (0 F, 9 M)	Mean: 18.7; SD: 1.0	VT
[221]	Koldenhoven, et al.	2020	Outdoor	Not Controlled	not controlled	3 runs	Rec.	16 (8 F, 8 M)	Mean: 23.5; SD: 5	AP, Res., Seg. Rot., Seg. Rot. Velocity
[116]	Macdermid, et al.	2017	Indoor	Treadmill	2.83 m/s	30 min	Comp.	6 (NS)	Mean: 29.8; SD: 13.0	Loading Rate, Shock-time, COM Disp.
[222]	McGregor, et al.	2009	Indoor	Treadmill	incremental from 0.56 m/s	2 runs to exhaustion	Non Comp.	7 (0 F, 7 M) 7 (NS)	Mean: 26.5; SD: 5.7	VT, AP, ML, Res.
[223]	Nüesch, et al.	2019	Indoor	Treadmill	self-selected maximal	15 min	Rec.	19 (11 F, 8 M)	Mean: 27.7; SD: 8.6	Joint ROM
[224]	Olcina, et al.	2019	NR Outdoor	Track Trail	not controlled	24 min	Comp.	10 (2 F, 8 M)	Mean: 25.7; SD: 8.9	COM Disp.
[225]	Rochat, et al.	2019	Outdoor	Trail	not controlled	4.1 km	Rec.	9 (0 F, 9 M)	Mean: 37.8; SD: 7	VT, COM Disp.
[226]	Ruder, et al.	2019	Outdoor	Pavement	not controlled	15 km	Rec.	222 (103 F, 119 M)	Mean: 44.1; SD: 10.8	VT
[227]	Ryan, et al.	2021	Outdoor	Not Controlled	not controlled	10–12 runs	Rec.	12 (0 F, 12 M)	NR; Range: 14–18	Res.
[228]	Strohrmann, et al.	2012	Indoor	Treadmill	85% of maximal	45 min	Rec.	21 (NS)	NR	Res., Joint ω, Seg. Rot., COM Disp.
			Outdoor	Track	85% of maximal	45 min				

Table 5. Cont.

Ref.	Author	Year	Location	Surface	Speed	Distance/Duration	Type	Number (Sex)	Overall Age	Metric(s)
[209]	Ueberschar, et al.	2019	Outdoor	Pavement	3.64 and 6.67 m/s	10.7 km	Comp.	2 (0 F, 2 M)	Mean: 17.6; SD: 1.13	VT
[229]	Van den Berghe, et al.	2020	Indoor	Track	3.2 m/s	24.5 min	Rec.	10 (5 F, 5 M)	Mean: 33; SD: 9	VT
[230]	Vanwanseele, et al.	2020	Indoor Outdoor	Treadmill	2.22, 3.33, and 4.44 m/s	3 min	Rec.	68 (NS)	Mean: 29.5; SD: 8.1	VT, AP, ML
[231]	Willis, et al.	2019	Indoor	Treadmill	not controlled 2.50, 2.78, 3.61, and 4.17 m/s	3 month training period 10 min	Comp.	12 (NS)	Mean: 33.6; SD: 4.3	Stiffness

Note: NR = not reported; Pavement = pavement or sidewalk; Floor = floor or platform; Rec. = recreational; Comp. = competitive; Non = non-runners; Disp. = displacement; Δv = change in velocity; Sym. or Reg. = symmetry or regularity; Res. = resultant magnitude; VT = vertical/axial magnitude; AP = anterior-posterior magnitude; ML = medial-lateral magnitude; Seg. Rot. = segment rotation; Shock—time attenuation—time domain; Shock—frequency = shock attenuation—frequency domain; Joint ROM = joint angles or range of motion; Joint ω = joint angular velocity; Freq. = frequency content.

Table 6. Study characteristics where the analyzed distance is not reported.

Ref.	Author	Year	Location	Surface	Speed	Distance/Duration	Type	Number (Sex)	Overall Age	Metric(s)
[232]	Bielik	2019	Outdoor	Track	2.78, 3.33, and 4.17 m/s	15 min	Rec.	73 (24 F, 49 M)	Mean: 29.2; SD: 4.1	COM Disp.
[233]	Bielik and Clementis	2017	Outdoor Indoor	Treadmill Treadmill	incremental from 0.28 m/s incremental from 2.22 m/s	run to exhaustion run to exhaustion	Comp. Rec.	30 (NS)	NR	COM Disp.
[234]	Butler, et al.	2007	Indoor	Treadmill	self-selected	2 runs	Rec.	24 (NS)	Mean: 21.4; SD: 3.1	VT
[235]	Cooper, et al.	2009	Indoor	Treadmill	incremental from 0.45 m/s to 2.24 m/s	5 min	Non	7 (2 F, 5 M)	Mean: 30; SD: 6	Joint ROM

Table 6. *Cont.*

Ref.	Author	Year	Location	Surface	Speed	Distance/Duration	Type	Number (Sex)	Overall Age	Metric(s)
[236]	de Fontenay, et al.	2020	Indoor	Treadmill	self-selected	NR	Non	32 (13 F, 19 M)	Mean: 27.0; SD: 5.5	AP, Loading Rate, Joint ROM, COM Disp.
[237]	Dufek, et al.	2008	Indoor	Treadmill	self-selected	90 s	Rec.	31 (31 F, 0 M)	Mean: 26.7; SD: 3.8	VT, Shock-time
[238]	Garrett, et al.	2019	NR	NR	6.25 m/s	450 m	Comp.	23 (0 F, 23 M)	Mean: 22.4; SD: 3.6	PlayerLoad
[239]	Gurchiek, et al.	2017	Indoor	Floor	sprint	NR	Non	15 (3 F, 12 M)	Mean: 23.2; SD: 2.11	Seg. Rot.
[240]	Sheerin, et al.	2020	Indoor Outdoor	Treadmill Track	comfortable	800 m run to exhaustion	Rec.	18 (7 F, 11 M)	Mean: 35.2; SD: 9.6	Res.
[241]	Ueberschar, et al.	2019	Indoor	Treadmill	incremental	36 physical training sessions	Comp.	53 (18 F, 35 M)	Mean: 20.07; SD: 3.65	VT, Shock-time
[242]	Zadeh, et al.	2020	Outdoor	Not Controlled	not controlled		Non	55 (16 F, 39 M)	Mean: 20.8; SD: 3.32	VT, Res., Loading Rate

Note: NR = not reported; Pavement = pavement or sidewalk; Floor = floor or platform; Rec. = recreational; Comp. = competitive; Non = non-runners; Disp. = displacement; ∆v = change in velocity; Sym. or Reg. = symmetry or regularity; Res. = resultant magnitude; VT = vertical/axial magnitude; AP = anterior-posterior magnitude; ML = medial-lateral magnitude; Seg. Rot. = segment rotation; Shock—time = shock attenuation—time domain; Shock—frequency = shock attenuation—frequency domain; Joint ROM = joint angles or range of motion; Joint ω = joint angular velocity; Freq. = frequency content.

3.2.1. Conditions

Across the 231 included studies, running gait was analyzed in 286 different conditions; however, for 24 conditions, the analyzed distance, speed and/or location could not be classified due to lack of information. The 262 running conditions that could be classified consisted of 27 unique combinations of the specified categories for analyzed distance (one step or stride, <200 m, 200–1000 m, >1000 m single trial, >1000 m multiple trials), speed (exact, calculated, subjective, not controlled) and location (indoor, outdoor) (Figure 2).

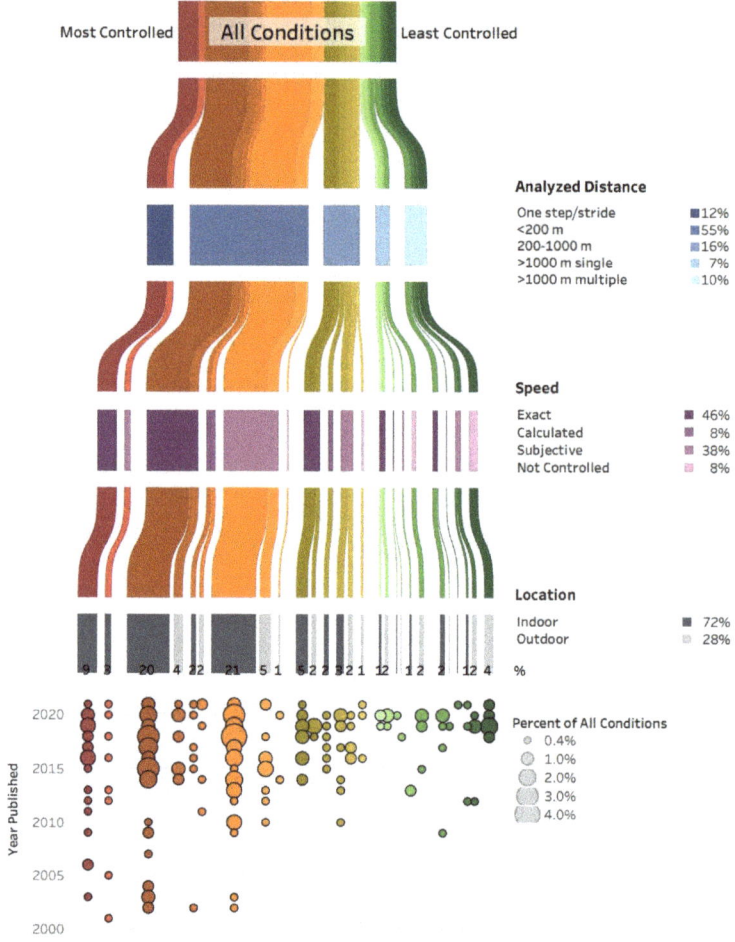

Figure 2. All conditions (262 across 231 studies) are grouped according to the analyzed distance, speed, and location. The condition groups are ranked from most controlled (red, on the left) to least controlled (green, on the right), and the width of each line corresponds to the percent of all conditions within that group. The degree of control is based on the analyzed distance (one step/stride is more controlled than >1000 m), speed (exact is more controlled than not controlled), and location (indoor is more controlled than outdoor). The percent of all conditions for each category of analyzed distance (shades of blue), speed (shades of purple), and location (shades of grey) is reported. In the bottom panel, the percent of all conditions within each group are further separated by year the study was published, with larger circles corresponding to a greater percent of all conditions. Note: 24 conditions that could not be categorized due to lack of information are not included in this figure.

The most common running condition was indoors at an exact speed with <200 m analyzed, accounting for 21% of all 262 conditions. Indoor running at a subjective speed with <200 m analyzed was the second most common condition at 20%. Indoor running at an exact or subjective speed with one step or stride analyzed accounted for 12% of all conditions. Overall, 72% of all conditions were indoors; and in 67% of all conditions, the analyzed distance was one step or stride or <200 m. Most of those studies were published between 2015 and 2021.

Studies with less controlled running conditions were primarily published after 2018. A total of 17% of all conditions included runs of >1000 m in a single or multiple trials, and speed was not controlled in races or training runs for 8% of all conditions. The least controlled condition—outdoor running with speed not controlled for multiple trials > 1000 m—accounted for 4% of all conditions.

The running conditions were grouped by surface and location (Figure 3). Overall, 49% of all conditions were indoors on a treadmill, and an additional 16% were indoors on a floor or platform. Outdoor pavement or sidewalk, trail, grass, and not controlled running surfaces combined for 19% of all conditions.

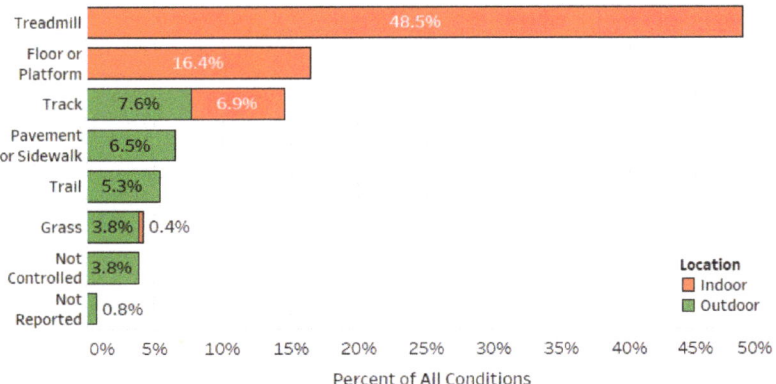

Figure 3. The percent of all conditions (262 across 231 studies) by running surface and location (indoor, outdoor).

3.2.2. Device(s)

There were 365 combinations of devices with specific sensor/axis composition and device locations on the body (Figure 4). The most common combination was a triaxial accelerometer on the shank (18% of all combinations) followed by a triaxial accelerometer on the lower back (13%). Across all sensors with any number of axes, the top three device locations were the shank, lower back and foot, accounting for 35%, 22% and 16% of all combinations, respectively. Across any number of axes, 70% of all combinations used an accelerometer only, and 22% of all combinations used all three sensors. A gyroscope was the only sensor for 1% of all combinations and was placed on the foot or shank.

Some studies used multiple devices, bringing the total number of devices to 251. Most devices (82%) were of research-grade. The remaining 18% of devices are commercially available and designed for public use and include adidas Run Genie, Catapult, DorsaVi, Garmin, Google Nexus, Lumo Run, Milestone Pod, Polar, RunScribe, Runteq Zoi, Stryd, and Zephyr BioHarness. These devices were commonly worn on the shoe or lower or upper back.

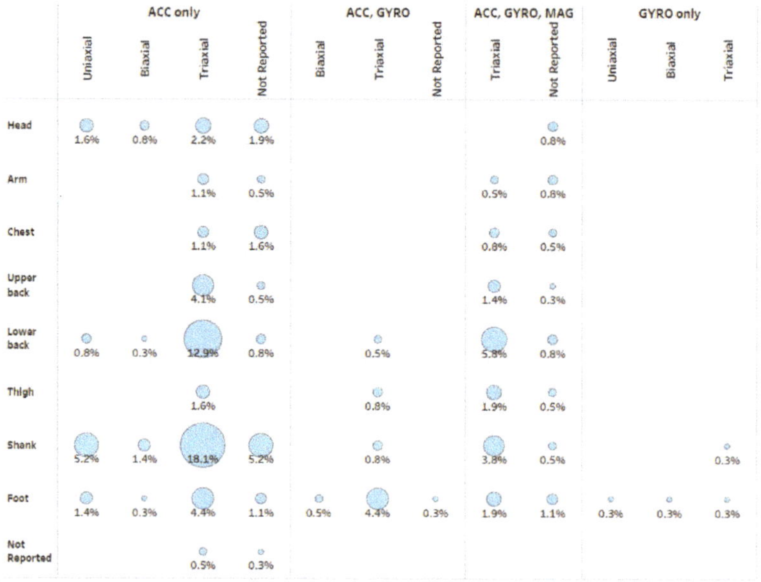

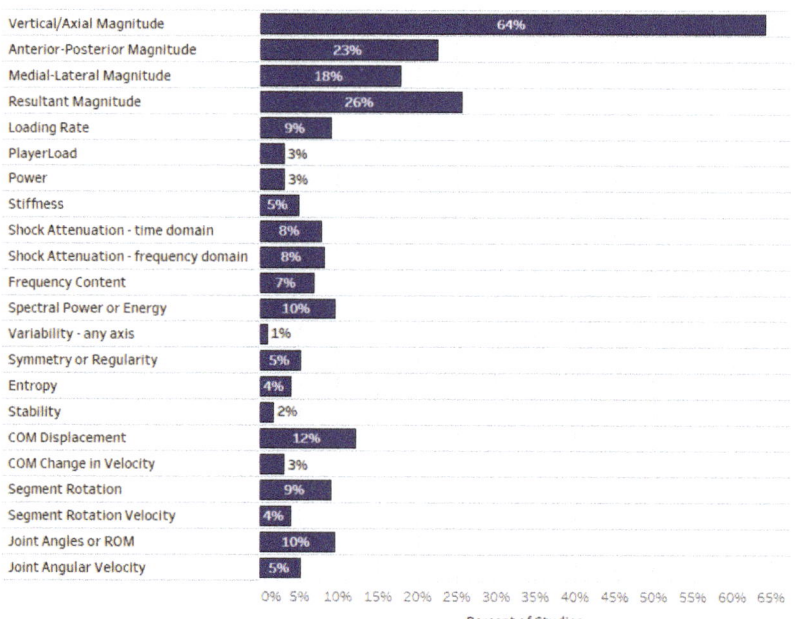

Figure 4. The percent of all combinations of devices and locations of devices on the body (365 combinations across 231 studies) by body location and sensor/axis composition. The circles are sized relative to percentage to provide visual comparisons for the frequency of device and location combinations. ACC = accelerometer, GYRO = gyroscope, and MAG = magnetometer.

Figure 5. The percent of all studies that reported each metric. Note: studies often reported multiple metrics, and therefore the sum of all percentages is greater than 100%. COM = center of mass; ROM = range of motion.

3.2.3. Analysis

The reported metrics across all studies are shown in Figure 5. The most common metric was accelerometer magnitude, with vertical/axial, anterior–posterior, medial–lateral and resultant magnitude reported in 64%, 23%, 18% and 26% of all studies, respectively. (Note: studies often reported multiple metrics, and therefore the sum of the percentages is greater than 100%.) The acceleration quantity was also reported in metrics such as loading rate, PlayerLoad, power and stiffness, with loading rate being the most common (9% of all studies). Shock attenuation was reported in 7% of all studies using time domain calculations and in 8% of all studies using frequency domain calculations. Signal frequency content was reported in 7% of all studies and the spectral power or energy was reported in 9% of all studies. Signal consistency, represented by metrics such as variability, symmetry or regularity, entropy, and stability, was reported in 5% or less of all studies, each. Segment (including center of mass) or joint kinematics were reported in up to 12% of studies, with measures of displacement more common than measures of velocity.

In terms of a statistical approach, 91% of all studies used inferential statistics, 2% used machine learning, and 7% presented results descriptively. The most common metrics reported in studies that used a machine learning statistical approach were vertical/axial magnitude, anterior–posterior magnitude, and joint angles or range of motion.

3.2.4. Participants

Half of the studies included male and female participants, 35% included males only, 3% included females only, and the sex of participants was not specified in 12% of all studies. Participants were uninjured in 99% of all studies. The mean participant age within a study ranged from 5 to 59 years, with an average of 27 years across all studies.

Recreational runners, non-runners and competitive runners were participants in 56%, 30% and 17% of all studies, respectively. (Note: some studies included multiple participant types, and therefore the sum of the percentages is greater than 100%.) The average number of participants reported for each participant type and sex is shown in Figure 6. With an average of 25 participants per study, recreational runners had the greatest number of participants per study, followed by non-runners (n = 20) then competitive runners (n = 14). This pattern was consistent when separated by males and females, and the average number of male recreational and competitive runners was greater than the average number of females in each group.

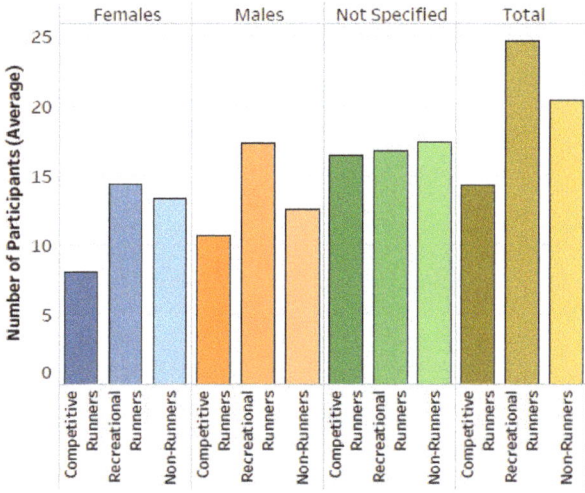

Figure 6. The average number of participants for each participant type and sex. Averages are reported across studies that included the given participant type and sex.

3.2.5. Study Details

Studies were conducted in 27 different countries. The USA had the most studies (29%), followed by Canada at 9%. In total, 39% of studies were conducted in 11 European countries.

One-quarter of the studies had interventions: 24% were quasi-experimental and 1% were randomized controlled trials. Two-thirds of the interventions (17% of all studies) were equipment-based and one-third (9% of all studies) involved training interventions. The remaining 75% of studies were observational, and 95% of observational studies (71% of all studies) used a cross-sectional study design. Prospective and retrospective cohorts accounted for 2% and <1% of studies, respectively, and 2% of studies were case studies or case control. The most common purpose (22% of studies) was to determine the validity or reliability of metrics, and 16% of studies compared metrics. In 20% of studies, the purpose was to identify changes in conditions not related to fatigue or different sessions. Differences in gait due to group membership, fatigue and sessions were reported in 13%, 12% and 2% of studies, respectively. Associations of gait metrics with performance and injury were reported for less than 2% of studies, each. (Note: some studies had multiple purposes, and therefore the sum of the percentages is greater than 100%).

3.3. Quality Assessment

There was an adequate amount of information provided for the conditions (92% of studies), devices (91%), analysis (93%), participants (83%) and study details (100%). Additionally, the relevance to running and IMUs was deemed appropriate for the conditions (99% of studies), devices (100%), analysis (100%), participants (98%) and study details (99%).

4. Discussion

The primary purpose of this review was to systematically identify how IMUs are used to record running biomechanics across real-world settings and describe the conditions in which IMU data were collected. Identifying the characteristics of IMU-based running biomechanical studies serves to mark the progress made and the steps that remain for analyzing running gait in real-world settings.

4.1. Running Environments

Laboratory-based conditions are controlled and are often different from typical running conditions, as most runners complete their runs outdoors [243]. Additionally, loads vary with each stride and a runner's load capacity changes throughout a running session [244], suggesting that assigning the same estimated load to each stride is not a suitable approximation for the cumulative load in a running session. Therefore, it is important to monitor running in actual real-world conditions, including over long distances. Yet, despite the portability of IMUs [6,7], one of the main findings of this review is that running biomechanics are mainly recorded with IMUs indoors, on a treadmill, at prescribed speeds, and over small distances. Furthermore, the majority of studies that investigated running in artificial environments have been published recently; there has not been a trend away from laboratory-based conditions over time. It is unclear why researchers are using IMUs to record running, but still have participants running in the laboratory, at controlled speeds, on treadmills and/or over short distances. If the purpose of these devices is to capture real-world running, we suggest that the research in this area should move out of the lab to less controlled environments.

Several of the included studies compared running quality between surfaces, and the findings underscore the need to observe runners in their actual running environment. More unstable surfaces lead to less regularity and greater variability during running [5,142], and the variance in outdoor data cannot be explained by indoor measures [31,95]. Moreover, it is likely that not all metrics differ between the running conditions [245]. For example, there was no difference in running power on a track compared to a treadmill [166]. Among the four studies that compared tibial acceleration between treadmill and outdoor running, the acceleration magnitude was either lower [241], greater [31,95], or not different [84,241] in outdoor conditions compared to on the treadmill, but in only one case did the outdoor conditions represent an uncontrolled running environment [95]. We suggest that rather than estimating what it is like to run outdoors, it would be helpful to use IMUs during actual training runs, over longer distances and on surfaces that represent real-world running.

To our point, starting from 2015, some studies have followed athletes for uncontrolled training runs or races [188,200–202,206,207,210–213,220,221,225–227,230]. A myriad of external factors, such as weather, traffic, and surface conditions, could influence how someone runs and therefore, it is crucial to capture running patterns in the same settings that runners *actually* run. Additionally, just as multiple trials are often used in a laboratory setting, multiple runs are needed to establish running patterns in uncontrolled settings [213].

4.2. IMU Considerations

The ability to collect accurate and useful metrics from IMUs depends on the desired metrics, the sensor specifications, device placement, running styles, and user capabilities [4]. IMUs intended for long term monitoring need to be user-friendly. The commercial devices in the included studies were worn on the foot or upper or lower back. In contrast, the most common position for devices among all included studies was on the shank, where tibial acceleration in one or multiple axes was recorded. Tibial accelerations have been used in the context of stress fractures as well as to gauge impact forces at the shank and how they are distributed along the kinetic chain [32]. While devices designed for consumer use have not been developed for placement on the shank, a research-grade device was used to record tibial accelerations of nearly 200 runners during a marathon [95]. Future investigations of impact forces in actual running conditions should consider devices and placement that can be easily applied during long-term monitoring.

The metrics reported from accelerometer sensors, such as the magnitude of acceleration, loading rate and shock attenuation, are similar to metrics obtained from force plates. When the gyroscope and/or magnetometer sensors in an IMU are used, the reported metrics provide information on the kinematics, including segment and joint rotations [28,48,51,53,55,76,102,106,113–115,127–129,134,140,144,145,148,157,181,183,186,188, 190,192,200,201,210–213,216,217,219,221,228,235]. While it is typical for IMUs to contain multiple sensors, most included studies only used an accelerometer sensor, limiting the reported metrics to those that resemble force plate metrics.

Many of the included studies were conducted in indoor settings because the purpose of the study was to evaluate the validity and reliability of IMU-based metrics compared to metrics from force plates or motion capture systems. Assessing strength of the validity and reliability was not within the scope of this review; however, devices that demonstrate adequate validity and reliability can be used in the field. Additionally, while metrics reported from an IMU are often chosen to be similar to metrics from force plates and motion capture systems, it is possible to report metrics specific to IMU signals (e.g., entropy, regularity, and symmetry) that monitor movement quality [246].

4.3. Changing Running Biomechanics

It is expected that equipment or training interventions that lead to changes in running biomechanics are needed to change injury rates. However, there is limited or conflicting evidence on the relationship between modifications of running biomechanics and running injuries [6,72,73]. It is also possible that lack of clarity on running injury risk factors is related to evaluation of biomechanical metrics in a laboratory setting before and after an intervention or injury observation, and not in the runner's natural environment [2].

Short-term changes, observed within a laboratory session, may show how training or equipment interventions can change running patterns [72,151]. Some studies use an intervention that is more long term to allow for adaptation and assess movement patterns at baseline and follow up to observe changes [20,154]. If biomechanics are only recorded in a single session, or at baseline and follow up, it is possible to use laboratory equipment (e.g., force plates and motion capture), but this does not reflect how runners run during real-world conditions. The benefit of IMUs is that movement patterns can be measured during the intervention period in actual running settings to monitor changes over time. Yet just two of the intervention studies from this review analyzed metrics from IMUs during an intervention (i.e., not just pre- and post-intervention) that was greater than one session, plus the intervention runs were conducted on a treadmill in both studies [154,218].

IMUs can also be used to observe changes in running patterns throughout a single run. In studies investigating changes in running biomechanics due to fatigue, it is common to have participants run to the point of exhaustion. Reaching a state of exhaustion as defined in a study may occur in some training runs or races, but it is likely not a typical running strategy for all runners. Thus, it is important to look at how running patterns change during actual training runs. More prospective or retrospective studies are also needed that look at how running patterns change over time, especially when those changes precede an injury [4,8]. Only five of the included studies included injured runners [24,144,152,208,221]. Due to pain, running in an injured state is likely not representative of running prior to injury. While some included studies involved runners that were previously injured and others looked at runners that were eventually injured, the data on the running patterns were only observed at a point when the runners were not injured. Regardless, IMUs can facilitate continuous monitoring that will allow for observation of changes in running patterns that lead to injury.

4.4. Participant Characteristics

Over 75% of runners use wearables, and most runners use wearable technology to monitor spatiotemporal parameters, such as distance or speed [247–249]. Competitive runners are more likely to use wearables to monitor running form or biomechanics than recreational runners [249]. Even if runners are not personally using IMUs that monitor their biomechanics, based on the results of survey studies, runners have a large appetite for using and consuming data from wearable technology [247,249]. Yet the number of participants in the included studies is low. Considering the popularity of running and runners' attitudes towards wearable technology, investigations of real-world running biomechanics should be able to recruit large numbers of participants. A bigger pool of participants will enable better comparisons across participant types and consider sex differences as injury rates differ between sexes [250]. Based on race participation statistics, there are more female than male runners [251]. However, consistent with previous findings that show females are underrepresented in sport and exercise medicine research [252], we found that the running and IMU literature is also heavily focused on male runners, with only 3% of studies being female specific.

4.5. Limitations

There are some limitations to this review, based on the exclusion criteria. First, the only type of wearable technology considered was IMUs. Limiting the search to only IMUs excluded studies that only utilized GPS devices, which are very common among runners [249]. Additional types of wearable technology that were not included in this review are heart rate monitors, mobile phone apps that did not utilize the phone's IMU sensors, and pressure-sensing insoles. Second, studies were excluded if they only reported spatiotemporal metrics. IMUs can be used to derive valid and reliable spatiotemporal stride parameters that capture running quantity [253]; however, load magnitude and distribution are also needed on a per stride basis to evaluate injury risk [244]. Finally, we excluded studies that focused on the development of new technology or methods, which eliminated some studies that reported novel machine learning algorithms. Whilst wearable technology is a growing field, future advancements will hopefully improve our ability to monitor real-world running.

There was no meta-analysis or formal quality assessment of each study as these are not expected for a scoping review. Based on our subjective evaluation, nearly all studies were appropriate to the topic of running and IMUs and contained adequate information for inclusion in this scoping review. Most likely, a more rigorous evaluation of study quality would have revealed overall weak levels of evidence across this field of study. We leave it to future systematic reviews and meta-analyses of specific outcomes and populations to use objective protocols for evaluating study quality.

5. Conclusions

Despite the portability of IMUs, one of the main findings of this review is that running biomechanics are mainly recorded with IMUs indoors, on a treadmill, at prescribed speeds, and over small distances. While it is challenging to collect data in real-world conditions due to the myriad of extrinsic factors such as weather, traffic, and surface conditions, our results indicate the vast majority of studies do not capture running biomechanical data in the same settings that runners actually run. Moreover, while it is typical for IMUs to contain multiple sensors, most included studies only used data derived from the accelerometer sensor and most studies involved placement of the IMU at the shank. Finally, the number of participants in the included studies is low and our findings show that research is still heavily focused on male runners, with only 3% of studies being female specific. Overall, considering that the purpose of IMU devices is to capture real-world running, we suggest that future research in this area should move out of the lab to less controlled and more real-world environments.

Author Contributions: Conceptualization, L.C.B., A.M.R., C.A.C. and R.F.; methodology, L.C.B., A.M.R., C.A.C. and R.F.; formal analysis, L.C.B., A.M.R. and C.A.C.; data curation, L.C.B.; writing—original draft preparation, L.C.B. and A.M.R.; writing—review and editing, L.C.B., A.M.R., C.A.C. and R.F.; visualization, L.C.B. All authors have read and agreed to the published version of the manuscript.

Funding: This study was partially funded by the NSERC CREATE Wearable Technology Research and Collaboration (We-TRAC) Training Program (Project No. CREATE/511166-2018).

Institutional Review Board Statement: Not applicable.

Informed Consent Statement: Not applicable.

Data Availability Statement: All data are available within this manuscript.

Acknowledgments: This research did not receive any specific grant from funding agencies in the public, commercial, or not-for-profit sectors.

Conflicts of Interest: The authors declare no conflict of interest.

References

1. Benson, L.C.; Räisänen, A.M.; Volkova, V.G.; Pasanen, K.; Emery, C.A. Workload a-WEAR-ness: Monitoring Workload in Team Sports with Wearable Technology. A Scoping Review. *J. Orthop. Sports Phys. Ther.* **2020**, *50*, 549–563. [CrossRef] [PubMed]
2. Willy, R.W. Innovations and pitfalls in the use of wearable devices in the prevention and rehabilitation of running related injuries. *Phys. Ther. Sport* **2018**, *29*, 26–33. [CrossRef] [PubMed]
3. Moore, I.S.; Willy, R.W. Use of Wearables: Tracking and Retraining in Endurance Runners. *Curr. Sports Med. Rep.* **2019**, *18*, 437–444. [CrossRef] [PubMed]
4. Johnston, W.; Heiderscheit, B. Mobile Technology in Running Science and Medicine: Are We Ready? *J. Orthop. Sports Phys. Ther.* **2019**, *49*, 122–125. [CrossRef]
5. Benson, L.C.; Clermont, C.A.; Ferber, R. New Considerations for Collecting Biomechanical Data Using Wearable Sensors: The Effect of Different Running Environments. *Front. Bioeng. Biotechnol.* **2020**, *8*, 86. [CrossRef]
6. Van Hooren, B.; Goudsmit, J.; Restrepo, J.; Vos, S. Real-time feedback by wearables in running: Current approaches, challenges and suggestions for improvements. *J. Sports Sci.* **2020**, *38*, 214–230. [CrossRef]
7. Napier, C.; Esculier, J.-F.; Hunt, M.A. Gait retraining: Out of the lab and onto the streets with the benefit of wearables. *Br. J. Sports Med.* **2017**, *51*, 1642–1643. [CrossRef]
8. Benson, L.C.; Clermont, C.A.; Bošnjak, E.; Ferber, R. The use of wearable devices for walking and running gait analysis outside of the lab: A systematic review. *Gait Posture* **2018**, *63*, 124–138. [CrossRef]
9. Watari, R.; Hettinga, B.; Osis, S.; Ferber, R. Validation of a Torso-Mounted Accelerometer for Measures of Vertical Oscillation and Ground Contact Time During Treadmill Running. *J. Appl. Biomech.* **2016**, *32*, 306–310. [CrossRef]

10. Benson, L.C.; Clermont, C.A.; Watari, R.; Exley, T.; Ferber, R. Automated accelerometer-based gait event detection during multiple running conditions. *Sensors* **2019**, *19*, 1483. [CrossRef]
11. Lenhart, R.L.; Thelen, D.G.; Wille, C.M.; Chumanov, E.S.; Heiderscheit, B.C. Increasing Running Step Rate Reduces Patellofemoral Joint Forces. *Med. Sci. Sports Exerc.* **2014**, *46*, 557–564. [CrossRef] [PubMed]
12. Hafer, J.; Brown, A.M.; DeMille, P.; Hillstrom, H.J.; Garber, C. The effect of a cadence retraining protocol on running biomechanics and efficiency: A pilot study. *J. Sports Sci.* **2015**, *33*, 724–731. [CrossRef] [PubMed]
13. Bood, R.J.; Nijssen, M.; van der Kamp, J.; Roerdink, M. The Power of Auditory-Motor Synchronization in Sports: Enhancing Running Performance by Coupling Cadence with the Right Beats. *PLoS ONE* **2013**, *8*, e70758. [CrossRef] [PubMed]
14. Billat, V.L.; Mille-Hamard, L.; Petit, B.; Koralsztein, J.P. The Role of Cadence on the V˙O2 Slow Component in Cycling and Running in Triathletes. *Int. J. Sports Med.* **1999**, *20*, 429–437. [CrossRef] [PubMed]
15. Aubol, K.G.; Hawkins, J.L.; Milner, C.E. Tibial Acceleration Reliability and Minimal Detectable Difference During Overground and Treadmill Running. *J. Appl. Biomech.* **2020**, *36*, 457–459. [CrossRef]
16. Blackah, N.; Bradshaw, E.J.; Kemp, J.G.; Shoushtarian, M. The Effect of Exercise-Induced Muscle Damage on Shock Dissipation during Treadmill Running. *Asian J. Exerc. Sports Sci.* **2013**, *10*, 16–30.
17. Boyer, K.A.; Nigg, B.M. Soft tissue vibrations within one soft tissue compartment. *J. Biomech.* **2006**, *39*, 645–651. [CrossRef]
18. Chadefaux, D.; Gueguen, N.; Thouze, A.; Rao, G. 3D propagation of the shock-induced vibrations through the whole lower-limb during running. *J. Biomech.* **2019**, *96*, 109343. [CrossRef]
19. Clansey, A.C.; Hanlon, M.; Wallace, E.S.; Lake, M.J. Effects of Fatigue on Running Mechanics Associated with Tibial Stress Fracture Risk. *Med. Sci. Sports Exerc.* **2012**, *44*, 1917–1923. [CrossRef]
20. Crowell, H.P.; Davis, I.S. Gait retraining to reduce lower extremity loading in runners. *Clin. Biomech.* **2011**, *26*, 78–83. [CrossRef]
21. Edwards, S.; White, S.; Humphreys, S.; Robergs, R.; O'Dwyer, N. Caution using data from triaxial accelerometers housed in player tracking units during running. *J. Sports Sci.* **2018**, *37*, 810–818. [CrossRef]
22. Gil-Rey, E.; Deere, K.C.; Maldonado-Martín, S.; Palacios-Samper, N.; Azpeitia, A.; Gorostiaga, E.M.; Tobias, J. Investigation of the Relationship Between Peak Vertical Accelerations and Aerobic Exercise Intensity During Graded Walking and Running in Postmenopausal Women. *J. Aging Phys. Act.* **2021**, *29*, 71–79. [CrossRef] [PubMed]
23. Hagen, M.; Hennig, E.M. Effects of different shoe-lacing patterns on the biomechanics of running shoes. *J. Sports Sci.* **2009**, *27*, 267–275. [CrossRef] [PubMed]
24. Havens, K.L.; Cohen, S.C.; Pratt, K.A.; Sigward, S.M. Accelerations from wearable accelerometers reflect knee loading during running after anterior cruciate ligament reconstruction. *Clin. Biomech.* **2018**, *58*, 57–61. [CrossRef] [PubMed]
25. Higgins, S.; Higgins, L.Q.; Vallabhajosula, S. Site-specific Concurrent Validity of the ActiGraph GT9X Link in the Estimation of Activity-related Skeletal Loading. *Med. Sci. Sports Exerc.* **2021**, *53*, 951–959. [CrossRef]
26. Lam, W.-K.; Liebenberg, J.; Woo, J.; Park, S.-K.; Yoon, S.-H.; Cheung, R.T.H.; Ryu, J. Do running speed and shoe cushioning influence impact loading and tibial shock in basketball players? *PeerJ* **2018**, *6*, e4753. [CrossRef]
27. Laughton, C.A.; Davis, I.M.; Hamill, J. Effect of Strike Pattern and Orthotic Intervention on Tibial Shock during Running. *J. Appl. Biomech.* **2003**, *19*, 153–168. [CrossRef]
28. Mavor, M.P.; Ross, G.B.; Clouthier, A.L.; Karakolis, T.; Graham, R.B. Validation of an IMU Suit for Military-Based Tasks. *Sensors* **2020**, *20*, 4280. [CrossRef]
29. Meinert, I.; Brown, N.; Alt, W. Effect of Footwear Modifications on Oscillations at the Achilles Tendon during Running on a Treadmill and Over Ground: A Cross-Sectional Study. *PLoS ONE* **2016**, *11*, e0152435. [CrossRef]
30. Mercer, J.A.; Bezodis, N.E.; Russell, M.; Purdy, A.; Delion, D. Kinetic consequences of constraining running behavior. *J. Sports Sci. Med.* **2005**, *4*, 144–152.
31. Milner, C.E.; Hawkins, J.L.; Aubol, K.G. Tibial Acceleration during Running Is Higher in Field Testing Than Indoor Testing. *Med. Sci. Sports Exerc.* **2020**, *52*, 1361–1366. [CrossRef]
32. Milner, C.E.; Ferber, R.; Pollard, C.D.; Hamill, J.; Davis, I.S. Biomechanical Factors Associated with Tibial Stress Fracture in Female Runners. *Med. Sci. Sports Exerc.* **2006**, *38*, 323–328. [CrossRef]
33. Nedergaard, N.J.; Verheul, J.; Drust, B.; Etchells, T.; Lisboa, P.; Robinson, M.A.; Vanrenterghem, J. The feasibility of predicting ground reaction forces during running from a trunk accelerometry driven mass-spring-damper model. *PeerJ* **2018**, *6*, e6105. [CrossRef]
34. Ogon, M.; Aleksiev, A.R.; Spratt, K.F.; Pope, M.H.; Saltzman, C.L. Footwear Affects the Behavior of Low Back Muscles When Jogging. *Int. J. Sports Med.* **2001**, *22*, 414–419. [CrossRef]
35. Rowlands, A.; Stiles, V. Accelerometer counts and raw acceleration output in relation to mechanical loading. *J. Biomech.* **2012**, *45*, 448–454. [CrossRef]
36. Sayer, T.A.; Hinman, R.S.; Paterson, K.L.; Bennell, K.L.; Hall, M.; Allison, K.; Bryant, A.L. Running-related muscle activation patterns and tibial acceleration across puberty. *J. Electromyogr. Kinesiol.* **2020**, *50*, 102381. [CrossRef]
37. Sinclair, J.; Dillon, S. The Influence of Energy Boost and Springblade Footwear on The Kinetics and Kinematics of Running. *Hum. Mov.* **2016**, *17*, 112–118. [CrossRef]
38. Sinclair, J.; Sant, B. The effects of cross-fit footwear on the kinetics and kinematics of running. *Footwear Sci.* **2016**, *9*, 41–48. [CrossRef]

39. Sinclair, J.; Fau-Goodwin, J.; Richards, J.; Shore, H. The influence of minimalist and maximalist footwear on the kinetics and kinematics of running. *Footwear Sci.* **2016**, *8*, 33–39. [CrossRef]
40. Sinclair, J.; Naemi, R.; Chockalingam, N.; Taylor, P.J.; Shore, H. The effects of shoe temperature on the kinetics and kinematics of running. *Footwear Sci.* **2015**, *7*, 173–180. [CrossRef]
41. Sinclair, J.; Rooney, E.; Naemi, R.; Atkins, S.; Chockalingam, N. Effects of Footwear Variations on Three-Dimensional Kinematics and Tibial Accelerations of Specific Movements in American Football. *J. Mech. Med. Biol.* **2017**, *17*, 1750026. [CrossRef]
42. Thompson, M.; Seegmiller, J.; McGowan, C.P. Impact Accelerations of Barefoot and Shod Running. *Int. J. Sports Med.* **2016**, *37*, 364–368. [CrossRef]
43. Trama, R.; Blache, Y.; Hautier, C. Effect of rocker shoes and running speed on lower limb mechanics and soft tissue vibrations. *J. Biomech.* **2019**, *82*, 171–177. [CrossRef]
44. Berghe, P.V.D.; Six, J.; Gerlo, J.; Leman, M.; De Clercq, D. Validity and reliability of peak tibial accelerations as real-time measure of impact loading during over-ground rearfoot running at different speeds. *J. Biomech.* **2019**, *86*, 238–242. [CrossRef]
45. Wundersitz, D.W.T.; Netto, K.J.; Aisbett, B.; Gastin, P.B. Validity of an upper-body-mounted accelerometer to measure peak vertical and resultant force during running and change-of-direction tasks. *Sports Biomech.* **2013**, *12*, 403–412. [CrossRef]
46. Adams, D.; Pozzi, F.; Carroll, A.; Rombach, A.; Zeni, J. Validity and Reliability of a Commercial Fitness Watch for Measuring Running Dynamics. *J. Orthop. Sports Phys. Ther.* **2016**, *46*, 471–476. [CrossRef]
47. Adams, D.; Pozzi, F.; Willy, R.W.; Carrol, A.; Zeni, J. Altering Cadence or Vertical Oscillation During Running: Effects on Running Related Injury Factors. *Int. J. Sports Phys. Ther.* **2018**, *13*, 633–642. [CrossRef]
48. Bayram, H.A.; Yalcin, B. The influence of biofeedback on physiological and kinematic variables of treadmill running. *Int. J. Perform. Anal. Sport* **2021**, *21*, 156–169. [CrossRef]
49. Armitage, M.; Beato, M.; McErlain-Naylor, S.A. Inter-unit reliability of IMU Step metrics using IMeasureU Blue Trident inertial measurement units for running-based team sport tasks. *J. Sports Sci.* **2021**, *39*, 1512–1518. [CrossRef]
50. Backes, A.; Skejø, S.D.; Gette, P.; Nielsen, R.Ø.; Sørensen, H.; Morio, C.; Malisoux, L. Predicting cumulative load during running using field-based measures. *Scand. J. Med. Sci. Sports* **2020**, *30*, 2399–2407. [CrossRef]
51. Bailey, G.P.; Harle, R.K. Sampling Rates and Sensor Requirements for Kinematic Assessment During Running Using Foot Mounted IMUs. *Interakt. Syst.* **2015**, *556*, 42–56. [CrossRef]
52. Barnes, M.; Guy, J.; Elsworthy, N.; Scanlan, A. A Comparison of PlayerLoad^{TM} and Heart Rate during Backwards and Forwards Locomotion during Intermittent Exercise in Rugby League Players. *Sports* **2021**, *9*, 21. [CrossRef]
53. Bastiaansen, B.; Wilmes, E.; Brink, M.; De Ruiter, C.J.; Savelsbergh, G.J.; Steijlen, A.; Jansen, K.; Van Der Helm, F.C.; Goedhart, E.A.; Van Der Laan, D.; et al. An Inertial Measurement Unit Based Method to Estimate Hip and Knee Joint Kinematics in Team Sport Athletes on the Field. *J. Vis. Exp.* **2020**, e60857. [CrossRef]
54. Benson, L.C.; Clermont, C.A.; Osis, S.T.; Kobsar, D.; Ferber, R. Classifying running speed conditions using a single wearable sensor: Optimal segmentation and feature extraction methods. *J. Biomech.* **2018**, *71*, 94–99. [CrossRef]
55. Bergamini, E.; Picerno, P.; Pillet, H.; Natta, F.; Thoreux, P.; Camomilla, V. Estimation of temporal parameters during sprint running using a trunk-mounted inertial measurement unit. *J. Biomech.* **2012**, *45*, 1123–1126. [CrossRef]
56. Boey, H.; Aeles, J.; Schütte, K.; Vanwanseele, B. The effect of three surface conditions, speed and running experience on vertical acceleration of the tibia during running. *Sports Biomech.* **2016**, *16*, 166–176. [CrossRef]
57. Boyer, K.A.; Nigg, B.M. Quantification of the input signal for soft tissue vibration during running. *J. Biomech.* **2007**, *40*, 1877–1880. [CrossRef]
58. Boyer, K.A.; Nigg, B.M. Muscle activity in the leg is tuned in response to impact force characteristics. *J. Biomech.* **2004**, *37*, 1583–1588. [CrossRef]
59. Brayne, L.; Barnes, A.; Heller, B.; Wheat, J. Using a wireless consumer accelerometer to measure tibial acceleration during running: Agreement with a skin-mounted sensor. *Sports Eng.* **2018**, *21*, 487–491. [CrossRef]
60. Buchheit, M.; Gray, A.; Morin, J.-B. Assessing Stride Variables and Vertical Stiffness with GPS-Embedded Accel-erometers: Preliminary Insights for the Monitoring of Neuromuscular Fatigue on the Field. *J. Sports Sci. Med.* **2015**, *14*, 698–701.
61. Butler, R.J.; Davis, I.M.; Laughton, C.M.; Hughes, M. Dual-Function Foot Orthosis: Effect on Shock and Control of Rearfoot Motion. *Foot Ankle Int.* **2003**, *24*, 410–414. [CrossRef] [PubMed]
62. Camelio, K.; Gruber, A.H.; Powell, D.W.; Paquette, M.R. Influence of Prolonged Running and Training on Tibial Acceleration and Movement Quality in Novice Runners. *J. Athl. Train.* **2020**, *55*, 1292–1299. [CrossRef] [PubMed]
63. Carrier, B.; Creer, A.; Williams, L.R.; Holmes, T.M.; Jolley, B.D.; Dahl, S.; Weber, E.; Standifird, T. Validation of Garmin Fenix 3 HR Fitness Tracker Biomechanics and Metabolics (VO2max). *J. Meas. Phys. Behav.* **2020**, *3*, 331–337. [CrossRef]
64. Castillo, E.R.; Lieberman, D.E. Shock attenuation in the human lumbar spine during walking and running. *J. Exp. Biol.* **2018**, *221*, jeb177949. [CrossRef]
65. Chen, C.-H.; Yang, W.-W.; Chen, Y.-P.; Chen, V.C.-F.; Liu, C.; Shiang, T.-Y. High vibration frequency of soft tissue occurs during gait in power-trained athletes. *J. Sports Sci.* **2021**, *39*, 439–445. [CrossRef]
66. Cheung, R.T.H.; An, W.W.; Au, I.P.H.; Zhang, J.H.; Chan, Z.Y.S.; MacPhail, A.J. Control of impact loading during distracted running before and after gait retraining in runners. *J. Sports Sci.* **2017**, *36*, 1497–1501. [CrossRef]
67. Cheung, R.T.H.; Zhang, J.H.; Chan, Z.Y.S.; An, W.W.; Au, I.P.; MacPhail, A.; Davis, I.S. Shoe-mounted accelerometers should be used with caution in gait retraining. *Scand. J. Med. Sci. Sports* **2019**, *29*, 835–842. [CrossRef]

68. Ching, E.; An, W.W.-K.; Au, I.P.H.; Zhang, J.H.; Chan, Z.Y.; Shum, G.; Cheung, R.T. Impact Loading During Distracted Running Before and After Auditory Gait Retraining. *Int. J. Sports Med.* **2018**, *39*, 1075–1080. [CrossRef]
69. Chu, J.J.; Caldwell, G.E. Stiffness and Damping Response Associated with Shock Attenuation in Downhill Running. *J. Appl. Biomech.* **2004**, *20*, 291–308. [CrossRef]
70. Clark, R.A.; Bartold, S.; Bryant, A.L. Tibial acceleration variability during consecutive gait cycles is influenced by the menstrual cycle. *Clin. Biomech.* **2010**, *25*, 557–562. [CrossRef]
71. Creaby, M.W.; Smith, M.M.F. Retraining running gait to reduce tibial loads with clinician or accelerometry guided feedback. *J. Sci. Med. Sport* **2016**, *19*, 288–292. [CrossRef] [PubMed]
72. Crowell, H.P.; Milner, C.E.; Hamill, J.; Davis, I.S. Reducing Impact Loading During Running With the Use of Real-Time Visual Feedback. *J. Orthop. Sports Phys. Ther.* **2010**, *40*, 206–213. [CrossRef] [PubMed]
73. Day, E.M.; Alcantara, R.S.; McGeehan, M.A.; Grabowski, A.M.; Hahn, M.E. Low-pass filter cutoff frequency affects sacral-mounted inertial measurement unit estimations of peak vertical ground reaction force and contact time during treadmill running. *J. Biomech.* **2021**, *119*, 110323. [CrossRef]
74. De La Fuente, C.; Henriquez, H.; Andrade, D.C.; Yañez, A. Running Footwear with Custom Insoles for Pressure Distribution Are Appropriate to Diminish Impacts After Shin Splints. *Asian J. Sports Med.* **2019**, *10*, 1–7. [CrossRef]
75. Deflandre, D.; Miny, K.; Schwartz, C.; Dardenne, N.; Leclerc, A.F.; Bury, T. Myotest efficiency in the mechanical analysis of the stride. *Gazzetta Medica Ital. Arch. Sci. Mediche* **2018**, *177*, 293–300. [CrossRef]
76. DeJong, M.A.F.; Hertel, J. Validation of Foot-Strike Assessment Using Wearable Sensors During Running. *J. Athl. Train.* **2020**, *55*, 1307–1310. [CrossRef] [PubMed]
77. Derrick, T.R.; Dereu, D.; McLean, S.P. Impacts and kinematic adjustments during an exhaustive run. *Med. Sci. Sports Exerc.* **2002**, *34*, 998–1002. [CrossRef]
78. Dufek, J.S.; Mercer, J.A.; Griffin, J.R. The Effects of Speed and Surface Compliance on Shock Attenuation Characteristics for Male and Female Runners. *J. Appl. Biomech.* **2009**, *25*, 219–228. [CrossRef]
79. Eggers, T.M.; Massard, T.I.; Clothier, P.J.; Lovell, R. Measuring Vertical Stiffness in Sport With Accelerometers: Exercise Caution! *J. Strength Cond. Res.* **2018**, *32*, 1919–1922. [CrossRef]
80. Encarnación-Martínez, A.; Sanchis-Sanchis, R.; Pérez-Soriano, P.; García-Gallart, A. Relationship between muscular extensibility, strength and stability and the transmission of impacts during fatigued running. *Sports Biomech.* **2020**, 1–17. [CrossRef]
81. Encarnación-Martínez, A.; García-Gallart, A.; Gallardo, A.M.; Sánchez-Sáez, J.A.; Sánchez-Sánchez, J. Effects of structural components of artificial turf on the transmission of impacts in football players. *Sports Biomech.* **2017**, *17*, 251–260. [CrossRef] [PubMed]
82. Encarnación-Martínez, A.; Pérez-Soriano, P.; Sanchis-Sanchis, R.; García-Gallart, A.; Berenguer-Vidal, R. Validity and Reliability of an Instrumented Treadmill with an Accelerometry System for Assessment of Spatio-Temporal Parameters and Impact Transmission. *Sensors* **2021**, *21*, 1758. [CrossRef]
83. Friesenbichler, B.; Stirling, L.M.; Federolf, P.; Nigg, B.M. Tissue vibration in prolonged running. *J. Biomech.* **2011**, *44*, 116–120. [CrossRef] [PubMed]
84. Fu, W.; Fang, Y.; Liu, D.M.S.; Wang, L.; Ren, S.; Liu, Y. Surface effects on in-shoe plantar pressure and tibial impact during running. *J. Sport Health Sci.* **2015**, *4*, 384–390. [CrossRef]
85. Gantz, A.M.; Derrick, T.R. Kinematics and metabolic cost of running on an irregular treadmill surface. *J. Sports Sci.* **2017**, *36*, 1103–1110. [CrossRef] [PubMed]
86. Garcia, M.C.; Gust, G.; Bazett-Jones, D.M. Tibial acceleration and shock attenuation while running over different surfaces in a trail environment. *J. Sci. Med. Sport* **2021**, *24*, 1161–1165. [CrossRef]
87. García-Pérez, J.A.; Pérez-Soriano, P.; Belloch, S.L.; Lucas, A.; Sánchez-Zuriaga, D. Effects of treadmill running and fatigue on impact acceleration in distance running. *Sports Biomech.* **2014**, *13*, 259–266. [CrossRef]
88. Giandolini, M.; Poupard, T.; Gimenez, P.; Horvais, N.; Millet, G.; Morin, J.-B.; Samozino, P. A simple field method to identify foot strike pattern during running. *J. Biomech.* **2014**, *47*, 1588–1593. [CrossRef]
89. Giandolini, M.; Horvais, N.; Farges, Y.; Samozino, P.; Morin, J.-B. Impact reduction through long-term intervention in recreational runners: Midfoot strike pattern versus low-drop/low-heel height footwear. *Eur. J. Appl. Physiol.* **2013**, *113*, 2077–2090. [CrossRef]
90. Glassbrook, D.J.; Fuller, J.T.; Alderson, J.A.; Doyle, T.L.A. Foot accelerations are larger than tibia accelerations during sprinting when measured with inertial measurement units. *J. Sports Sci.* **2019**, *38*, 248–255. [CrossRef]
91. Gullstrand, L.; Halvorsen, K.; Tinmark, F.; Eriksson, M.; Nilsson, J. Measurements of vertical displacement in running, a methodological comparison. *Gait Posture* **2009**, *30*, 71–75. [CrossRef]
92. Hardin, E.C.; Hamill, J. The Influence of Midsole Cushioning on Mechanical and Hematological Responses during a Prolonged Downhill Run. *Res. Q. Exerc. Sport* **2002**, *73*, 125–133. [CrossRef] [PubMed]
93. Iosa, M.; Morelli, D.; Nisi, E.; Sorbara, C.; Negrini, S.; Gentili, P.; Paolucci, S.; Fusco, A. Assessment of upper body accelerations in young adults with intellectual disabilities while walking, running, and dual-task running. *Hum. Mov. Sci.* **2014**, *34*, 187–195. [CrossRef] [PubMed]
94. Morelli, D.; Marro, T.; Paolucci, S.; Fusco, A.; Iosa, M. Ability and Stability of Running and Walking in Children with Cerebral Palsy. *Neuropediatrics* **2013**, *44*, 147–154. [CrossRef]

95. Johnson, C.D.; Outerleys, J.; Jamison, S.T.; Tenforde, A.S.; Ruder, M.; Davis, I.S. Comparison of Tibial Shock during Treadmill and Real-World Running. *Med. Sci. Sports Exerc.* **2020**, *52*, 1557–1562. [CrossRef] [PubMed]
96. Johnson, C.D.; Outerleys, J.; Davis, I.S. Relationships between tibial acceleration and ground reaction force measures in the medial-lateral and anterior-posterior planes. *J. Biomech.* **2021**, *117*, 110250. [CrossRef] [PubMed]
97. Johnson, C.D.; Outerleys, J.; Tenforde, A.S.; Davis, I.S. A comparison of attachment methods of skin mounted inertial measurement units on tibial accelerations. *J. Biomech.* **2020**, *113*, 110118. [CrossRef]
98. Kawabata, M.; Goto, K.; Fukusaki, C.; Sasaki, K.; Hihara, E.; Mizushina, T.; Ishii, N. Acceleration patterns in the lower and upper trunk during running. *J. Sports Sci.* **2013**, *31*, 1841–1853. [CrossRef]
99. Kenneally-Dabrowski, C.J.; Serpell, B.G.; Spratford, W. Are accelerometers a valid tool for measuring overground sprinting symmetry? *Int. J. Sports Sci. Coach.* **2017**, *13*, 270–277. [CrossRef]
100. Khassetarash, A.; Hassannejad, R.; Ettefagh, M.M.; Sari-Sarraf, V. Fatigue and soft tissue vibration during prolonged running. *Hum. Mov. Sci.* **2015**, *44*, 157–167. [CrossRef]
101. Kobsar, D.; Osis, S.T.; Hettinga, B.A.; Ferber, R. Classification accuracy of a single tri-axial accelerometer for training background and experience level in runners. *J. Biomech.* **2014**, *47*, 2508–2511. [CrossRef] [PubMed]
102. Koldenhoven, R.M.; Hertel, J. Validation of a Wearable Sensor for Measuring Running Biomechanics. *Digit. Biomark.* **2018**, *2*, 74–78. [CrossRef] [PubMed]
103. Le Bris, R.; Billat, V.; Auvinet, B.; Chaleil, D.; Hamard, L.; Barrey, E. Effect of fatigue on stride pattern continuously measured by an accelerometric gait recorder in middle distance runners. *J. Sports Med. Phys. Fit.* **2006**, *46*, 227–231.
104. LeDuc, C.; Tee, J.; Lacome, M.; Weakley, J.; Cheradame, J.; Ramirez, C.; Jones, B. Convergent Validity, Reliability, and Sensitivity of a Running Test to Monitor Neuromuscular Fatigue. *Int. J. Sports Physiol. Perform.* **2020**, *15*, 1067–1073. [CrossRef]
105. Lee, J.B.; Sutter, K.J.; Askew, C.D.; Burkett, B.J. Identifying symmetry in running gait using a single inertial sensor. *J. Sci. Med. Sport* **2010**, *13*, 559–563. [CrossRef]
106. Lee, Y.-S.; Ho, C.-S.; Shih, Y.; Chang, S.-Y.; Róbert, F.J.; Shiang, T.-Y. Assessment of walking, running, and jumping movement features by using the inertial measurement unit. *Gait Posture* **2015**, *41*, 877–881. [CrossRef]
107. Lin, S.-P.; Sung, W.-H.; Kuo, F.-C.; Kuo, T.B.; Chen, J.-J. Impact of Center-of-Mass Acceleration on the Performance of Ultramarathon Runners. *J. Hum. Kinet.* **2014**, *44*, 41–52. [CrossRef]
108. Lindsay, T.R.; Yaggie, J.A.; McGregor, S.J. A wireless accelerometer node for reliable and valid measurement of lumbar accelerations during treadmill running. *Sports Biomech.* **2016**, *15*, 11–22. [CrossRef]
109. Lindsay, T.R.; Yaggie, J.A.; McGregor, S.J. Contributions of lower extremity kinematics to trunk accelerations during moderate treadmill running. *J. Neuroeng. Rehabilit.* **2014**, *11*, 162. [CrossRef]
110. Lucas-Cuevas, A.G.; Encarnación-Martínez, A.; Camacho-García, A.; Llana-Belloch, S.; Pérez-Soriano, P. The location of the tibial accelerometer does influence impact acceleration parameters during running. *J. Sports Sci.* **2016**, *35*, 1734–1738. [CrossRef]
111. Lucas-Cuevas, A.G.; Quesada, J.I.P.; Giménez, J.V.; Aparicio, I.; Jimenez-Perez, I.; Pérez-Soriano, P. Initiating running barefoot: Effects on muscle activation and impact accelerations in habitually rearfoot shod runners. *Eur. J. Sport Sci.* **2016**, *16*, 1145–1152. [CrossRef] [PubMed]
112. Lucas-Cuevas, A.G.; García, A.C.; Llinares, R.; Quesada, J.I.P.; Llana-Belloch, S.; Pérez-Soriano, P. Influence of custom-made and prefabricated insoles before and after an intense run. *PLoS ONE* **2017**, *12*, e0173179. [CrossRef] [PubMed]
113. Macadam, P.; Nuell, S.; Cronin, J.B.; Diewald, S.; Neville, J. Thigh positioned wearable resistance improves 40 m sprint performance: A longitudinal single case design study. *J. Aust. Strength Cond.* **2019**, *27*, 39–45.
114. Macadam, P.; Cronin, J.B.; Uthoff, A.M.; Nagahara, R.; Zois, J.; Diewald, S.; Tinwala, F.; Neville, J. Thigh loaded wearable resistance increases sagittal plane rotational work of the thigh resulting in slower 50-m sprint times. *Sports Biomech.* **2020**, 1–12. [CrossRef] [PubMed]
115. Macadam, P.; Nuell, S.; Cronin, J.B.; Diewald, S.; Rowley, R.; Forster, J.; Fosch, P. Load effects of thigh wearable resistance on angular and linear kinematics and kinetics during non-motorised treadmill sprint-running. *Eur. J. Sport Sci.* **2021**, *21*, 531–538. [CrossRef] [PubMed]
116. Macdermid, P.W.; Fink, P.W.; Stannard, S.R. Shock attenuation, spatio-temporal and physiological parameter comparisons between land treadmill and water treadmill running. *J. Sport Health Sci.* **2015**, *6*, 482–488. [CrossRef]
117. Mangubat, A.L.S.; Zhang, J.H.; Chan, Z.Y.-S.; MacPhail, A.J.; Au, I.P.-H.; Cheung, R.T.-H. Biomechanical Outcomes Due to Impact Loading in Runners While Looking Sideways. *J. Appl. Biomech.* **2018**, *34*, 483–487. [CrossRef]
118. Masci, I.; Vannozzi, G.; Bergamini, E.; Pesce, C.; Getchell, N.; Cappozzo, A. Assessing locomotor skills development in childhood using wearable inertial sensor devices: The running paradigm. *Gait Posture* **2013**, *37*, 570–574. [CrossRef]
119. McGregor, S.J.; Busa, M.A.; Skufca, J.; Yaggie, J.A.; Bollt, E.M. Control entropy identifies differential changes in complexity of walking and running gait patterns with increasing speed in highly trained runners. *Chaos Interdiscip. J. Nonlinear Sci.* **2009**, *19*, 026109. [CrossRef]
120. Mercer, J.A.; Chona, C. Stride length–velocity relationship during running with body weight support. *J. Sport Health Sci.* **2015**, *4*, 391–395. [CrossRef]
121. Mercer, J.A.; Vance, J.; Hreljac, A.; Hamill, J. Relationship between shock attenuation and stride length during running at different velocities. *Graefe's Arch. Clin. Exp. Ophthalmol.* **2002**, *87*, 403–408. [CrossRef] [PubMed]

122. Mercer, J.A.; Devita, P.; Derrick, T.R.; Bates, B.T. Individual Effects of Stride Length and Frequency on Shock Attenuation during Running. *Med. Sci. Sports Exerc.* **2003**, *35*, 307–313. [CrossRef] [PubMed]
123. Mercer, J.A.; Dufek, J.S.; Mangus, B.C.; Rubley, M.D.; Bhanot, K.; Aldridge, J.M. A Description of Shock Attenuation for Children Running. *J. Athl. Train.* **2010**, *45*, 259–264. [CrossRef] [PubMed]
124. Mercer, J.A.; Bates, B.T.; Dufek, J.; Hreljac, A. Characteristics of shock attenuation during fatigued running. *J. Sports Sci.* **2003**, *21*, 911–919. [CrossRef]
125. Meyer, U.; Ernst, D.; Schott, S.; Riera, C.; Hattendorf, J.; Romkes, J.; Granacher, U.; Göpfert, B.; Kriemler, S. Validation of two accelerometers to determine mechanical loading of physical activities in children. *J. Sports Sci.* **2015**, *33*, 1702–1709. [CrossRef] [PubMed]
126. Meyer, C.; Mohr, M.; Falbriard, M.; Nigg, S.R.; Nigg, B.M. Influence of footwear comfort on the variability of running kinematics. *Footwear Sci.* **2017**, *10*, 29–38. [CrossRef]
127. Mitschke, C.; Öhmichen, M.; Milani, T.L. A Single Gyroscope Can Be Used to Accurately Determine Peak Eversion Velocity during Locomotion at Different Speeds and in Various Shoes. *Appl. Sci.* **2017**, *7*, 659. [CrossRef]
128. Mitschke, C.; Zaumseil, F.; Milani, T.L. The influence of inertial sensor sampling frequency on the accuracy of measurement parameters in rearfoot running. *Comput. Methods Biomech. Biomed. Eng.* **2017**, *20*, 1502–1511. [CrossRef]
129. Mitschke, C.; Kiesewetter, P.; Milani, T.L. The Effect of the Accelerometer Operating Range on Biomechanical Parameters: Stride Length, Velocity, and Peak Tibial Acceleration during Running. *Sensors* **2018**, *18*, 130. [CrossRef]
130. Montgomery, G.; Abt, G.; Dobson, C.; Smith, T.; Ditroilo, M. Tibial impacts and muscle activation during walking, jogging and running when performed overground, and on motorised and non-motorised treadmills. *Gait Posture* **2016**, *49*, 120–126. [CrossRef]
131. Moran, M.; Rickert, B.J.; Greer, B.K. Tibial Acceleration and Spatiotemporal Mechanics in Distance Runners During Reduced-Body-Weight Conditions. *J. Sport Rehabil.* **2017**, *26*, 221–226. [CrossRef] [PubMed]
132. Morrow, M.M.B.; Hurd, W.J.; Fortune, E.; Lugade, V.; Aufman, K.R.K. Accelerations of the Waist and Lower Extremities over a Range of Gait Velocities to Aid in Activity Monitor Selection for Field-Based Studies. *J. Appl. Biomech.* **2014**, *30*, 581–585. [CrossRef]
133. Neugebauer, J.M.; Hawkins, D.A.; Beckett, L. Estimating Youth Locomotion Ground Reaction Forces Using an Accelerometer-Based Activity Monitor. *PLoS ONE* **2012**, *7*, e48182. [CrossRef] [PubMed]
134. Nüesch, C.; Roos, E.; Pagenstert, G.; Muendermann, A. Measuring joint kinematics of treadmill walking and running: Comparison between an inertial sensor based system and a camera-based system. *J. Biomech.* **2017**, *57*, 32–38. [CrossRef] [PubMed]
135. O'Connor, K.M.; Hamill, J. Does Running on a Cambered Road Predispose a Runner to Injury? *J. Appl. Biomech.* **2002**, *18*, 3–14. [CrossRef]
136. Provot, T.; Chiementin, X.; Oudin, E.; Bolaers, F.; Murer, S. Validation of a High Sampling Rate Inertial Measurement Unit for Acceleration During Running. *Sensors* **2017**, *17*, 1958. [CrossRef]
137. Provot, T.; Chiementin, X.; Bolaers, F.; Murer, S. Effect of running speed on temporal and frequency indicators from wearable MEMS accelerometers. *Sports Biomech.* **2021**, *20*, 831–843. [CrossRef]
138. Rabuffetti, M.; Scalera, G.M.; Ferrarin, M. Effects of Gait Strategy and Speed on Regularity of Locomotion Assessed in Healthy Subjects Using a Multi-Sensor Method. *Sensors* **2019**, *19*, 513. [CrossRef]
139. Raper, D.P.; Witchalls, J.; Philips, E.J.; Knight, E.; Drew, M.K.; Waddington, G. Use of a tibial accelerometer to measure ground reaction force in running: A reliability and validity comparison with force plates. *J. Sci. Med. Sport* **2018**, *21*, 84–88. [CrossRef]
140. Reenalda, J.; Maartens, E.; Buurke, J.H.; Gruber, A.H. Kinematics and shock attenuation during a prolonged run on the athletic track as measured with inertial magnetic measurement units. *Gait Posture* **2019**, *68*, 155–160. [CrossRef]
141. Schütte, K.H.; Maas, E.A.; Exadaktylos, V.; Berckmans, D.; Venter, R.; Vanwanseele, B. Wireless Tri-Axial Trunk Accelerometry Detects Deviations in Dynamic Center of Mass Motion Due to Running-Induced Fatigue. *PLoS ONE* **2015**, *10*, e0141957. [CrossRef] [PubMed]
142. Schütte, K.H.; Aeles, J.; De Beéck, T.O.; van der Zwaard, B.C.; Venter, R.; Vanwanseele, B. Surface effects on dynamic stability and loading during outdoor running using wireless trunk accelerometry. *Gait Posture* **2016**, *48*, 220–225. [CrossRef] [PubMed]
143. Schütte, K.H.; Sackey, S.; Venter, R.; Vanwanseele, B. Energy cost of running instability evaluated with wearable trunk accelerometry. *J. Appl. Physiol.* **2018**, *124*, 462–472. [CrossRef] [PubMed]
144. Setuain, I.; Lecumberri, P.; Izquierdo, M. Sprint mechanics return to competition follow-up after hamstring injury on a professional soccer player: A case study with an inertial sensor unit based methodological approach. *J. Biomech.* **2017**, *63*, 186–191. [CrossRef]
145. Setuain, I.; Lecumberri, P.; Ahtiainen, J.P.; Mero, A.A.; Häkkinen, K.; Izquierdo, M. Sprint mechanics evaluation using inertial sensor-based technology: A laboratory validation study. *Scand. J. Med. Sci. Sports* **2017**, *28*, 463–472. [CrossRef]
146. Sheerin, K.R.; Besier, T.; Reid, D.; Hume, P.A. The one-week and six-month reliability and variability of three-dimensional tibial acceleration in runners. *Sports Biomech.* **2017**, *17*, 531–540. [CrossRef]
147. Sheerin, K.R.; Besier, T.; Reid, D. The influence of running velocity on resultant tibial acceleration in runners. *Sports Biomech.* **2020**, *19*, 750–760. [CrossRef]
148. Shiang, T.-Y.; Hsieh, T.-Y.; Lee, Y.-S.; Wu, C.-C.; Yu, M.-C.; Mei, C.-H.; Tai, I.-H. Determine the Foot Strike Pattern Using Inertial Sensors. *J. Sens.* **2016**, *2016*, 1–6. [CrossRef]
149. Simoni, L.; Pancani, S.; Vannetti, F.; Macchi, C.; Pasquini, G. Relationship between Lower Limb Kinematics and Upper Trunk Acceleration in Recreational Runners. *J. Healthc. Eng.* **2020**, *2020*, 1–7. [CrossRef]

150. Stickford, A.S.; Chapman, R.F.; Johnston, J.D.; Stager, J.M. Lower-Leg Compression, Running Mechanics, and Economy in Trained Distance Runners. *Int. J. Sports Physiol. Perform.* **2015**, *10*, 76–83. [CrossRef]
151. TenBroek, T.M.; Rodrigues, P.A.; Frederick, E.C.; Hamill, J. Midsole Thickness Affects Running Patterns in Habitual Rearfoot Strikers During a Sustained Run. *J. Appl. Biomech.* **2014**, *30*, 521–528. [CrossRef] [PubMed]
152. Tenforde, A.S.; Hayano, T.; Jamison, S.T.; Outerleys, J.; Davis, I.S. Tibial Acceleration Measured from Wearable Sensors Is Associated with Loading Rates in Injured Runners. *PM&R* **2020**, *12*, 679–684. [CrossRef]
153. Thomas, J.M.; Derrick, T.R. Effects of Step Uncertainty on Impact Peaks, Shock Attenuation, and Knee/Subtalar Synchrony in Treadmill Running. *J. Appl. Biomech.* **2003**, *19*, 60–70. [CrossRef]
154. Tirosh, O.; Steinberg, N.; Nemet, D.; Eliakim, A.; Orland, G. Visual feedback gait re-training in overweight children can reduce excessive tibial acceleration during walking and running: An experimental intervention study. *Gait Posture* **2019**, *68*, 101–105. [CrossRef] [PubMed]
155. Tirosh, O.; Orland, G.; Eliakim, A.; Nemet, D.; Steinberg, N. Tibial impact accelerations in gait of primary school children: The effect of age and speed. *Gait Posture* **2017**, *57*, 265–269. [CrossRef] [PubMed]
156. Tirosh, O.; Orland, G.; Eliakim, A.; Nemet, D.; Steinberg, N. Attenuation of Lower Body Acceleration in Overweight and Healthy-Weight Children During Running. *J. Appl. Biomech.* **2020**, *36*, 33–38. [CrossRef]
157. Van Werkhoven, H.; Farina, K.; Langley, M.H. Using A Soft Conformable Foot Sensor to Measure Changes in Foot Strike Angle During Running. *Sports* **2019**, *7*, 184. [CrossRef]
158. Walsh, G.S. Dynamics of Modular Neuromotor Control of Walking and Running during Single and Dual Task Conditions. *Neurosci.* **2021**, *465*, 1–10. [CrossRef]
159. Waite, N.; Goetschius, J.; Lauver, J.D. Effect of Grade and Surface Type on Peak Tibial Acceleration in Trained Distance Runners. *J. Appl. Biomech.* **2021**, *37*, 2–5. [CrossRef]
160. Winter, S.C.; Lee, J.B.; Leadbetter, R.I.; Gordon, S.J. Validation of a Single Inertial Sensor for Measuring Running Kinematics Overground during a Prolonged Run. *J. Fit. Res.* **2016**, *5*, 14–23.
161. Wixted, A.; Billing, D.C.; James, D. Validation of trunk mounted inertial sensors for analysing running biomechanics under field conditions, using synchronously collected foot contact data. *Sports Eng.* **2010**, *12*, 207–212. [CrossRef]
162. Wood, C.M.; Kipp, K. Use of audio biofeedback to reduce tibial impact accelerations during running. *J. Biomech.* **2014**, *47*, 1739–1741. [CrossRef] [PubMed]
163. Wundersitz, D.; Gastin, P.B.; Richter, C.; Robertson, S.J.; Netto, K. Validity of a trunk-mounted accelerometer to assess peak accelerations during walking, jogging and running. *Eur. J. Sport Sci.* **2015**, *15*, 382–390. [CrossRef] [PubMed]
164. Zhang, J.H.; Chan, Z.Y.-S.; Au, I.P.-H.; An, W.W.; Shull, P.B.; Cheung, R.T.-H. Transfer Learning Effects of Biofeedback Running Retraining in Untrained Conditions. *Med. Sci. Sports Exerc.* **2019**, *51*, 1904–1908. [CrossRef] [PubMed]
165. Zhang, J.H.; An, W.W.; Au, I.P.; Chen, T.L.; Cheung, R.T. Comparison of the correlations between impact loading rates and peak accelerations measured at two different body sites: Intra- and inter-subject analysis. *Gait Posture* **2016**, *46*, 53–56. [CrossRef]
166. Aubry, R.L.; Power, G.A.; Burr, J.F. An Assessment of Running Power as a Training Metric for Elite and Recreational Runners. *J. Strength Cond. Res.* **2018**, *32*, 2258–2264. [CrossRef]
167. Austin, C.L.; Hokanson, J.F.; McGinnis, P.M.; Patrick, S. The Relationship between Running Power and Running Economy in Well-Trained Distance Runners. *Sports* **2018**, *6*, 142. [CrossRef]
168. Barrett, S.; Midgley, A.; Lovell, R. PlayerLoad™: Reliability, Convergent Validity, and Influence of Unit Position during Treadmill Running. *Int. J. Sports Physiol. Perform.* **2014**, *9*, 945–952. [CrossRef]
169. De Brabandere, A.; De Beéck, T.O.; Schütte, K.H.; Meert, W.; Vanwanseele, B.; Davis, J. Data fusion of body-worn accelerometers and heart rate to predict VO2max during submaximal running. *PLoS ONE* **2018**, *13*, e0199509. [CrossRef]
170. Cher, P.H.; Worringham, C.J.; Stewart, I.B. Human runners exhibit a least variable gait speed. *J. Sports Sci.* **2016**, *35*, 2211–2219. [CrossRef]
171. Clansey, A.C.; Lake, M.J.; Wallace, E.S.; Feehally, T.; Hanlon, M. Can Trained Runners Effectively Attenuate Impact Acceleration During Repeated High-Intensity Running Bouts? *J. Appl. Biomech.* **2016**, *32*, 261–268. [CrossRef]
172. Clermont, C.A.; Benson, L.C.; Osis, S.T.; Kobsar, D.; Ferber, R. Running patterns for male and female competitive and recreational runners based on accelerometer data. *J. Sports Sci.* **2019**, *37*, 204–211. [CrossRef] [PubMed]
173. Clermont, C.A.; Pohl, A.J.; Ferber, R. Fatigue-Related Changes in Running Gait Patterns Persist in the Days Following a Marathon Race. *J. Sport Rehabilit.* **2020**, *29*, 934–941. [CrossRef] [PubMed]
174. Dériaz, O.; Najafi, B.; Ballabeni, P.; Crettenand, A.; Gobelet, C.; Aminian, K.; Rizzoli, R.; Gremion, G. Proximal tibia volumetric bone mineral density is correlated to the magnitude of local acceleration in male long-distance runners. *J. Appl. Physiol.* **2010**, *108*, 852–857. [CrossRef] [PubMed]
175. Enders, H.; von Tscharner, V.; Nigg, B.M. The effects of preferred and non-preferred running strike patterns on tissue vibration properties. *J. Sci. Med. Sport* **2014**, *17*, 218–222. [CrossRef]
176. Garcia-Byrne, F.; Wycherley, T.; Bishop, C.; Schwerdt, S.; Porter, J.; Buckley, J. Accelerometer detected lateral sway during a submaximal running test correlates with endurance exercise performance in elite Australian male cricket players. *J. Sci. Med. Sport* **2019**, *23*, 519–523. [CrossRef]
177. Giandolini, M.; Horvais, N.; Rossi, J.; Millet, G.; Samozino, P.; Morin, J.-B. Foot strike pattern differently affects the axial and transverse components of shock acceleration and attenuation in downhill trail running. *J. Biomech.* **2016**, *49*, 1765–1771. [CrossRef]

178. Giandolini, M.; Horvais, N.; Rossi, J.; Millet, G.; Morin, J.-B.; Samozino, P. Effects of the foot strike pattern on muscle activity and neuromuscular fatigue in downhill trail running. *Scand. J. Med. Sci. Sports* **2016**, *27*, 809–819. [CrossRef]
179. Horvais, N.; Samozino, P.; Chiementin, X.; Morin, J.-B.; Giandolini, M. Cushioning perception is associated with both tibia acceleration peak and vibration magnitude in heel-toe running. *Footwear Sci.* **2019**, *11*, 35–44. [CrossRef]
180. Hughes, T.; Jones, R.K.; Starbuck, C.; Sergeant, J.C.; Callaghan, M. The value of tibial mounted inertial measurement units to quantify running kinetics in elite football (soccer) players. A reliability and agreement study using a research orientated and a clinically orientated system. *J. Electromyogr. Kinesiol.* **2019**, *44*, 156–164. [CrossRef]
181. Koska, D.; Gaudel, J.; Hein, T.; Maiwald, C. Validation of an inertial measurement unit for the quantification of rearfoot kinematics during running. *Gait Posture* **2018**, *64*, 135–140. [CrossRef] [PubMed]
182. Melo, C.C.; Carpes, F.P.; Vieira, T.M.; Mendes, T.T.; de Paula, L.V.; Chagas, M.H.; Peixoto, G.H.; de Andrade, A.G.P. Correlation between running asymmetry, mechanical efficiency, and performance during a 10 km run. *J. Biomech.* **2020**, *109*, 109913. [CrossRef] [PubMed]
183. Moltó, I.N.; Albiach, J.P.; Amer-Cuenca, J.J.; Segura-Ortí, E.; Gabriel, W.; Martínez-Gramage, J. Wearable Sensors Detect Differences between the Sexes in Lower Limb Electromyographic Activity and Pelvis 3D Kinematics during Running. *Sensors* **2020**, *20*, 6478. [CrossRef] [PubMed]
184. Morio, C.; Sevrez, V.; Chavet, P.; Berton, E.; Nicol, C. Neuro-mechanical adjustments to shod versus barefoot treadmill runs in the acute and delayed stretch-shortening cycle recovery phases. *J. Sports Sci.* **2016**, *34*, 738–745. [CrossRef]
185. Murray, A.M.; Ryu, J.H.; Sproule, J.; Turner, A.P.; Graham-Smith, P.; Cardinale, M. A Pilot Study Using Entropy as a Noninvasive Assessment of Running. *Int. J. Sports Physiol. Perform.* **2017**, *12*, 1119–1122. [CrossRef]
186. Navalta, J.W.; Montes, J.; Bodell, N.G.; Aguilar, C.D.; Radzak, K.; Manning, J.W.; DeBeliso, M. Reliability of Trail Walking and Running Tasks Using the Stryd Power Meter. *Int. J. Sports Med.* **2019**, *40*, 498–502. [CrossRef]
187. Olin, E.D.; Gutierrez, G.M. EMG and tibial shock upon the first attempt at barefoot running. *Hum. Mov. Sci.* **2013**, *32*, 343–352. [CrossRef]
188. Perrotin, N.; Gardan, N.; Lesprillier, A.; Le Goff, C.; Seigneur, J.-M.; Abdi, E.; Sanudo, B.; Taiar, R. Biomechanics of Trail Running Performance: Quantification of Spatio-Temporal Parameters by Using Low Cost Sensors in Ecological Conditions. *Appl. Sci.* **2021**, *11*, 2093. [CrossRef]
189. Provot, T.; Munera, M.; Bolaers, F.; Vitry, G.; Chiementin, X. Intra and Inter Test Repeatability of Accelerometric Indicators Measured While Running. *Procedia Eng.* **2016**, *147*, 573–577. [CrossRef]
190. Reenalda, J.; Maartens, E.; Homan, L.; Buurke, J. (Jaap) Continuous three dimensional analysis of running mechanics during a marathon by means of inertial magnetic measurement units to objectify changes in running mechanics. *J. Biomech.* **2016**, *49*, 3362–3367. [CrossRef]
191. Seeley, M.K.; Evans-Pickett, A.; Collins, G.Q.; Tracy, J.B.; Tuttle, N.J.; Rosquist, P.G.; Merrell, A.J.; Christensen, W.F.; Fullwood, D.T.; Bowden, A.E. Predicting vertical ground reaction force during running using novel piezoresponsive sensors and accelerometry. *J. Sports Sci.* **2020**, *38*, 1844–1858. [CrossRef] [PubMed]
192. Shih, Y.; Ho, C.-S.; Shiang, T.-Y. Measuring kinematic changes of the foot using a gyro sensor during intense running. *J. Sports Sci.* **2013**, *32*, 550–556. [CrossRef] [PubMed]
193. Tirosh, O.; Orland, G.; Eliakim, A.; Nemet, D.; Steinberg, N. Repeatability of tibial acceleration measurements made on children during walking and running. *J. Sci. Med. Sport* **2019**, *22*, 91–95. [CrossRef] [PubMed]
194. Ueberschär, O.; Fleckenstein, D.; Wüstenfeld, J.C.; Warschun, F.; Falz, R.; Wolfarth, B. Running on the hypogravity treadmill AlterG® does not reduce the magnitude of peak tibial impact accelerations. *Sports Orthop. Traumatol.* **2019**, *35*, 423–434. [CrossRef]
195. Berghe, P.V.D.; Lorenzoni, V.; Derie, R.; Six, J.; Gerlo, J.; Leman, M.; De Clercq, D. Music-based biofeedback to reduce tibial shock in over-ground running: A proof-of-concept study. *Sci. Rep.* **2021**, *11*, 4091. [CrossRef]
196. van der Bie, J.; Kröse, B. Happy Running? *Hybrid Learn. Educ.* **2015**, *9425*, 357–360. [CrossRef]
197. Weich, C.; Jensen, R.L.; Vieten, M. Triathlon transition study: Quantifying differences in running movement pattern and precision after bike-run transition. *Sports Biomech.* **2017**, *18*, 215–228. [CrossRef]
198. Bigelow, E.M.; Elvin, N.G.; Elvin, A.A.; Arnoczky, S.P. Peak Impact Accelerations during Track and Treadmill Running. *J. Appl. Biomech.* **2013**, *29*, 639–644. [CrossRef]
199. Brahms, C.M.; Zhao, Y.; Gerhard, D.; Barden, J.M. Long-range correlations and stride pattern variability in recreational and elite distance runners during a prolonged run. *Gait Posture* **2020**, *92*, 487–492. [CrossRef]
200. Clermont, C.A.; Benson, L.C.; Edwards, W.B.; Hettinga, B.A.; Ferber, R. New Considerations for Wearable Technology Data: Changes in Running Biomechanics During a Marathon. *J. Appl. Biomech.* **2019**, *35*, 401–409. [CrossRef]
201. DeJong, M.A.F.; Hertel, J. Outdoor Running Activities Captured Using Wearable Sensors in Adult Competitive Runners. *Int. J. Athl. Ther. Train.* **2020**, *25*, 76–85. [CrossRef]
202. Giandolini, M.; Pavailler, S.; Samozino, P.; Morin, J.-B.; Horvais, N. Foot strike pattern and impact continuous measurements during a trail running race: Proof of concept in a world-class athlete. *Footwear Sci.* **2015**, *7*, 127–137. [CrossRef]
203. Gómez-Carmona, C.D.; Bastida-Castillo, A.; González-Custodio, A.; Olcina, G.; Pino-Ortega, J. Using an Inertial Device (WIMU PRO) to Quantify Neuromuscular Load in Running: Reliability, Convergent Validity, and Influence of Type of Surface and Device Location. *J. Strength Cond. Res.* **2020**, *34*, 365–373. [CrossRef] [PubMed]

204. Hoenig, T.; Hamacher, D.; Braumann, K.-M.; Zech, A.; Hollander, K. Analysis of running stability during 5000 m running. *Eur. J. Sport Sci.* **2019**, *19*, 413–421. [CrossRef] [PubMed]
205. Provot, T.; Chiementin, X.; Bolaers, F.; Munera, M. A time to exhaustion model during prolonged running based on wearable accelerometers. *Sports Biomech.* **2021**, *20*, 330–343. [CrossRef] [PubMed]
206. Rojas-Valverde, D.; Sánchez-Ureña, B.; Pino-Ortega, J.; Gómez-Carmona, C.; Gutierrez-Vargas, R.; Timón, R.; Olcina, G. External Workload Indicators of Muscle and Kidney Mechanical Injury in Endurance Trail Running. *Int. J. Environ. Res. Public Health* **2019**, *16*, 3909. [CrossRef]
207. Rojas-Valverde, D.; Timón, R.; Sánchez-Ureña, B.; Pino-Ortega, J.; Martínez-Guardado, I.; Olcina, G. Potential Use of Wearable Sensors to Assess Cumulative Kidney Trauma in Endurance Off-Road Running. *J. Funct. Morphol. Kinesiol.* **2020**, *5*, 93. [CrossRef]
208. Schütte, K.H.; Seerden, S.; Venter, R.; Vanwanseele, B. Influence of outdoor running fatigue and medial tibial stress syndrome on accelerometer-based loading and stability. *Gait Posture* **2018**, *59*, 222–228. [CrossRef]
209. Ueberschär, O.; Fleckenstein, D.; Warschun, F.; Walter, N.; Hoppe, M.W. Case report on lateral asymmetries in two junior elite long-distance runners during a high-altitude training camp. *Sports Orthop. Traumatol.* **2019**, *35*, 399–406. [CrossRef]
210. Ahamed, N.U.; Kobsar, D.; Benson, L.C.; Clermont, C.A.; Osis, S.T.; Ferber, R. Subject-specific and group-based running pattern classification using a single wearable sensor. *J. Biomech.* **2019**, *84*, 227–233. [CrossRef]
211. Ahamed, N.U.; Kobsar, D.; Benson, L.; Clermont, C.; Kohrs, R.; Osis, S.T.; Ferber, R. Using wearable sensors to classify subject-specific running biomechanical gait patterns based on changes in environmental weather conditions. *PLoS ONE* **2018**, *13*, e0203839. [CrossRef]
212. Ahamed, N.U.; Benson, L.C.; Clermont, C.A.; Pohl, A.J.; Ferber, R. New Considerations for Collecting Biomechanical Data Using Wearable Sensors: How Does Inclination Influence the Number of Runs Needed to Determine a Stable Running Gait Pattern? *Sensors* **2019**, *19*, 2516. [CrossRef] [PubMed]
213. Benson, L.C.; Ahamed, N.U.; Kobsar, D.; Ferber, R. New considerations for collecting biomechanical data using wearable sensors: Number of level runs to define a stable running pattern with a single IMU. *J. Biomech.* **2019**, *85*, 187–192. [CrossRef]
214. Cartón-Llorente, A.; García-Pinillos, F.; Royo-Borruel, J.; Rubio-Peirotén, A.; Jaén-Carrillo, D.; Roche-Seruendo, L.E. Estimating Functional Threshold Power in Endurance Running from Shorter Time Trials Using a 6-Axis Inertial Measurement Sensor. *Sensors* **2021**, *21*, 582. [CrossRef] [PubMed]
215. Cerezuela-Espejo, V.; Hernández-Belmonte, A.; Courel-Ibáñez, J.; Conesa-Ros, E.; Martínez-Cava, A.; Pallarés, J.G. Running power meters and theoretical models based on laws of physics: Effects of environments and running conditions. *Physiol. Behav.* **2020**, *223*, 112972. [CrossRef] [PubMed]
216. Colapietro, M.; Fraser, J.J.; Resch, J.E.; Hertel, J. Running mechanics during 1600 meter track runs in young adults with and without chronic ankle instability. *Phys. Ther. Sport* **2019**, *42*, 16–25. [CrossRef]
217. Gregory, C.J.; Koldenhoven, R.M.; Higgins, M.; Hertel, J. External ankle supports alter running biomechanics: A field-based study using wearable sensors. *Physiol. Meas.* **2019**, *40*, 044003. [CrossRef]
218. Hollander, K.; Hamacher, D.; Zech, A. Running barefoot leads to lower running stability compared to shod running - results from a randomized controlled study. *Sci. Rep.* **2021**, *11*, 4376. [CrossRef]
219. Hollis, C.R.; Koldenhoven, R.M.; Resch, J.E.; Hertel, J. Running biomechanics as measured by wearable sensors: Effects of speed and surface. *Sports Biomech.* **2021**, *20*, 521–531. [CrossRef]
220. Kiernan, D.; Hawkins, D.A.; Manoukian, M.A.; McKallip, M.; Oelsner, L.; Caskey, C.F.; Coolbaugh, C.L. Accelerometer-based prediction of running injury in National Collegiate Athletic Association track athletes. *J. Biomech.* **2018**, *73*, 201–209. [CrossRef]
221. Koldenhoven, R.M.; Virostek, M.A.; DeJong, M.A.F.; Higgins, M.; Hertel, J. Increased Contact Time and Strength Deficits in Runners With Exercise-Related Lower Leg Pain. *J. Athl. Train.* **2020**, *55*, 1247–1254. [CrossRef] [PubMed]
222. McGregor, S.J.; Busa, M.A.; Yaggie, J.A.; Bollt, E.M. High Resolution MEMS Accelerometers to Estimate VO2 and Compare Running Mechanics between Highly Trained Inter-Collegiate and Untrained Runners. *PLoS ONE* **2009**, *4*, e7355. [CrossRef] [PubMed]
223. Nüesch, C.; Roos, E.; Egloff, C.; Pagenstert, G.; Mündermann, A. The effect of different running shoes on treadmill running mechanics and muscle activity assessed using statistical parametric mapping (SPM). *Gait Posture* **2019**, *69*, 1–7. [CrossRef] [PubMed]
224. Olcina, G.; Perez-Sousa, M. Ángel; Escobar-Alvarez, J.A.; Timón, R. Effects of Cycling on Subsequent Running Performance, Stride Length, and Muscle Oxygen Saturation in Triathletes. *Sports* **2019**, *7*, 115. [CrossRef]
225. Rochat, N.; Seifert, L.; Guignard, B.; Hauw, D. An enactive approach to appropriation in the instrumented activity of trail running. *Cogn. Process.* **2019**, *20*, 459–477. [CrossRef]
226. Ruder, M.; Jamison, S.T.; Tenforde, A.; Mulloy, F.; Davis, I.S. Relationship of Foot Strike Pattern and Landing Impacts during a Marathon. *Med. Sci. Sports Exerc.* **2019**, *51*, 2073–2079. [CrossRef]
227. Ryan, M.R.; Napier, C.; Greenwood, D.; Paquette, M.R. Comparison of different measures to monitor week-to-week changes in training load in high school runners. *Int. J. Sports Sci. Coach.* **2021**, *16*, 370–379. [CrossRef]
228. Strohrmann, C.; Harms, H.; Kappeler-Setz, C.; Troster, G. Monitoring Kinematic Changes with Fatigue in Running Using Body-Worn Sensors. *IEEE Trans. Inf. Technol. Biomed.* **2012**, *16*, 983–990. [CrossRef]
229. Berghe, P.V.D.; Gosseries, M.; Gerlo, J.; Lenoir, M.; Leman, M.; De Clercq, D. Change-Point Detection of Peak Tibial Acceleration in Overground Running Retraining. *Sensors* **2020**, *20*, 1720. [CrossRef]

230. Vanwanseele, B.; De Beéck, T.O.; Schütte, K.; Davis, J. Accelerometer Based Data Can Provide a Better Estimate of Cumulative Load During Running Compared to GPS Based Parameters. *Front. Sports Act. Living* **2020**, *2*, 575596. [CrossRef]
231. Willis, S.J.; Gellaerts, J.; Mariani, B.; Basset, P.; Borrani, F.; Millet, G.P. Level Versus Uphill Economy and Mechanical Responses in Elite Ultratrail Runners. *Int. J. Sports Physiol. Perform.* **2019**, *14*, 1001–1005. [CrossRef] [PubMed]
232. Bielik, V. Gender differences of running kinematics and economy in trained distance runners. *Gazz. Med. Ital. Arch. Sci. Med.* **2019**, *178*, 403–410. [CrossRef]
233. Bielik, V.; Clementis, M. Running mechanics in recreational runners, soccer and tennis players. *Gazz. Med. Ital. Arch. Sci. Med* **2017**, *176*, 461–466. [CrossRef]
234. Butler, R.J.; Hamill, J.; Davis, I. Effect of footwear on high and low arched runners' mechanics during a prolonged run. *Gait Posture* **2007**, *26*, 219–225. [CrossRef]
235. Cooper, G.; Sheret, I.; McMillan, L.; Siliverdis, K.; Sha, N.; Hodgins, D.; Kenney, L.; Howard, D. Inertial sensor-based knee flexion/extension angle estimation. *J. Biomech.* **2009**, *42*, 2678–2685. [CrossRef]
236. de Fontenay, B.P.; Roy, J.S.; Dubois, B.; Bouyer, L.; Esculier, J.F. Validating Commercial Wearable Sensors for Running Gait Parameters Estimation. *IEEE Sens. J.* **2020**, *20*, 7783–7791. [CrossRef]
237. Dufek, J.S.; Mercer, J.A.; Teramoto, K.; Mangus, B.C.; Freedman, J.A. Impact attenuation and variability during running in females: A lifespan investigation. *J. Sport Rehabilit.* **2008**, *17*, 230–242. [CrossRef]
238. Garrett, J.; Graham, S.R.; Eston, R.G.; Burgess, D.J.; Garrett, L.J.; Jakeman, J.; Norton, K. A Novel Method of Assessment for Monitoring Neuromuscular Fatigue in Australian Rules Football Players. *Int. J. Sports Physiol. Perform.* **2019**, *14*, 598–605. [CrossRef]
239. Gurchiek, R.D.; McGinnis, R.; Needle, A.R.; McBride, J.M.; van Werkhoven, H. The use of a single inertial sensor to estimate 3-dimensional ground reaction force during accelerative running tasks. *J. Biomech.* **2017**, *61*, 263–268. [CrossRef]
240. Sheerin, K.R.; Reid, D.; Taylor, D.; Besier, T.F. The effectiveness of real-time haptic feedback gait retraining for reducing resultant tibial acceleration with runners. *Phys. Ther. Sport* **2020**, *43*, 173–180. [CrossRef]
241. Ueberschär, O.; Fleckenstein, D.; Warschun, F.; Kränzler, S.; Walter, N.; Hoppe, M.W. Measuring biomechanical loads and asymmetries in junior elite long-distance runners through triaxial inertial sensors. *Sports Orthop. Traumatol.* **2019**, *35*, 296–308. [CrossRef]
242. Zadeh, A.; Taylor, D.; Bertsos, M.; Tillman, T.; Nosoudi, N.; Bruce, S. Predicting Sports Injuries with Wearable Technology and Data Analysis. *Inf. Syst. Front.* **2021**, *23*, 1023–1037. [CrossRef]
243. Taunton, J.E.; Ryan, M.B.; Clement, D.B.; McKenzie, D.C.; Lloyd-Smith, D.R.; Zumbo, B.D. A prospective study of running injuries: The Vancouver Sun Run "In Training" clinics. *Br. J. Sports Med.* **2003**, *37*, 239–244. [CrossRef] [PubMed]
244. Bertelsen, M.L.; Hulme, A.; Petersen, J.; Brund, R.K.; Sørensen, H.; Finch, C.F.; Parner, E.; Nielsen, R.O. A framework for the etiology of running-related injuries. *Scand. J. Med. Sci. Sports* **2017**, *27*, 1170–1180. [CrossRef] [PubMed]
245. Van Hooren, B.; Fuller, J.T.; Buckley, J.D.; Miller, J.R.; Sewell, K.; Rao, G.; Barton, C.; Bishop, C.; Willy, R.W. Is Motorized Treadmill Running Biomechanically Comparable to Overground Running? A Systematic Review and Meta-Analysis of Cross-Over Studies. *Sports Med.* **2020**, *50*, 785–813. [CrossRef]
246. Moe-Nilssen, R.; Helbostad, J.L. Estimation of gait cycle characteristics by trunk accelerometry. *J. Biomech.* **2004**, *37*, 121–126. [CrossRef]
247. Janssen, M.; Scheerder, J.; Thibaut, E.; Brombacher, A.; Vos, S. Who uses running apps and sports watches? Determinants and consumer profiles of event runners' usage of running-related smartphone applications and sports watches. *PLoS ONE* **2017**, *12*, e0181167. [CrossRef]
248. Pobiruchin, M.; Suleder, J.; Zowalla, R.; Wiesner, M.; Wilson, G.; Mauriello, M.L.; Cena, F. Accuracy and Adoption of Wearable Technology Used by Active Citizens: A Marathon Event Field Study. *JMIR mHealth uHealth* **2017**, *5*, e24. [CrossRef]
249. Clermont, C.A.; Duffett-Leger, L.; Hettinga, B.A.; Ferber, R. Runners' Perspectives on 'Smart' Wearable Technology and Its Use for Preventing Injury. *Int. J. Hum.-Comput. Interact.* **2019**, *36*, 31–40. [CrossRef]
250. Aderem, J.; Louw, Q.A. Biomechanical risk factors associated with iliotibial band syndrome in runners: A systematic review. *BMC Musculoskelet. Disord.* **2015**, *16*, 356. [CrossRef]
251. Andersen, J.J. The State of Running 2019. Available online: https://runrepeat.com/state-of-running?fbclid=IwAR3x_Z4MeyKxCaLBwOTBL8uSqcAnz64s5H_Lh8aGHbsm72GxRz_G4Su1zcU (accessed on 26 May 2021).
252. Costello, J.; Bieuzen, F.; Bleakley, C. Where are all the female participants in Sports and Exercise Medicine research? *Eur. J. Sport Sci.* **2014**, *14*, 847–851. [CrossRef] [PubMed]
253. Horsley, B.J.; Tofari, P.J.; Halson, S.L.; Kemp, J.G.; Dickson, J.; Maniar, N.; Cormack, S.J. Does Site Matter? Impact of Inertial Measurement Unit Placement on the Validity and Reliability of Stride Variables During Running: A Systematic Review and Meta-analysis. *Sports Med.* **2021**, *51*, 1449–1489. [CrossRef] [PubMed]

MDPI
St. Alban-Anlage 66
4052 Basel
Switzerland
www.mdpi.com

Sensors Editorial Office
E-mail: sensors@mdpi.com
www.mdpi.com/journal/sensors

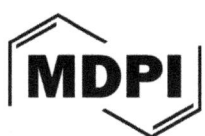

Disclaimer/Publisher's Note: The statements, opinions and data contained in all publications are solely those of the individual author(s) and contributor(s) and not of MDPI and/or the editor(s). MDPI and/or the editor(s) disclaim responsibility for any injury to people or property resulting from any ideas, methods, instructions or products referred to in the content.

www.ingramcontent.com/pod-product-compliance
Lightning Source LLC
LaVergne TN
LVHW070445100526
838202LV00014B/1668